T0331152

Linear Differential Equations and Oscillators

Mathematics and Physics for Science and Technology
Series Editor: L.M.B.C. Campos
Director of the Center for Aeronautical
and Space Science and Technology
Lisbon University

Volumes in the series:

Topic A – Theory of Functions and Potential Problems

Volume I (Book 1) – Complex Analysis with Applications to Flows and Fields
L.M.B.C. Campos

Volume II (Book 2) – Elementary Transcendentals with Applications to Solids and Fluids
L.M.B.C. Campos

Volume III (Book 3) – Generalized Calculus with Applications to Matter and Forces
L.M.B.C. Campos

Topic B – Boundary and Initial-Value Problems

Volume IV – Ordinary Differential Equations with Applications to Trajectories and Vibrations
L.M.B.C. Campos

Book 4 – Linear Differential Equations and Oscillators
L.M.B.C. Campos

Book 5 – Non-Linear Differential Equations and Dynamical Systems
L.M.B.C. Campos

Book 6 – Higher-Order Differential Equations and Elasticity
L.M.B.C. Campos

Book 7 – Simultaneous Differential Equations and Multi-Dimensional Vibrations
L.M.B.C. Campos

Book 8 – Singular Differential Equations and Special Functions
L.M.B.C. Campos

Book 9 – Classification and Examples of Differential Equations and their Applications
L.M.B.C. Campos

For more information about this series, please visit: https://www.crcpress.com/Mathematics-and-Physics-for-Science-and-Technology/book-series/CRCMATPHYSCI

Mathematics and Physics for Science and Technology

Volume IV

Ordinary Differential Equations with Applications to Trajectories and Vibrations

Book 4

Linear Differential Equations and Oscillators

By

L.M.B.C. Campos

Director of the Center for Aeronautical and Space Science and Technology

Lisbon University

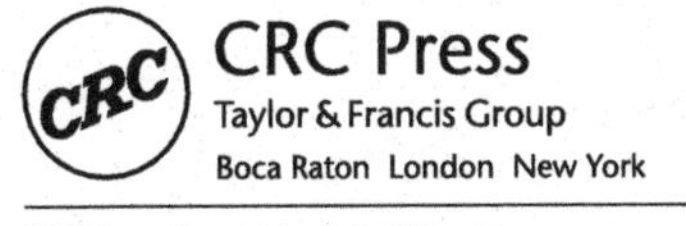

CRC Press is an imprint of the
Taylor & Francis Group, an **informa** business

CRC Press
Taylor & Francis Group
6000 Broken Sound Parkway NW, Suite 300
Boca Raton, FL 33487-2742

Printed on acid-free paper

International Standard Book Number-13: 978-0-367-13718-2 (Hardback)

Library of Congress Cataloging-in-Publication Data

Names: Campos, Luis Manuel Braga da Costa, author.
Title: Linear differential equations and oscillators / Luis Manuel Braga da Campos.
Description: Boca Raton : Taylor & Francis, a CRC title, part of the Taylor & Francis imprint, a member of the Taylor & Francis Group, the academic division of T&F Informa, plc, 2018. | Includes bibliographical references and index.
Identifiers: LCCN 2018046413| ISBN 9780367137182 (hardback : acid-free paper) | ISBN 9780429028984 (ebook)
Subjects: LCSH: Vibrators–Mathematical models. | Mechanical movements–Mathematical models. | Oscillations–Mathematical models. | Differential equations, Linear.
Classification: LCC TJ208 .C36 2018 | DDC 621.8–dc23
LC record available at https://lccn.loc.gov/2018046413

DOI: 10.1201/9780429028984

Visit the Taylor & Francis Web site at
http://www.taylorandfrancis.com

and the CRC Press Web site at
http://www.crcpress.com

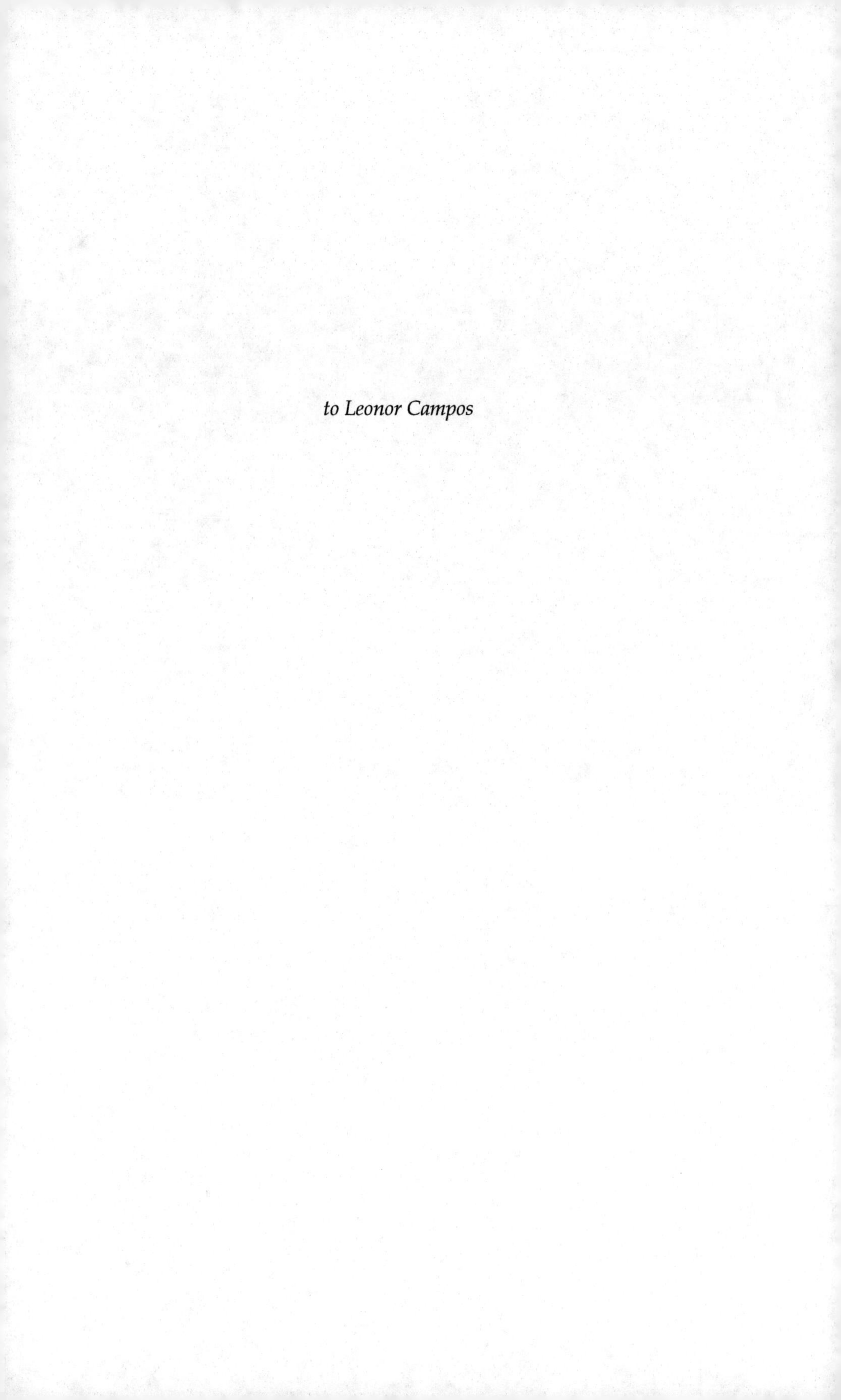

to Leonor Campos

Contents

Diagrams, Notes, and Tables

Diagrams

Notes

Tables

Series Preface

The aim of the "Mathematics and Physics for Science and Technology" series is to describe the mathematical methods as they are applied to model natural physical phenomena and solve scientific and technological problems. The primary emphasis is on the application, including formulation of the problem, detailed solution, and interpretation of results. Mathematical methods are presented in sufficient detail to justify every step of solution, and to avoid superfluous assumptions.

The main areas of physics are covered, namely:

- Mechanics of particles, rigid bodies, deformable solids, and fluids;
- Electromagnetism, thermodynamics, and statistical physics, as well as their classical, relativistic, and quantum formulations;
- Interactions and combined effects (e.g., thermal stresses, magnetohydrodynamics, plasmas, piezoelectricity, and chemically reacting and radiating flows).

The examples and problems chosen include natural phenomena in our environment, geophysics, and astrophysics; the technological implications in various branches of engineering—aerospace, mechanical, civil, electrical, chemical, computer; and other mathematical models in biological, economic, and social sciences.

The coverage of areas of mathematics and branches of physics is sufficient to lay the foundations of all branches of engineering, namely:

- Mechanical—including machines, engines, structures, and vehicles;
- Civil—including structures and hydraulics;
- Electrical—including circuits, waves, and quantum effects;
- Chemical—including transport phenomena and multiphase media;
- Computer—including analytical and numerical methods and associated algorithms.

Particular emphasis is given to interdisciplinary areas, such as electromechanics and aerospace engineering. These require combined knowledge of several areas and have an increasing importance in modern technology.

Analogies are applied in an efficient and concise way, across distinct disciplines, but also stressing the differences and aspects specific to each area, for example:

- Potential flow, electrostatics, magnetostatics, gravity field, steady heat conduction, plane elasticity, and viscous flow;
- Acoustic, elastic, electromagnetic, internal, and surfaces waves;
- Diffusion of mass, electricity, and momentum.

The acoustic, internal, inertial, and magnetic waves appear combined as magneto-acoustic-gravity-inertial (MAGI) waves in a compressible, ionized, stratified, and rotating fluid. The simplest exact solutions of the MAGI wave equation require special functions. Thus, the topic of MAGI waves combines six subjects: gravity field, fluid mechanics, and electromagnetism, and uses complex analysis, differential equations, and special functions. This is not such a remote subject since many astrophysical phenomena do involve this combination of several of these effects, as does the technology of controlled nuclear fusion. The latter is the main source of energy in stars and in the universe; if harnessed, it would provide a clean and inexhaustible source of energy on Earth. Closer to our everyday experience, there is a variety of electromechanical and control systems that use modern interdisciplinary technology. The ultimate aim of the present series is to build up knowledge seamlessly from undergraduate to research level, across a range of subjects, to cover contemporary or likely interdisciplinary needs. This requires a consistent treatment of all subjects so that their combination fits together as a whole.

The approach followed in the present series is a combined study of mathematics, physics, and engineering, so that the practical motivation develops side by side with the theoretical concepts; the mathematical methods are applied without delay to "real" problems, not just to exercises. The electromechanical and other analogies stimulate the ability to combine different disciplines, which is the basis of much of modern interdisciplinary science and technology. Starting with the simpler mathematical methods, and then consolidating them with the detailed solutions of physical and engineering problems, gradually widens the range of topics that can be covered. The traditional method of separate monodisciplinary study remains possible, selecting mathematical disciplines (e.g., complex functions) or sets of applications (e.g., fluid mechanics). The combined multidisciplinary method of study has the advantage of connecting mathematics, physics, and technology at an earlier stage. Moreover, preserving that link provides a broader view of the subject and the ability to innovate. Innovation requires an understanding of the aims, the physical phenomena that can implement them, and the mathematical methods that quantify the expected results. The combined interdisciplinary approach to the study of mathematics, physics, and engineering is thus a direct introduction to a professional experience in scientific discovery and technological innovation.

Preface to Volume IV

Relationship with Previous Volumes of the Series

Topic A was concerned with the theory of functions: (volume I) starting with complex functions of a complex variable; (volume II) proceeding to the elementary transcendental functions in the complex plane; (volume III) extending to any dimension via the generalized functions, like the Dirac delta, derivatives, and primitives. The applications of the theory of functions in topic A were mostly potential fields, that is, solutions of the Laplace and Poisson equations that arise in various domains such as: (volume I) potential flow, gravity field, electrostatics, magnetostatics, and steady heat conduction in two dimensions; (volume II) still in two dimensions, solutions of the unforced and forced Laplace and biharmonic partial differential equations, including some vortical, compressible, rotating and viscous flows, plane elasticity, torsion of bars, deflection of membranes, and capillarity; (volume III) extension of potential fields to three and higher dimensions, including irrotational and/or incompressible flows, electro- and magnetostatics and one-dimensional elastic bodies like strings, bars, and beams.

The applications of the theory of functions in topic A already include many boundary and initial-value problems; the latter are the focus of topic B, starting from the solution of ordinary and partial differential equations, which uses the theory of functions in topic A. In particular, the mechanical oscillators, electrical circuits, and elastic bodies already briefly considered in topic A become the main focus of the first volume, IV, of topic B on *Ordinary Differential Equations with Applications to Trajectories and Oscillations*. Thus, the present volume, IV, of the series *"Mathematics and Physics Applied to Science and Technology"* covers, on the mathematical side: (i) the solution of single ordinary differential equations or simultaneous systems, non-linear or linear, the latter with constant and variable coefficients and special functions; (iv) existence, unicity, bifurcations, and other properties of the solutions as particular, general, complete, and special integrals. On the application side: (iii) single or multiple oscillators, without or with damping and/or forcing in linear and non-linear cases, including harmonic and parametric resonance; (iv) one (two)-dimensional bodies like bars (plates) without or with axial tension (in-plane stresses), as concerns elastic deformations, static stability, and unsteady wave motions.

Objectives and Contents of Volume IV

A large number and wide variety of problems in mathematics, physics, engineering, and other quantitative sciences involve the solution of differential equations. The most common ordinary differential equations are (i) linear with constant coefficients, whose unforced solutions are determined by the roots of a characteristic polynomial. The characteristic polynomial also exists (chapter 1) in the case of (ii) linear differential equations with power coefficients leading to homogeneous derivatives, and (iii) linear finite difference equations with constant coefficients. The extension of (i) to (iii) to simultaneous systems of equations (chapter 7) leads to a matrix whose determinant is the characteristic polynomial. The characteristic polynomial specifies the unforced (forced) solutions through its roots (as an inverse operator of derivatives). The single (simultaneous systems) of linear differential equations with constant coefficients [chapter 1(7)] apply to one (multi)-dimensional linear oscillators, including cases without or with damping and with forcing, leading to beats or ordinary resonance [chapter 2 (8)]. The extension from one to two characteristic polynomials with ordinary or homogeneous derivatives leads to special functions (chapter 9).

The non-linear oscillations (chapter 4), due to non-linear restoring or dissipative effects, can lead to bifurcations that are associated with some non-linear differential equations (chapter 3). Whereas discrete oscillators are described by second-order ordinary differential equations, continuous systems without (with) stiffness, like elastic strings (bars) in one-dimension, and membranes (plates) in two dimensions, lead to second (fourth)-order differential equations (chapter 6). The differential equations of higher orders (chapter 5), like those of first-order, can have special integrals not included in the general integral. The combination of spatial and time dependences leads to the vibrations of solids like strings, membranes, bars and plates; waves in fluids like sound or water waves; and also electromagnetic waves in matter or vacuo (chapters 6 and 7). The last odd-numbered chapter 9 addresses more general issues, like the existence and unicity of solutions, the stability of equilibrium positions, and the solution of linear differential equations with variable coefficients; the solution of the latter as infinite series, parametric integrals, and continued fractions lead to a variety of special functions, among which are chosen as preferred examples: (i) the generalized Bessel, Neumann, and Hankel functions; (ii) the Gaussian, confluent, generalized, and extended hypergeometric functions.

Organization and Presentation of the Subject Matter

Volume IV (*Ordinary Differential Equations with Applications to Trajectories and Oscillations*) is organized like the preceding three volumes of the series, *Mathematics and Physics Applied to Science and Technology*: (volume III) *Generalized Calculus with Applications to Matter and Forces*; (volume II) *Elementary Transcendentals with Applications to Solids and Fluids*; and (volume I) *Complex Analysis with Applications to Flows and Fields*. Volume IV consists of ten chapters: (i) the odd-numbered chapters present mathematical developments; (ii) the even-numbered chapters contain physical and engineering applications; (iii) the last chapter is a set of 20 detailed examples of (i) and (ii). The chapters are divided into sections and subsections, for example, chapter 1, section 1.1, and subsection 1.1.1. The formulas are numbered by chapters in curved brackets, for example (1.2) is equation 2 of chapter 1. When referring to volume I the symbol I is inserted at the beginning, for example: (i) chapter I.36, section I.36.1, subsection I.36.1.2; (ii) equation (I.36.33a). The final part of each chapter includes: (i) a conclusion referring to the figures as a kind of visual summary; (ii) the notes, lists, tables, diagrams, and classifications as additional support. The latter (ii) appear at the end of each chapter, and are numbered within the chapter (for example, diagram—D2.1, note—N1.1, table—T2.1); if there is more than one diagram, note, or table, they are numbered sequentially (for example, notes—N2.1 to N2.13). The chapter starts with an introductory preview, and related topics may be mentioned in the notes at the end. The lists of mathematical symbols and physical quantities appear before the main text, and the index of subjects and bibliography are found at the end of the book.

The contents of volume IV, *Ordinary Differential Equations with Applications to Trajectories and Oscillations,* are divided into six books, with the first book, *"Linear Differential Equations and Oscillators,"* corresponding to chapters 1 and 2, which focus on the simpler methods and problems. After a brief introduction to general ordinary differential equations, chapter 1 focuses on linear equations of any order with (i) constant or (ii) homogeneous power coefficients that have a characteristic polynomial; the method of characteristic polynomials also applies (iii) to linear finite difference equations of any order with constant coefficients, and in all cases (i, ii, iii) can be used to obtain free and forced solutions.

The linear second-order oscillators, such as the mechanical mass-damper-spring-force system and the electrical self-resistor-capacitor-battery circuit, lead to linear differential equations with constant coefficients. The solution without forcing specifies free oscillations, including damping and amplification; the forced solutions include beats and resonance. Besides the method of the characteristic polynomial others used include the variation of parameters, the Green's function, the Fourier series, and integrals and Laplace transforms.

Acknowledgments

The fourth volume of the series justifies renewing some of the acknowledgments made in the first three volumes. Thank you to those who contributed more directly to the final form of this volume: Ms. Ana Moura, L. Sousa, and S. Pernadas for help with the manuscripts; Mr. J. Coelho for all the drawings; and at last, but not least, to my wife, my companion in preparing this work.

About the Author

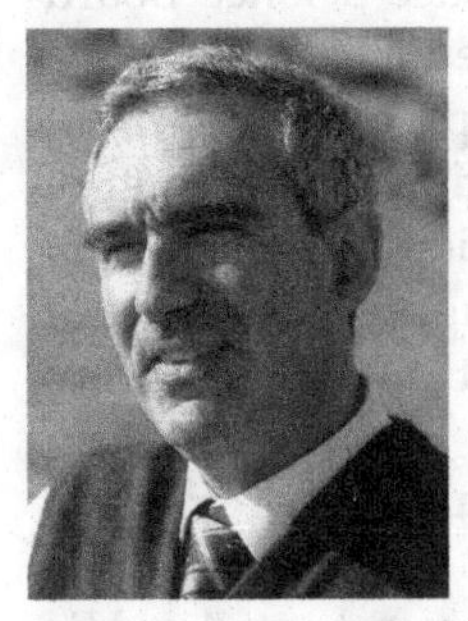

L.M.B.C. Campos was born on March 28, 1950, in Lisbon, Portugal. He graduated in 1972 as a mechanical engineer from the Instituto Superior Tecnico (IST) of Lisbon Technical University. The tutorials as a student (1970) were followed by a career at the same institution (IST) through all levels: assistant (1972), assistant with tenure (1974), assistant professor (1978), associate professor (1982), chair of Applied Mathematics and Mechanics (1985). He has served as the coordinator of undergraduate and postgraduate degrees in Aerospace Engineering since the creation of the programs in 1991. He is the coordinator of the Scientific Area of Applied and Aerospace Mechanics in the Department of Mechanical Engineering. He is also the director and founder of the Center for Aeronautical and Space Science and Technology.

In 1977, Campos received his doctorate on "waves in fluids" from the Engineering Department of Cambridge University, England. Afterwards, he received a Senior Rouse Ball Scholarship to study at Trinity College, while on leave from IST. In 1984, his first sabbatical was as a Senior Visitor at the Department of Applied Mathematics and Theoretical Physics of Cambridge University, England. In 1991, he spent a second sabbatical as an Alexander von Humboldt scholar at the Max-Planck Institut fur Aeronomic in Katlenburg-Lindau, Germany. Further sabbaticals abroad were excluded by major commitments at the home institution. The latter were always compatible with extensive professional travel related to participation in scientific meetings, individual or national representation in international institutions, and collaborative research projects.

Campos received the von Karman medal from the Advisory Group for Aerospace Research and Development (AGARD) and Research and Technology Organization (RTO). Participation in AGARD/RTO included serving as a vice-chairman of the System Concepts and Integration Panel, and chairman of the Flight Mechanics Panel and of the Flight Vehicle Integration Panel. He was also a member of the Flight Test Techniques Working Group. Here he was involved in the creation of an independent flight test capability, active in Portugal during the last 30 years, which has been used in national and international projects, including Eurocontrol and the European Space Agency. The participation in the European Space Agency (ESA) has afforded Campos the opportunity to serve on various program boards at the levels of national representative and Council of Ministers.

His participation in activities sponsored by the European Union (EU) has included: (i) 27 research projects with industry, research, and academic institutions; (ii) membership of various Committees, including Vice-Chairman of the Aeronautical Science and Technology Advisory Committee; (iii) participation on the Space Advisory Panel on the future role of EU in space. Campos has been a member of the Space Science Committee of the European Science Foundation, which works with the Space Science Board of the National Science Foundation of the United States. He has been a member of the Committee for Peaceful Uses of Outer Space (COPUOS) of the United Nations. He has served as a consultant and advisor on behalf of these organizations and other institutions. His participation in professional societies includes member and vice-chairman of the Portuguese Academy of Engineering, fellow of the Royal Aeronautical Society, Astronomical Society and Cambridge Philosophical Society, associate fellow of the American Institute of Aeronautics and Astronautics, and founding and life member of the European Astronomical Society.

Campos has published and worked on numerous books and articles. His publications include 10 books as a single author, one as an editor, and one as a co-editor. He has published 152 papers (82 as the single author, including 12 reviews) in 60 journals, and 254 communications to symposia. He has served as reviewer for 40 different journals, in addition to 23 reviews published in *Mathematics Reviews*. He is or has been member of the editorial boards of several journals, including *Progress in Aerospace Sciences, International Journal of Aeroacoustics, International Journal of Sound and Vibration*, and *Air & Space Europe*.

Campos's areas of research focus on four topics: acoustics, magnetohydrodynamics, special functions, and flight dynamics. His work on acoustics has concerned the generation, propagation, and refraction of sound in flows with mostly aeronautical applications. His work on magnetohydrodynamics has concerned magneto-acoustic-gravity-inertial waves in solar-terrestrial and stellar physics. His developments on special functions have used differintegration operators, generalizing the ordinary derivative and primitive to complex order; they have led to the introduction of new special functions. His work on flight dynamics has concerned aircraft and rockets, including trajectory optimization, performance, stability, control, and atmospheric disturbances.

The range of topics from mathematics to physics and engineering fits with the aims and contents of the present series. Campos's experience in university teaching and scientific and industrial research has enhanced his ability to make the series valuable to students from undergraduate level to research level.

Campos's professional activities on the technical side are balanced by other cultural and humanistic interests. Complementary non-technical interests include classical music (mostly orchestral and choral), plastic arts (painting, sculpture, architecture), social sciences (psychology and biography), history (classical, renaissance and overseas expansion) and technology (automotive, photo, audio). Campos is listed in various biographical publications, including *Who's Who in the World* since 1986, *Who's Who in Science and Technology* since 1994, and *Who's Who in America* since 2011.

Mathematical Symbols

The mathematical symbols presented are those of more common use in the context of: (i) sets, quantifiers, and logic; (ii) numbers, ordering, and bounds; (iii) operations, limits, and convergence; (iv) vectors, functions, and the calculus. This section includes a list of functional spaces, not all of which appear in the present volume. The section where the symbol first appears may be indicated after a colon, for example: "IV.10.2" means section 10.2, of the present volume IV; "II.1.1.4" means subsection 1.1.4 of the volume II; "N.IV.9.42" means note 9.42 of the present volume IV; and "N.III.9.38" means note 9.38 of the volume III.

1 Sets, Quantifiers, and Logic

1.1 Sets

$A \equiv \{x:\ldots\}$ — set A whose elements x have the property…

$A \cup B$ — union of sets A and B

$A \cap B$ — intersection of sets A and B

$A \supset B$ — set A contains set B

$A \subset B$ — set A is contained in set B

1.2 Quantifiers

$\forall_{x\varepsilon A}$ — for all x belonging to A holds…

$\exists_{x\varepsilon A}$ — there exists at least one x belonging to A such that…

$\exists^1_{x\varepsilon A}$ — there exists one and only one x belonging to A such that…

$\exists^\infty_{x\varepsilon A}$ — there exist infinitely many x belonging to A such that…

1.3 Logic

$a \wedge b$ — a and b

$a \vee b$ — or (inclusive): a or b or both

$a \dot{\vee} b$ — or (exclusive): a or b but not both

$a \Rightarrow b$ — implication: a implies b

$a \Leftrightarrow b$ — equivalence: a implies b and b implies a
$a \not\Rightarrow b$ — non-implication: a may not imply b

1.4 Constants

$e = 2.7182\ 81828\ 45904\ 52353\ 60287$
$\pi = 3.1415\ 92653\ 58979\ 32384\ 62643$
$\gamma = 0.5772\ 15664\ 90153\ 28606\ 06512$
$\log 10 = 2.3025\ 85092\ 99404\ 56840\ 179915$

2 Numbers, Ordering, and Operations

2.1 Types of Numbers

$|C$ — complex numbers: I.1.2
$|C^n$ — ordered sets of n complex numbers
$|F$ — transfinite numbers: II.9.8
$|H$ — hypercomplex numbers
$|I$ — irrational numbers: real non-rational numbers: I.1.2
$|L$ — rational numbers: ratios of integers: I.1.1
$|N$ — natural numbers: positive integers: I.1.1
$|N_0$ — non-negative integers: zero plus natural numbers: I.1.1
$|P$ — prime numbers: numbers without divisors
$|Q$ — quaternions: I.1.9
$|R$ — real numbers: I.1.2
$|R^n$ — ordered sets of n real numbers
$|Z$ — integer numbers: I.1.1

2.2 Complex Numbers

$|\ldots|$ — modulus of complex number...: I.1.4
$\arg(\ldots)$ — argument of complex number...: I.1.4
$\operatorname{Re}(\ldots)$ — real part of complex number...: I.1.3
$\operatorname{Im}(\ldots)$ — imaginary part of complex number...: I.1.3
$\ldots^*$ — conjugate of complex number...: I.1.6

2.3 Relations and Ordering

$a > b$ — a greater than b

$a \geq b$ — a greater or equal to b

$a = b$ — a equal to b

$a \leq b$ — a smaller or equal to b

$a < b$ — a smaller than b

sup (...) — supremum: smallest number larger or equal than all numbers in the set...

max (...) — maximum: largest number in set...

min (...) — minimum: smallest number in set...

inf (...) — infimum: largest number smaller or equal than all numbers in set...

2.4 Operations between Numbers

$a + b$ — sum: a plus b

$a - b$ — difference: a minus b

$a \times b$ — product: a times b

a/b — ratio: a divided by b (alternative a:b)

a^b — power: a to the power b

$\sqrt[b]{a}$ — root: root b of a

3 Functions, Limits, and Convergence

3.1 Limits and Values

lim — limit when x tends to a: $x \to a$: I.11.2

l.i.m. — limit in the mean

$a \sim O(b)$ — a is of order b: lim $b/a \neq 0, \infty$: I.19.7

$a \sim o(b)$ — b is of lower order than a: lim $b/a = 0$: I.19.7

$f(a)$ — value of function f at point a

$f(a + 0)$ — right-hand limit at a

$f(a - 0)$ — left-hand limit at a

$f_{(n)}(a)$ — residue at pole of order n at a: I.15.8

$\overline{B}$ or M — upper bound: $|f(z)| \leq \overline{B}$ for z in ...: I.39.2

$\underline{B}$ or m — lower bound: $|f(z)| \geq \underline{B}$ for z in ...: I.39.2

$f \circ g$ — composition of functions f and g: N.I.38.1

3.2 Iterated Sums and Products

$\sum_{a}$ — sum over a set

$\sum_{n=a}^{b}$ — sum from $n = a$ to $n = b$

$\sum_{n,m=a}^{b}$ — double sum over $n, m = a,\dots, b$

$\prod_{a}$ — product over a set

$\prod_{n=a}^{b}$ — product from $n = a$ to $n = b$

3.3 Convergence

A.C. — absolutely convergent: I.21.2
A.D. — absolutely divergent: I.21.2
C. — convergent: I.21.2
C.C. — conditionally convergent: I.21.2
Cn — converges to class n: $C0 \equiv C$
C1 — converges to class 1: II.9.6
D. — divergent: I.21.1
N.C. — non-convergent: divergent or oscillatory: I.21.1
O. — oscillatory: I.21.1
T.C. — totally convergent: I.21.7
U.C. — uniformly convergent: I.21.5
applies to:
— power series: I.21.1
— series of fractions: I.36.6, II.1.2
— infinite products: I.36.6, II.1.4
— continued fractions: II.1.6

3.4 Integrals

$\int \dots dx$ — primitive of … with regards to x: I.13.1

$\int^{y} \dots dx$ — indefinite integral of … at y: I.13.2

$\int_a^b \cdots dx$ — definite integral of ... between a and b: I.13.2

$⨍_a^b \cdots dx$ — principal value of integral: I.17.8

$\int^{(z+)}$ — integral along a loop around z in the positive (counterclockwise) direction: I.13.5

$\int^{(z-)}$ — idem in the negative (clockwise) direction: I.13.5

$\int_L$ — integral along a path L: I.13.2

$\int_C^{(+)}$ — integral along a closed path or loop C in the positive direction: I.13.5

$\int_C^{(-)}$ — integral along a closed path or loop C in the negative direction: I.13.5

4 Vectors, Matrices, and Tensors

4.1 Vectors

$\vec{A}.\vec{B}$ — inner product

$\vec{A} \wedge \vec{B}$ — outer product

$\vec{A}.\left(\vec{B} \wedge \vec{C}\right)$ — mixed product

$\vec{A} \wedge \left(\vec{B} \wedge \vec{C}\right)$ — double outer product

$\left|\vec{A}\right|$ — modulus

$\text{ang}\left(\vec{A},\vec{B}\right)$ — angle of vector $\vec{B}$ with vector $\vec{A}$

4.2 Matrices

δ_j^i — identity matrix: III.5.8

$\overset{c}{A}{}_j^i$ — matrix of co-factors: N.III.9.10

$\overset{I}{A}{}_j^i$ — inverse matrix: N.III.9.10

$Det\left(A_j^i\right)$ — determinant of matrix: N.III.9.11

$Ra\left(A_j^i\right)$ — rank of matrix: N.III.5.5.1

4.3 Tensors

$\overset{(\vartheta)}{T}{}^{i_1 \ldots i_p}_{j_1 \ldots j_q}$ — tensor with weight ϑ, contravariance p and covariance q: N.III.9.14

$\delta^{i_1 \ldots i_N}_{j_1 \ldots j_N}$ — identity symbol: N.III.9.9

$e_{i_1 \ldots i_N}$ — covariant permutation symbol: N.III.9.9

4.4 Operations

$T_{(i_1 \cdots i_p)}$ — mixing: N.III.9.12

$T_{[i_1 \cdots i_p]}$ — alternation: N.III.9.12

T^{ij}_{ik} — contraction: N.III.9.12

$T^i_{jk} S^j_{i\ell}$ — transvection: N.III.9.12

5 Derivatives and Differential Operators

5.1 Differentials and Derivatives

$\mathrm{d}\Phi$ — differential of Φ

$\mathrm{d}\Phi/\mathrm{d}t$ — derivative of Φ with regards to t

$\partial\Phi/\partial t \equiv \partial_t \Phi$ — partial derivative of Φ with regards to t

$\partial\Phi/\partial x_i \equiv \partial_i \Phi \equiv \Phi_{,i}$ — partial derivative of Φ with regards to x_i

$\partial^n\Phi/\partial x_{i_1} \ldots \partial x_{i_n} \equiv \partial_{i_1 \cdots i_n} \Phi \equiv \Phi_{,i_1 \cdots i_n}$ — n-order partial derivative of Φ with regards to $x_{i_1}, \ldots, x_{i_n}$.

5.2 Vector Operators

$\nabla\Phi = \partial_i \Phi$ — gradient of a scalar: III.6.1

$\nabla . \vec{A} = \partial_i A_i$ — divergence of a vector: III.6.1

$\nabla \wedge \vec{A} = e_{ijk}\, \partial_j A_k$ — curl of a vector: III.6.1,3.9.1

$H \equiv \vec{A}.\left(\nabla \wedge \vec{A}\right) = A_k e_{ijk}\, \partial_i A_j$ — helicity: IV.3.9.2

$\nabla^2 = \partial_{ii} = \partial_i \partial_i$ — Laplacian: III.6.1

$\bar{\nabla}^2$ — modified Laplacian: III.6.2

5.3 Tensor Operators

$\partial_{[i_{M+1}} U_{i_1 \cdots i_n]}$ — curl of a covariant M-vector: N.III.9.20

$\partial_{i_{M+1}} U^{i_1 \cdots i_{M+1}}$ — divergence of a contravariant (M + 1) – vector density: N.III.9.20.

5.4 Adjointness

$\{L(\partial/\partial x_i)\}\Phi$ — linear differential operator: III.7.6

$\{\bar{L}[(\partial/\partial x_i)]\}\Psi$ — adjoint differential operator: III.7.6

$W(\Phi,\Psi)$ — bilinear concomitant: III.7.6

6 Functional Spaces

The spaces of functions are denoted by calligraphic letters, in alphabetical order:

… (a, b) — set of functions over interval from a to b omission of interval: set of functions over real line $)-\infty, +\infty($

$\mathcal{A}$ (…) — analytic functions in …: I.27.1

$\bar{\mathcal{A}}$ (…) — monogenic functions in …: I.31.1

$\mathcal{B}$ (…) — bounded functions in …: $B \equiv B^0$: I.3.3

$\mathcal{B}^n$ (…) — functions with bounded n-th derivative in ….

$\mathcal{C}$ (…) — continuous functions in …: $C \equiv C^0$: I.12.2

$\mathcal{C}^n$ (…) — functions with continuous n-th derivative in …

$\bar{\mathcal{C}}$ (…) — piecewise continuous functions in …: $\bar{C} \equiv \bar{C}^0$

$\bar{\mathcal{C}}^n$ (…) — functions with piecewise continuous n-th derivative in …

$\tilde{\mathcal{C}}$ (…) — uniformly continuous functions in…: I.13.4

$\tilde{\mathcal{C}}^n$ (…) — functions with uniformly continuous n-th derivative in…

$\mathcal{D}$ (…) — differentiable functions in …: $D \equiv D^0$: I.12.2

$\mathcal{D}^n$ (…) — n-times differentiable functions in …

$\mathcal{D}^\infty$ (…) — infinitely differentiable functions or smooth in …: I.27.1

$\bar{\mathcal{D}}$ (…) — piecewise differentiable functions in …: $\bar{\mathcal{D}} \equiv \bar{\mathcal{D}}^0$

$\bar{\mathcal{D}}^n$ (…) — functions with piecewise continuous n-th derivative in …

$\mathcal{E}$ (…) — Riemann integrable functions in …: I.13.2

$\bar{\mathcal{E}}$ (…) — Lebesgue integrable functions in …

$\mathcal{F}$ (…) — functions of bounded oscillation (or bounded fluctuation or bounded variation) in …; $F \equiv E \equiv F^0$: I.5.7.5

$\mathcal{F}^n$ (…) — functions with n-th derivative of bounded oscillation (or fluctuation or variation) in ….

$\mathcal{G}$ (…) — generalized functions (or distributions) in …: III.3.4.1

$\mathcal{H}$ (…) — harmonic functions in …: I.11.4, II.4.6.4

$\mathcal{H}_2$ (…) — biharmonic functions in …: II.4.6.4

$\mathcal{H}_n$ (...) — multiharmonic functions of order ` in ...: II.4.6.6
$\mathcal{I}$ (...) — integral functions in ...: I.27.9, II.1.1.7
$\mathcal{I}_m$ (...) — rational-integral functions of degree m in... $I \equiv I_0$: I.27.9, II.1.1.9.
$\mathcal{J}$ (...) — square integrable functions with a complete orthogonal set of functions—*Hilbert space*
$\bar{\mathcal{K}}$ (...) — Lipshitz functions in ...: IV.9.1.5
$\mathcal{K}^n$ (...) — homogeneous functions of degree n in ...
$\mathcal{L}^1$ (...) — absolutely integrable functions in ...: N.III.3.7
$\mathcal{L}^2$ (...) — square integrable functions in ...: III.7.1.1
$\mathcal{L}^p$ (...) — functions with power p of modulus integrable in ...
—*normed* space: III.7.1.1
$\mathcal{M}^+$ (...) — monotonic increasing functions in ...: I.9.1.1
$\mathcal{M}_0^+$ (...) — monotonic non-decreasing functions in ...: I.9.1.1
$\mathcal{M}_0^-$ (...) — monotonic non-increasing functions in...: I 9.1.2
$\mathcal{M}^-$ (...) — monotonic decreasing functions in ...: I.9.1.2
$\mathcal{N}$ (...) — null functions in ...
$\mathcal{O}$ (...) — orthogonal systems of functions in ...: II.5.7.2
$\bar{\mathcal{O}}$ (...) — orthonormal systems of functions in ...: II.5.7.2
$\tilde{\mathcal{O}}$ (...) — complete orthogonal systems of functions in ...: II.5.7.5
$\mathcal{P}$ (...) — polynomials in ...: I.27.7, II.1.1.6
$\mathcal{P}_n$ (...) — polynomials of degree n in ...: I.27.7, II.1.1.6
$\mathcal{Q}$ (...) — rational functions in...: I.27.7, II.1.2.6
$\mathcal{Q}_n^m$ (...) — rational functions of degrees n, m in...
$\mathcal{R}$ (...) — real functions, that is, with the real line as the range
$\mathcal{S}$ (...) — complex functions, that with the complex plane as the range
$\mathcal{T}^0$ (...) — functions with compact support, that is which vanish outside a finite interval: III.3.3.2
$\mathcal{T}^n$ (...) — excellent functions of order n: n-times differentiable functions with compact support: III.3.3.2
$\mathcal{T}^\infty$ (...) — excellent functions: smooth or infinitely differentiable functions with compact support: II.3.3.6
$\mathcal{V}$ (...) — single-valued functions in...: I.9.1
$\tilde{\mathcal{V}}$ (...) — injective functions in...: I.9.1
$\bar{\mathcal{V}}$ (...) — surjective functions: I.9.1
$\bar{\tilde{\mathcal{V}}}$ (...) — bijective functions: I.9.1
$\mathcal{V}_n$ (...) — multivalued functions with n branches in...: I.6.1
$\mathcal{V}_\infty$ (...) — many-valued functions in...: I.6.2

$\mathcal{U}^1$ (...) — univalent functions, in ...: I.37.4

$\mathcal{U}^m$ (...) — multivalent functions taking m values in...: I.37.4

$\mathcal{U}^\infty$ (...) — many-valued functions in ...: N.I.37.4

$\mathcal{U}_n^m$ (...) — multivalued multivalent functions with n branches and m values in ...: N.I.37.4

$\mathcal{V}$ (...) — good functions that is with slow decay at infinity faster than some power: III.3.3.1

$\mathcal{V}^n$ (...) — good or slow decay functions of degree n, that is, with decay at infinity faster than the inverse of a polynomial of degree n: III.3.3.1

$\mathcal{V}$ (...) — fairly good or slow growth functions, that is, with growth at infinity slower than some power: III.3.3.1

$\mathcal{V}_n$ (...) — fairly good or slow growth functions of degree n, that is, with growth at infinity slower than a polynomial of degree n: III.3.3.1

$\mathcal{V}_\infty$ (...) — very good or fast decay functions, that is, with faster decay at infinity than any power: II.3.3.1

V_∞^∞ (...) — optimal functions, that is, smooth functions with compact support: II.3.3.6

$\mathcal{W}_q^p$ (...) — functions with generalized derivatives of orders up to q such that for all the power p of the modulus is integrable ... — *Sobolev space*

$\mathcal{X}_0$ (...) — self-inverse linear functions in ....: II.37.5

$\mathcal{X}_1$ (...) — linear functions in ...: I.35.2

$\mathcal{X}_2$ (...) — bilinear, homographic, or Mobius functions in ...: I.35.4

$\mathcal{X}_3$ (...) — self-inverse bilinear functions in ...: II.37.5

$\mathcal{X}_a$ (...) — automorphic functions in ...: I.37.6

$\mathcal{X}_m$ (...) — isometric mappings in ...: I.35.1

$\mathcal{X}_r$ (...) — rotation mappings in ...: II.35.1

$\mathcal{X}_t$ (...) — translation mappings in ...: II.35.1

$\mathcal{Y}$(...) — meromorphic functions in...: I.37.9, II.1.1.10

$\mathcal{Z}$ (...) — polymorphic functions in...: I.37.9, II.1.1.10

7 Geometries with *N* Dimensions

$\mathfrak{A}_N$ — rectilinear: N.III.9.6

$\mathfrak{W}_N$ — metric: N.III.9.34

$\mathfrak{N}_N$ — orthogonal: N.III.9.38
$\mathfrak{O}_N$ — orthogonal: N.III.9.38
$\mathfrak{X}_N$ — curvilinear: N.III.9.6
$\mathfrak{X}_N^2$ — curvilinear with curvature: N.III.9.17

8 Generalized Functions

$H(x)$ — Heaviside unit jump: III.1.2
$G(x;\xi)$ — Green's function: N1.5
$\delta(x)$ —Dirac unit impulse: III.1.3
sgn(x) — sign function: I.36.4.1, III.1.7.1

9 Auxiliary Functions

erf(x) — error function: III.1.2.2
$\sin(x;k)$ — elliptic sine of modulus k: I.39.9.2
$\tilde{y}(k)$ — Fourier transform of $y(x)$; N.IV.1.11
$\bar{y}(s)$ — Laplace transform of $y(x)$: N.IV.1.15
$W(y_1,\ldots,y_N)$ — Wronskian of a set of functions: IV.1.2.3
$\psi(x)$ — Digamma function: I.29.5.2
$\Gamma(x)$ — Gamma function: N.III.1.8.

Physical Quantities

The location of first appearance is indicated, for example, "2.7" means *section 2.7;* "6.8.4" means *subsection 6.8.4;* "N8.8" means *note 8.8;* and "E10.13.1" means *example 10.13.1.*

1 Small Arabic Letters

a — acceleration: 2.1.1
— amplitude of oscillation: 2.2.11
c — speed of light in vacuo: 2.1.9
c_{em} — speed of electromagnetic waves: 2.1.11
f —forcing function: 2.1.8
h — friction force: 2.1.1
j — restoring force: 2.1.1
— electric current: 2.1.6
$\vec{j}$ — convective electric current vector: 2.1.9
k — resilience of a point translational spring: 2.1.2
m — mass of a particle or body: 2.1.1
q — electric charge: 2.1.6
t — time: 2.1.1
— time of reception: 2.1.11
t_0 — time of emission: 2.1.11
v — velocity: 2.1.1
x — independent variable in ordinary differential equation: 1.1.1
— Cartesian coordinate: 2.1.1
$\vec{x}$ — position vector of observer: 2.1.11
y — dependent variable in ordinary differential equation: 1.1.1
— Cartesian coordinate: 2.1
$\vec{y}$ — position vector of source: 2.1.11

2 Capital Arabic Letters

A — Activity or power: 2.1.4
$\vec{A}$ — vector magnetic potential: 2.1.10
$\vec{B}$ — magnetic induction vector: 2.1.9
C — constant of integration: 1.1.1
— capacity of an electric condenser: 2.1.6
$\vec{D}$ — electric displacement vector: 2.1.9
$\vec{E}$ — electric field vector: 2.1.9
E_e — electric energy: 2.1.7
E_{em} — electromagnetic energy: 2.1.7
E_m — magnetic energy: 2.1.7
E_t — total energy: 2.1.4
E_v — kinetic energy: 2.1.4
F_e — electromotive force: 2.1.6
F_m — mechanical force: 2.1.1
H — friction force on a belt: 2.5.1
$\vec{H}$ — magnetic field vector: 2.1.9
$\vec{J}$ — electric current vector: 2.1.9
L — induction of a coil or self: 2.1.6
M — friction moment on a cam: 2.5.4
R — electrical resistance: 2.1.6, 4.7.1, 8.9.2
W — work: 2.2.2

3 Small Greek Letters

α — phase of an oscillator: 2.2.1
α_e — ohmic electrical diffusivity: 2.1.11
ε — dielectric permittivity: 2.1.9
λ — damping: 2.1.8
μ — kinematic friction coefficient: 2.1.3
— magnetic permeability: 2.1.9
σ — Ohmic electrical conductivity: 2.1.9

τ — period of oscillation 2.1.12

$\bar{\tau}$ — decay rate: 2.1.12

ω_0 — natural frequency: 2.1.8

$\bar{\omega}$ — oscillation frequency: 2.3.3, 2.4.1

$\tilde{\omega}$ — average of applied and natural frequencies: 2.7.5

ω_a — applied frequency of sinusoidal forcing: 2.7.1

4 Capital Greek Letters

Φ_e — scalar electric potential: 2.1.10

Φ_m — mechanical potential energy: 2.1.8

Ψ_e — dissipation by electrical resistance: 2.1.7

Ψ_m — dissipation by mechanical friction: 2.1.4, 8.1.2

1

Three Cases of Characteristic Polynomials

A differential equation of order N is a (section 1.1) relation between a function y, its variable x, and the derivatives $y', \ldots, y^{(N)}$ up to order N; the most general solution, called the **general integral**, involves N arbitrary constants of integration. If the equation is linear in $y, \ldots, y^{(N)}$ and not forced, then it satisfies the **principle of superposition**, stating that a (section 1.2) linear combination of solutions is a solution; thus, given N linearly independent particular integrals, a linear combination of them supplies the general integral, because it is a solution involving N arbitrary constants. If the equation is linear and forced, that is it has a term not involving the **dependent variable**, then its complete integral is the sum of the general integral of the unforced equation plus a **particular integral** of the forced equation. In the case of a linear equation with constant coefficients all particular integrals are elementary functions, both for the unforced equation (section 1.3), and for the forced equation (section 1.4) with forcing by an elementary function; the complete integral can be derived from the roots of characteristic polynomial (section 1.5). A characteristic polynomial is also associated with a linear differential equation with variable coefficients, that is reducible to one with constant coefficients, namely the **homogeneous or Euler type** (section 1.6); in the latter the coefficient of the n-th derivative $y^{(n)}(x)$ is a constant times a power x^n, with exponent equal to the order of derivation. The characteristic polynomial can be used to obtain solutions of the homogeneous linear differential equation with power coefficients, both unforced (section 1.6) and forced (section 1.7). The characteristic polynomial exists not only for linear ordinary differential equations with constant (homogeneous power) coefficients (sections 1.3–1.5, 1.6–1.8), but also for a linear finite difference equation with constant coefficients (section 1.9); the latter relates the elements of a sequence of functions $y_1(x), \ldots, y_N(x)$, and is the third case of the use of a characteristic polynomial to obtain unforced and forced (section 1.9) solutions. The three types of linear equations with a characteristic polynomial are suitable starting cases since they can be solved for arbitrary orders, in terms of elementary functions alone.

1.1 Equation of Order N and Initial Conditions

The general solution of an ordinary differential equation (subsection 1.1.1) involves arbitrary constants (subsection 1.1.2) determined from initial values (subsection 1.1.3), as shown in an example (subsection 1.1.4). In the case of a first-order differential equation the general integral specifies one or more families of curves (subsection 1.1.5); a particular integral corresponds to the curve of the family passing through a given regular point. If several curves (no curve) pass(es) through a point it is a singular point of the second (first) kind of the differential equation [subsections 1.1.6 (1.1.7)]. Besides the general and particular integrals, a differential equation may have a special integral (subsection 1.1.8) distinct from both of the preceding that is not included in the general integral for any value of the arbitrary constant. The solution of a differential equation is a function that satisfies it; conversely given a differentiable function it is possible to construct one or more differential equations (subsection 1.1.9) that it satisfies. A differential equation may involve parameters (subsection 1.1.10), for example, in the coefficients; this leads to bifurcations if there is a different number of solutions for distinct values of the parameters (subsections 1.1.11–1.1.12). The special integrals and bifurcations can occur only for certain types of non-linear differential equations (subsection 1.1.13).

1.1.1 An Ordinary Differential Equation and its Integrals

An **ordinary differential equation of order** N is a relation (1.1b) between a function or **dependent variable** $y(x)$, and its derivatives (1.1a) of order $n = 1,\dots,N$ up to N, and its variable or **independent variable** x:

$$y^{(n)}(x) \equiv \frac{d^n y}{dx^n}: \qquad F\left(x, y, y', y'', \dots y^{(N)}\right) = 0. \qquad (1.1a, b)$$

The most general function $y(x)$ that when substituted into the differential equation (1.1b), satisfies it, is called the **general integral**; any solution of the differential equation (1.1b) that is contained in the general integral, is a **particular integral**. A solution of the differential equation (1.1b) that is not contained in the general integral is called a **special integral**; a special integral may exist for some, not all, forms of differential equation (subsection 1.1.8; sections 5.1–5.4). For example, the simplest differential equation of order N states that the n-th derivative is zero (1.2a):

$$y^{(N)}(x) = 0, \qquad y(x) = \sum_{m=0}^{N-1} C_m x^m, \qquad (1.2a, b)$$

and its general integral is a polynomial (1.2b) of degree $N-1$, with N arbitrary coefficients $C_1,...,C_N$; any set of particular values for the N coefficients of the polynomial (1.2b) specifies a particular integral of the differential equation. In this case there is no special integral, that is, all solutions of the differential equation (1.2a) are contained in (1.2b).

1.1.2 Arbitrary Constants in the General Integral

The example (1.2a, b) suggests that *a differential equation (1.1b) of order N, has a general integral:*

$$f(x,y;C_1,...,C_N)=0, \tag{1.3}$$

involving N arbitrary constants of integration $C_1,...,C_N$. The rigorous statement involves an **existence theorem**, whose proof is deferred to section 9.1. Next is given (subsection 1.1.2) a heuristic reasoning. Differentiating n times the (1.4a) general integral (1.3) with regard to the variable x, leads to the relations (1.4b):

$$n=1,...,N: \qquad y^{(n)}(x)=f_n(x;C_1,...,C_N). \tag{1.4a, b}$$

Eliminating the N constants of integration $C_1,...,C_N$, among the $N+1$ relations (1.3) and (1.4a, b), specifies a relation between $x,y,y',...y^{(N)}$, namely, the differential equation (1.1b). If the number M of constants of integration $C_1,...,C_M$ had been distinct $M\neq N$ from the order N of the equation, a contradiction would have been arrived at, because: (i) if $M>N$, then only N constants would be eliminated, and the remaining $M-N$ constants would appear in the differential equation; (ii) if $M<N$, then the $N+1$ equations for M unknowns would be generally incompatible; in the latter case (ii) compatibility would be assured by choosing $M+1$ equations for M unknowns, but this would lead to a differential equation of order $M<N$ inferior to (1.1b). The possibility remains, for particular forms of the differential equation (1.1b), of the existence special integral(s), not contained in the general integral (1.3), and involving less than N constants of integration, possibly even none at all.

1.1.3 Single- or Multi-Point or Mixed Boundary Values

In order to determine the N constants of integration $C_1,...,C_N$ in the general integral (1.3), it is necessary to impose N **boundary values**, for example, the values of the function and its first $N-1$ derivatives (1.5a) at (1.5b) point x_0:

$$m=0,...,N-1: \qquad y^{(m)}(x_0)=a_m, \qquad y(x_m)=b_m, \tag{1.5a–c}$$

or the value of the function at N distinct points (1.5c). The case (1.5b) is one of **single-point** x_0, and (1.5c) of **N-point** $x_0, ..., x_{N-1}$ boundary values; in the **mixed** case, the function y or a derivative of some order α_m is given (1.6b) at a set (1.6a) of coincident or distinct points $x_0, ..., x_{N-1}$:

$$m = 0, ..., N-1: \qquad y^{(\alpha_n)}(x_m) = c_m. \qquad (1.6a, b)$$

In all cases, the system of N equations (1.5b), or (1.5c), or (1.6b), should be solvable for $C_1, ..., C_N$, that requires that *the boundary conditions be compatible and independent*. For example, if some $M < N$ coincide, then not more than $N - M$ values (1.5c) are independent; if in (1.6b) all the derivatives are of order $\alpha_n \geq M$, among the N values there are $N - M$ that are either redundant or incompatible.

1.1.4 Example of a General Integral and of Initial Values

As an example, consider the differential equation of second order (1.7a):

$$y'' = \frac{1}{x}, \qquad y' = \log x + C_1, \qquad y = x \log x - x + C_1 x + C_2, \quad (1.7a, b, c)$$

that has general integral given (1.7b, c) by (1.8c):

$$A = C_1 - 1, \qquad B \equiv C_2: \qquad y(x; A, B) = x \log x + Ax + B, \qquad (1.8a–c)$$

where new constants of integration (1.8a, b) have been introduced. The latter can be determined, as indicated in the Table 1.1, where one-point, two-point, and mixed boundary values have been considered. The analytic preliminaries about the solution of differential equations of arbitrary order (subsections 1.1.1–1.1.4) can be illustrated geometrically for first-order equations (subsections 1.1.5–1.1.8).

1.1.5 Families of Integral Curves in the Plane

A differential equation of first order (1.9a) may in principle be solved for the slope (1.9b):

$$F(x, y, y') = 0 \qquad \Rightarrow \qquad y' = f(x, y). \qquad (1.9a, b)$$

Thus, it specifies (Figure 1.1) at each point of the plane a tangent direction. The general integral (1.10a) is a **parametric family of curves** whose tangents satisfy (1.9a) ≡ (1.9b):

$$y = y(x; C); \qquad y_0 = y(x_0; C_0), \qquad (1.10a, b)$$

TABLE 1.1

Boundary Conditions for a Differential Equation

Case	1-point	2-point	Mixed
boundary values	$y(1)=0$	$y(1)=0$	$y(1)=0$
	$y'(1)=0$	$y(2)=0$	$y'(2)=0$
relations	$A+B=0$	$A+B=0$	$A+B=0$
	$1+A=0$	$2\log 2+2A+B=0$	$\log 2+1+A=0$
constants	$A=-1$	$A=-2\log 2$	$A=-1-\log 2$
	$B=+1$	$B=2\log 2$	$B=1+\log 2$
solution	$y(x)=x\log x-x+1$	$x\log\frac{x}{4}+\log 4$	$x\log\frac{x}{2}-x+1+\log 2$

Note: The two arbitrary constants in the general integral (1.8c) of the second-order ordinary differential equation (1.7a) may be determined by three types of pairs of boundary conditions: (i) single-point, that is the values of the solution and its first derivative at the same point; (ii) two-point, that is the value of the solution at two distinct points; (iii) mixed, that is the value of the solution and its first derivative at two distinct points.

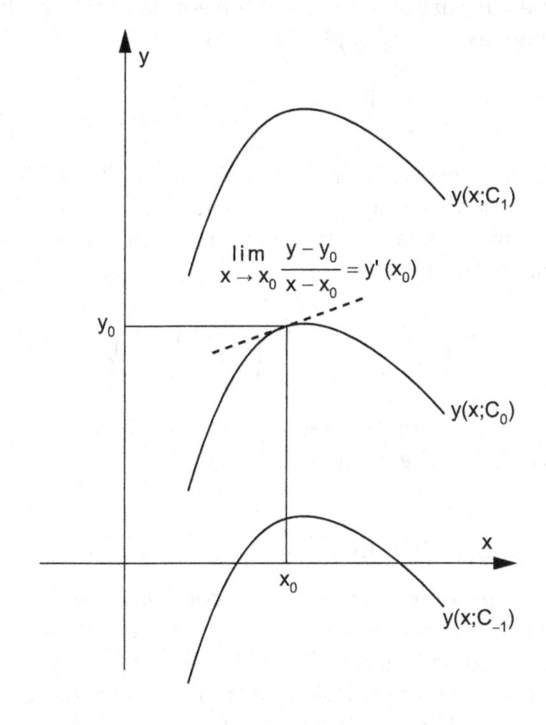

FIGURE 1.1
The general integral of a first-order ordinary differential equation is a one-parameter family of integral curves. Through each regular point passes one curve of the family specified by a particular value of the arbitrary constant. The differential equation specifies at each point the slope of the tangent to the integral curve passing through that point.

through a given point in the plane taken as the boundary condition (1.10b) passes one **integral curve** of the family corresponding to a particular value C_0 of the constant C, and hence to a particular integral. The points of the plane through which passes only one integral curve are called **regular points** of the differential equations. In specific cases non-regular or singular points (subsection 1.1.6) may occur.

1.1.6 Regular and Singular Points of a Differential Equation

Through a **singular point of the first (second) kind** of the differential equation (1.9a) either (i) passes no integral curve [or (ii) pass several integral curves, possibly even an infinite number]. As an example of the singular point of the first kind, (i) the differential equation (1.11a) has the general integral (1.11b):

$$y' = -\frac{1}{x^2}, \qquad y = \frac{1}{x} + C; \tag{1.11a, b}$$

the integral curves (Figure 1.2) consist of the equilateral hyperbolas (1.12a, b) with the coordinate axis as asymptotes (1.12b, c):

$$C = 0: \quad xy = 1; \qquad \lim_{x\to\infty} y = 0 = \lim_{y\to\infty} x, \tag{1.12a–d}$$

plus (1.12c, d) all their vertical translations by C along the y-axis. No curves of the family cross the y-axis that consists of singular point $x = 0$, in agreement with (1.13a); each hyperbola has two branches, and all are asymptotically tangent to the y-axis (1.12b):

$$\lim_{x\to 0} y' = 0; \qquad y\left(x = -\frac{1}{C}\right) = 0, \tag{1.13a, b}$$

all members of the family of integral curves cross the x-axis at (1.13b) except for $C = 0$, which also has the x-axis as asymptote.

1.1.7 Singular Points of Two Kinds

The case (ii) of a singular point of the second kind through which pass several integral curves corresponds to the first-order differential equation in implicit form (1.9a) that is non-linear in the derivative and has several roots (1.9b). For example, the simple quadratic first-order differential equation (1.14a) has roots (1.14b) specifying two families of integral curves (1.14c), which are straight lines with slopes $\pm a$:

$$y'^2 = a^2, \qquad y'_\pm = \pm a, \qquad y_\pm(x) = \pm ax + C_\pm. \tag{1.14a–c}$$

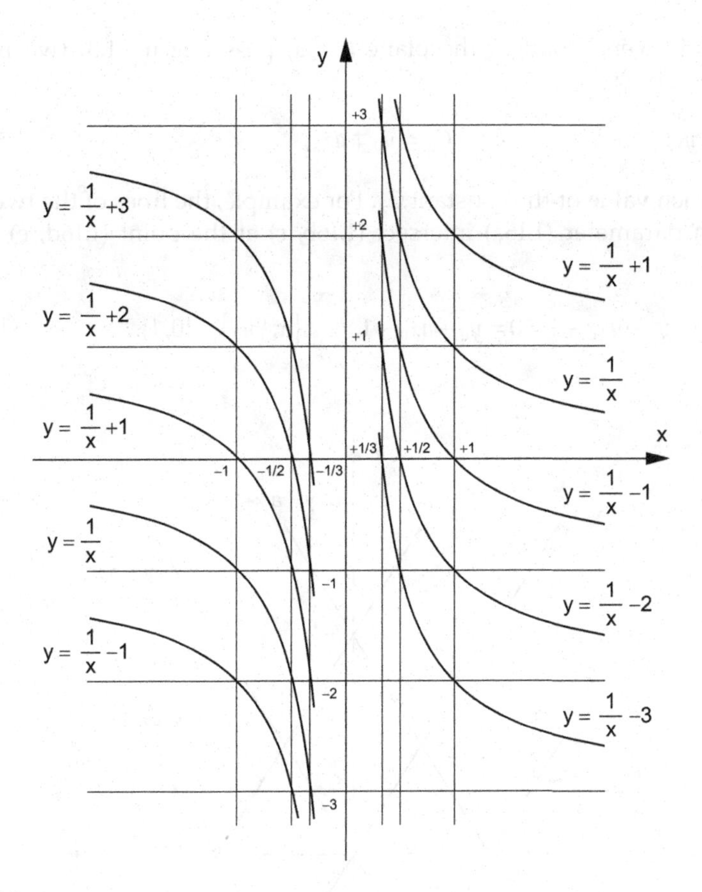

FIGURE 1.2
An ordinary differential equation may have singular point(s) of the first kind through which no integral curve passes. For example, if the integral curves are obtained by translation along the y-axis of a hyperbola tangent asymptotically to the x-axis and y-axis, then: (i) all integral curves are asymptotically tangent to the y-axis, that is the locus of singular points; (ii) all points outside the y-axis are regular points through which passes one integral curve.

Although two arbitrary constants $C_\pm$ appear in (1.14c) the general integral involves only one arbitrary constant C, as it should for a first-order differential equation:

$$0 = y_+(x)y_-(x) = (y - ax - C)(y + ax + C). \qquad (1.14d, e)$$

The general integral (1.14d) of the differential equation (1.14a) is the product of the two terms (1.14c), because if just one of them vanishes the differential equation is satisfied; thus, when substituting (1.14c) in (1.14d) the two constants $C_\pm$ may be replaced by one C.

Through every point of the plane (1.15a) pass (Figure 1.3) two integral curves (1.15b, c):

$$y_\pm(x_0) = y_0: \qquad C_\pm = y_0 \mp a x_0, \tag{1.15a–c}$$

one for each value of the constant $C_\pm$. For example, the lines of the two families with parameter (1.16a) intersect (1.16b, c) at the point (1.16d, e) on the y-axis:

$$C_\pm = 1: \qquad y_0 - a x_0 - 1 = 0 = y_0 + a x_0 - 1, \qquad \{x_0, y_0\} = \{0,1\}. \tag{1.16a–e}$$

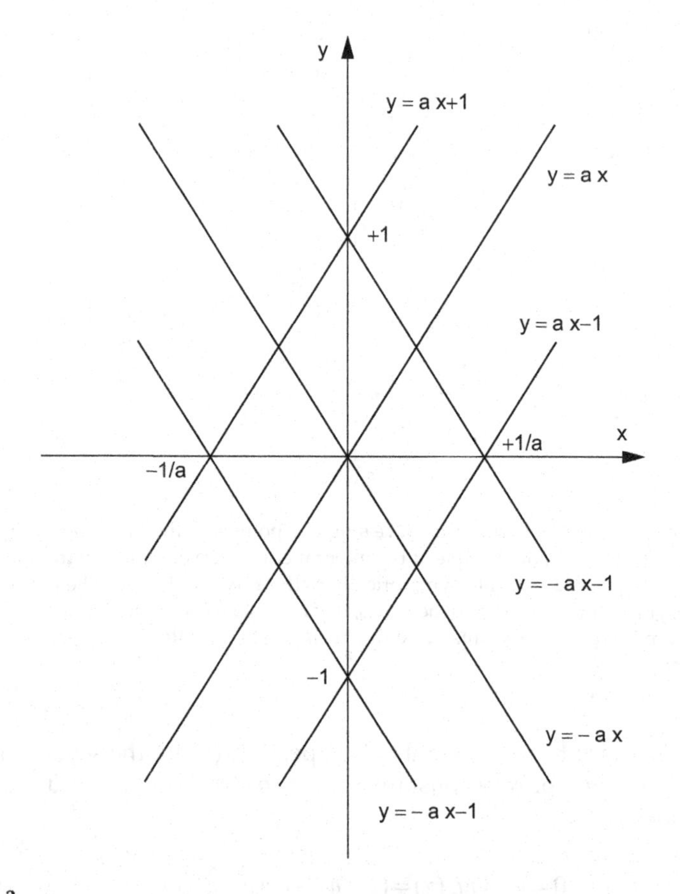

FIGURE 1.3
A non-linear ordinary differential equation may have singular point(s) of the second kind through which pass two or more, possibly an infinite number, of integral curves. In the case when the integral curves are straight lines with slopes $\pm a$ every point of the plane is a singular point through which pass two integral curves. The line vortex (source/sink) in a potential flow [Figure I.12.2b(a)] has a singular point of the first (second) kind at the center through which no (all) streamlines pass.

In the preceding cases (subsections 1.1.5–1.1.7) have been considered only the general (particular) integral of the first-order differential equation, corresponding to a family of integral curves (a particular curve of the set). Next are considered special integrals (subsection 1.1.8) that are not contained in the general integral, and thus do not coincide with a particular integral for any value of the arbitrary constant.

1.1.8 Envelope as an Example of a Special Integral

As an example of special integral consider the following case (Figure 1.4): (i) the integral curves (1.10a) have an **envelope**, that is there is a curve tangent to all members of the family and coincident with none of them; (ii) this curve has the same slope as the integral curves at the point of tangency and thus satisfies the differential equation (1.9a) ≡ (1.9b); (iii) it does not coincide with any integral curve, so it is not contained in the general integral, and must be a special integral. It has been shown that *if the family of integral curves (1.10a) of the first-order differential equation (1.9a) has an envelope* (Figure 1.4), *the latter is a special integral of the differential equation.* The converse is not true, that is there are special integrals of a differential equation that are not envelopes (sections 5.1–5.4).

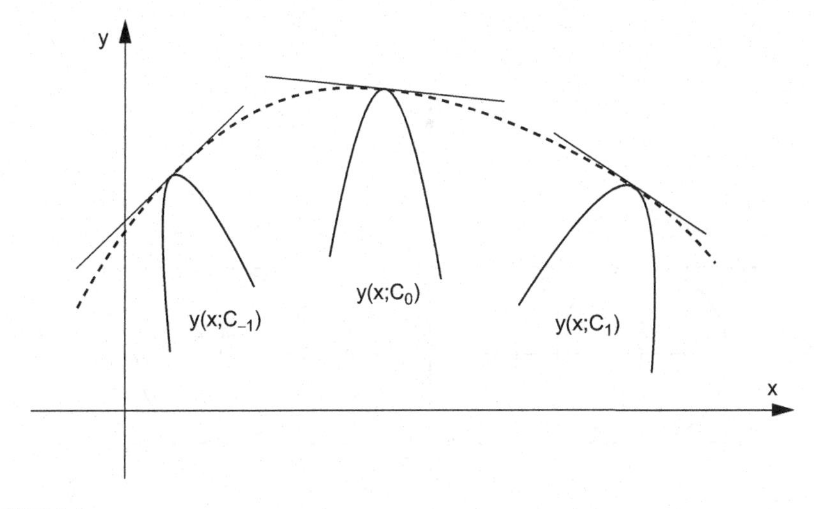

FIGURE 1.4
The general integral of an ordinary differential equation is a single-parameter family of integral curves with each value of the arbitrary constant of integration specifying an integral curve of the family. If the family of curves has an envelope it is also a solution of the differential equation, because it has the same slope at the common points of tangency. The envelope does not belong to the family of integral curves, and thus, specifies a special integral, which is not contained in the general integral for any value of the arbitrary constant. There may exist special integrals other than envelopes (Figures 5.1 to 5.14).

As an example, consider the family of circles with radius R and center at $(C,0)$ along the real axis (1.17a):

$$(x-C)^2+y^2=R^2; \qquad x-C+y'y=0. \tag{1.17a, b}$$

Differentiation gives the equation (1.17b) and elimination of $x-C$ with (1.17a), which leads to the differential equation (1.118a):

$$R^2=y^2\left(1+y'^2\right); \qquad y_{\pm}(x)=\pm R. \tag{1.18a, b}$$

A simple solution of (1.18a) is (1.18b), which does not involve the arbitrary constant C. The arbitrary constant C appears in the general integral (1.17a) of the differential equation (1.18a). The preceding results may be summarized (Figure 1.5) as follows: (i) the first-order differential equation (1.18a) has for the general integral (1.17a) specifying the integral curves that are the circles (1.17a) of radius R with center at $(C,0)$ on the real axis; (ii) each circle or integral curve corresponds to a particular integral for a given position $(C,0)$ of the center; (iii) all circles have the same radius and, thus, all integral curves are tangent to the horizontal lines (1.18b) that are the envelopes of the family of circles; (iv) the envelopes (1.18b) satisfy the

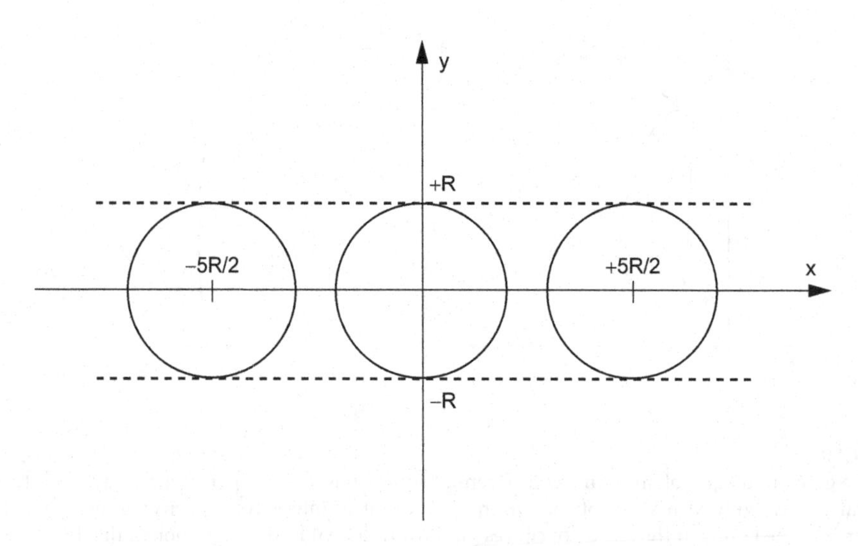

FIGURE 1.5
An example of envelope is the pair of horizontal straight lines to which are tangent the circles with the same radius and centers on the x-axis. The corresponding ordinary differential equation has the circles (straight lines) as the general (special) integral.

differential equation (1.18a) and are not contained in the general integral (1.17a) and, thus, are special integrals. In most of the preceding examples (subsections 1.1.1–1.1.7) the differential equation is given, and its solution is sought, which is the most general function that satisfies it. In the last case (subsection 1.1.8) the solution was given (1.17a) and a differential equation was found (1.18a) that it satisfies. This inverse problem to the solution of a differential equation is of less interest, but it is nevertheless briefly considered next (subsection 1.1.9).

1.1.9 Differential Equations Satisfied by a Function

Given a differentiable function, there are several differential equations of the first (or higher) order(s) obtained combining the independent x (dependent y) variable and the first y' (higher y'',...) order derivatives. For example, the function (1.19a) has derivative (1.19b):

$$y = x \log x, \qquad y' = 1 + \log x. \tag{1.19a, b}$$

Combining (1.19a, b) it is possible to form distinct differential equations of first order, for example:

$$y' = 1 + \frac{y}{x}, \qquad y' = 1 + \log y - \log(\log x), \tag{1.20a, b}$$

where (1.20a) [(1.20b)] follows from (1.19b) by substituting $\log x$ (x) from (1.19a). Proceeding as an example with the differential equation (1.20a) it is clear that (1.19a) is not the general integral, since it involves no constant of integration. To obtain the general integral, (1.20a) is rewritten as (1.21a):

$$x\,dy = x\,dx + y\,dx; \qquad 0 = \frac{dy}{x} - \frac{y}{x^2}dx - \frac{dx}{x} = d\left(\frac{y}{x} - \log x\right), \tag{1.21a, b}$$

dividing by x^2 leads to an exact differential (1.21b); thus, the general integral of the first-order differential equation (1.20a) is (1.22a):

$$y(x;C) = x(\log x + C), \qquad y(x;0) = x \log x, \tag{1.22a, b}$$

and the particular integral for $C = 0$ is (1.22b) $\equiv$ (1.19a). It has been shown that the same function (1.19a) can satisfy distinct differential equations (1.20a) and (1.20b). Conversely, the same differential equation can have a distinct number of solutions depending on the parameters and leading to bifurcations (subsection 1.1.10).

1.1.10 Parametric Differential Equations and Bifurcations

A differential equation (1.1b) may involve, in addition to the independent x variable and the dependent y variable, and the derivatives of the latter with regard to the former (1.1a) also a set of parameters (1.23a) that also appear in the general integral (1.23b):

$$F\left(x, y, y', \ldots, y^{(N)}; a_1, \ldots, a_M\right) = 0, \quad y = y\left(x; C_1, \ldots, C_N; a_1, \ldots, a_M\right), \quad (1.23\text{a, b})$$

and may appear, for example, in the coefficients. The solution may be (i) unique for each value of the parameters or (ii) there may be more than one solution for the same values of the parameters.

For example, the non-linear quadratic differential equation (1.14a) has two solutions (1.14c) for each value of the parameter a at all points (Figure 1.3). A more interesting case is when there is one solution for a range of the parameter, say $a < a_0$ and several solutions for another range, say $a > a_0$, so that $a = a_0$ is a **bifurcation** value of the parameter a. As an example, consider the non-linear second-order differential equation (1.24a):

$$0 = y'' + ay + y^3: \quad 0 = y''y' + y'y\left(a + y^3\right) = \frac{d}{dx}\left(\frac{y'^2}{2} + \frac{ay^2}{2} + \frac{y^4}{4}\right), \quad (1.24\text{a, b})$$

that on multiplication by y' becomes an exact differential (1.24b). Thus, the non-linear second-order differential equation (1.24a) has for **first integral** the non-linear first-order differential equation:

$$C = y'^2 + a\, y^2 + \frac{1}{2} y^4 \equiv \Psi(y, y'), \quad (1.25)$$

where C is an arbitrary constant. If it is shown next that the differential equation has one (three) solutions [subsection 1.1.11(1.1.12)] for $a > 0 (a < 0)$, then $a = 0$ is a bifurcation value of the parameter a.

1.1.11 Single Solution around Stable Equilibrium

The differential equation (1.25) can be rewritten (1.26a) involving a potential function (1.26b):

$$y'^2 = C - \Phi(y), \qquad \Phi(y) = y^2\left(a + \frac{1}{2} y^2\right), \quad (1.26\text{a, b})$$

whose first two derivatives are:

$$\Phi'(y) = 2y\left(a + y^2\right), \qquad \Phi''(y) = 2\left(a + 3y^2\right). \quad (1.27\text{a, b})$$

In the case (1.28a) the potential (1.26b) is a monotonic function (Figure 1.6a) with a minimum (1.28b, c) value zero (1.28d) at the origin, that is thus a position of stable equilibrium:

$$0 < a = |a|: \qquad \Phi'(0) = 0 < 2a = \Phi''(0), \qquad \Phi(y) \geq \Phi(0) = 0. \tag{1.28a–d}$$

This is confirmed by the paths (1.25) in the **phase plane** (y, y') that are (Figure 1.6b): (i) closed curves for $C \geq 0$; (ii) reduce to the origin $y = 0 = y'$ for $C = 0$: (iii) do not exist for $C < 0$. Using the **path diagram** with the arbitrary constant C as a third coordinate orthogonal to the phase plane (Figure 1.6c) the paths contract from closed curves to a point and disappear.

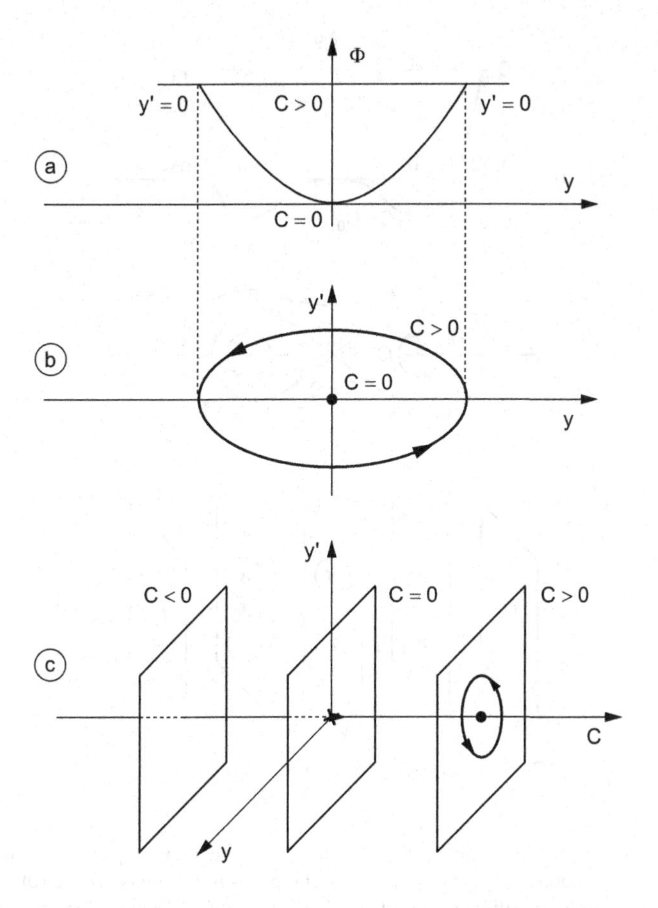

FIGURE 1.6
The monotonic potential (a) has a minimum at the origin, which is a position of stable equilibrium. The paths in the phase plane are (b) closed curves for $C > 0$, reduce to the origin for $C = 0$ and there is no solution for $C < 0$; this is shown in the path diagram (c) with C as third axis orthogonal to the phase plane.

1.1.12 Three Solutions around Stable/Unstable Equilibria

In the case (1.29a), the potential (1.26b) has three extrema (1.29b–d):

$$0 > a = -|a|: \quad \Phi'(y_{1-3}) = 0 \Rightarrow y_1 = 0, y_{2,3} = \pm\sqrt{-a} = \pm|a|^{1/2} \equiv \pm b, \tag{1.29a–d}$$

of which (Figure 1.7a) the origin (other two points) is a local maximum (minimum) and hence a position of unstable (stable) equilibrium (1.30a) [(1.30b)]:

$$\Phi''(y_1) = \Phi''(0) = 2a = -2|a| < 0, \tag{1.30a}$$

$$\Phi''(y_{2,3}) = 2\left[a + 3(y_{2,3})^2\right] = 2(a - 3a) = -4a = 4|a| > 0. \tag{1.30b}$$

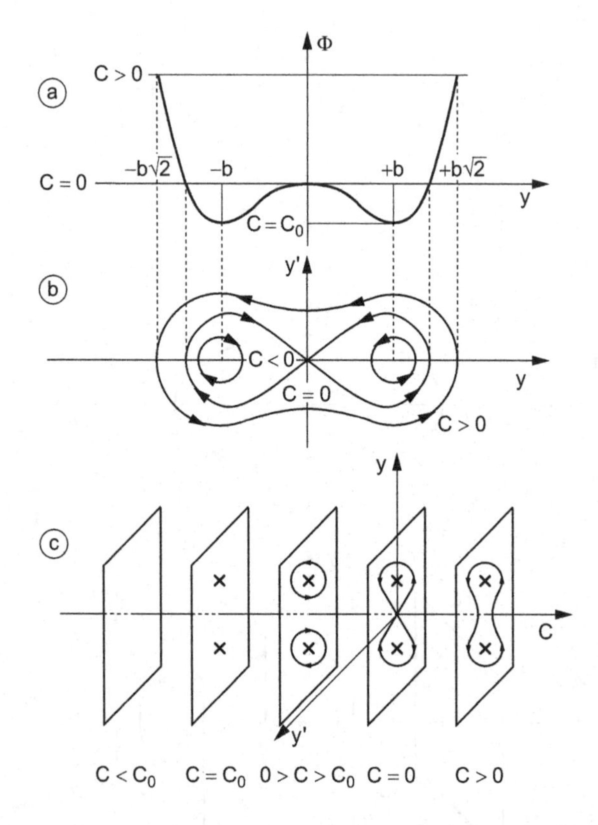

FIGURE 1.7
The potential (a) is not monotonic and has one local maximum (two global minima C_0) at the origin (at symmetric points outside the origin). The paths in the phase plane (b) may be: (i) a closed curve around all equilibrium points for $C > 0$; (ii) for $C = 0$ a curve passing through the position of unstable equilibrium at the origin and going round both positions of stable equilibrium; (iii) for $0 > C > C_0$ there are separate closed paths around each position of stable equilibrium. As seen in the path diagram (c) the paths reduce to the points of stable equilibrium for $C = C_0$, and for $C < C_0$ there are no solutions.

The potential is zero at the local maximum at the origin (1.30c) and takes a negative value at the absolute minima (1.30d):

$$\Phi(y_1)=\Phi(0)=0, \Phi(y_{2,3})=(y_{2,3})^2\left[a+\frac{1}{2}(y_{2,3})^2\right]=-a\left(a-\frac{a}{2}\right)=-\frac{|a|^2}{2}\equiv C_0<0. \tag{1.30c, d}$$

The curves in phase plane (y, y') intersect the y-axis at the points (1.31a), which are (1.26a, b) the roots (1.31c) of the quartic polynomial (1.31b).

$$y'(y_*)=0: \quad C=\Phi(y_*)=\frac{1}{2}(y_*)^4+a(y_*)^2, \quad (y_*)^2=-a\pm\sqrt{a^2+2C}. \tag{1.31a–c}$$

Thus, there are five cases (Figure 1.7b):

$$C=0: \qquad (y_*)^2=0,-2a=0,2|a|, \quad y_*=0,\pm\sqrt{2|a|}=0,\pm b\sqrt{2}; \tag{1.32a–c}$$

$$C>0: \quad 2|a|=-2a<(y_+)^2>0>(y_-)^2, \quad y_*=\pm y_+,\pm i|y_-|^2, \quad |y_+|>b\sqrt{2}, \tag{1.32d–g}$$

$$0>C>C_0: \qquad 2|a|=-2a>(y_+)^2>(y_-)^2>0, \quad y_*=\pm y_\pm, |y_*|<b\sqrt{2}. \tag{1.32h–k}$$

$$C=C_0=-\frac{a^2}{2}: \qquad (y_*)^2=-a=|a|, \quad y_*=\pm|a|^{1/2}=y_{2,3}; \tag{1.32l–n}$$

$$C<C_0=-\frac{a^2}{2}: \qquad (y_*)^2=-a\pm i|-2C-a^2|^{1/2}, \tag{1.32p, q}$$

namely, (Figure 1.7c). (i) In the case (1.32a) there are (1.32b) a double root at the origin and two real symmetric roots (1.32c), and the curve passes through the origin and the points $\pm b\sqrt{2}$ and thus, is lace-like, and is the **separatrix** of the cases (ii) and (iii); (ii) in the case (1.32d), there are (1.32e) a pair of conjugate imaginary roots and a pair of real symmetric roots (1.32f), and the single closed curve lies outside the separatrix; (iii) in the case (1.32h), there are (1.32i) two pairs of real symmetric roots (1.32j), and hence two closed symmetric curves inside the separatrix; (iv) the two curves reduce to two symmetric points (1.32n) in the case (1.32l) of a pair of double real symmetric roots; (v) in the remaining case (1.32p), all roots are complex (1.32q) and there is no real curve. The evolution as C changes from positive to negative is shown in three dimensions in the path diagram (Figure 1.7c) with the two-lobed closed path shrinking to a lace passing through the origin, then splitting into two closed curves that shrink to two points and disappear.

1.1.13 Poincaré (1892) Diagrams and Parametric Evolution

The value $a = 0$ of the parameter a corresponds to a bifurcation, as can be seen from the **Poincare (1892) diagram** (Figure 1.8) adding to the phase plane (Figures 1.6–1.7), a third orthogonal coordinate, namely the parameter a such that: (i) For $a > 0$ there is only one solution (Figure 1.6) around the minimum of the potential (Figure 1.6); (ii) For $a < 0$ there are three types of solutions around (i–1) each of the minima $\pm b$, and (ii–3) around both minima, with (ii–2) the separatrix passing through the local maximum at the origin.

The non-linear differential equation (1.24a) applies to a **anharmonic oscillator** (section 4.4). It has been shown that there is as great a variety of solutions of differential equations as for the functions that satisfy them. The non-linear differential equations may have special integrals (subsection 1.1.8) and bifurcations (subsection 1.1.10) that do not occur for linear differential equations; the latter are a simpler starting case considered next (section 1.2) for which the general integral contains all solutions and can be constructed from linearly independent particular integrals.

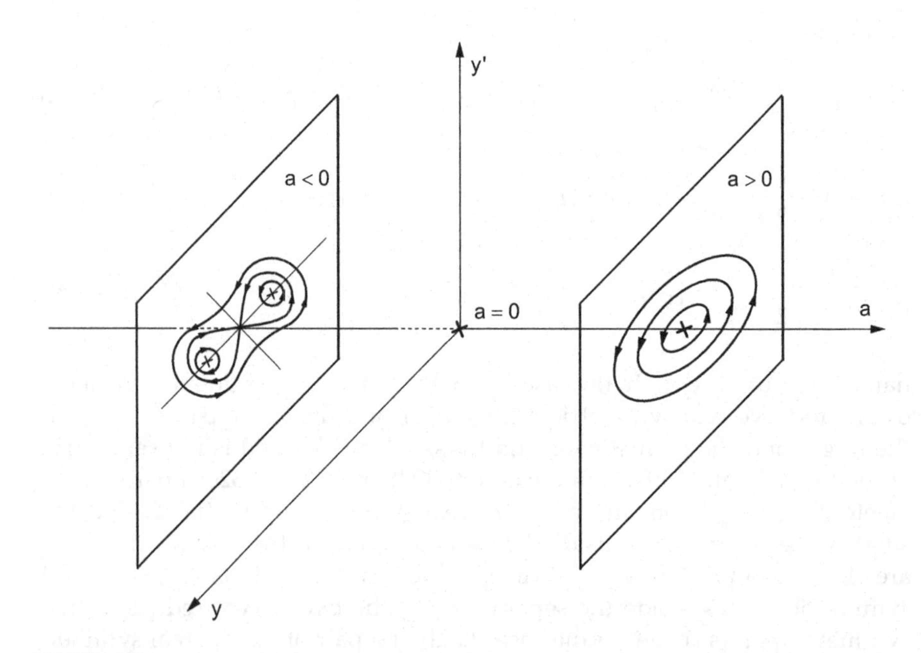

FIGURE 1.8
The two potentials in Figures 1.6a (1.7a) correspond to the same potential function with distinct values of a parameter a, namely positive $a > 0$ (negative $a < 0$) to which corresponds one (three) solutions [Figure 1.6b (1.7b)]. Thus $a = 0$ is a bifurcation value of the parameter across which (Figure 1.8) the qualitative nature of the solution of the differential equation changes from one to three solutions.

1.2 General, Particular, and Complete Integrals

A differential equation linear in the dependent variable and its derivatives (subsection 1.2.1) allows superposition of particular solutions (subsection 1.2.2); thus, its general integral in the unforced case is specified by (subsection 1.2.4) a linear combination of linearly independent (subsection 1.2.3) particular solutions. If the linear differential equation has a forcing term not involving the dependent variable (subsection 1.2.5) adding a particular integral to the general integral of the unforced equation specifies the complete integral of the forced equation (subsection 1.2.6).

1.2.1 Linear Unforced and Forced Differential Equations

The n-th order differential equation (1.1a, b) is **linear** if the dependent variable y and its derivatives $y',...,y^{(N)}$ appear linearly:

$$\sum_{n=0}^{N} A_n(x)\frac{d^n y}{dx^n} = B(x), \tag{1.33}$$

with coefficients $B, A_1,..., A_N$, that may depend on the independent variable x; thus, any powers or cross-products of the dependent variable and/or of its derivatives are excluded. The equation (1.33) may be written in the form (1.34a):

$$\left\{L\left(\frac{d}{dx}\right)\right\}y(x) = B(x), \qquad L\left(\frac{d}{dx}\right) \equiv \sum_{n=0}^{N} A_n(x)\frac{d^n}{dx^n}, \tag{1.34a, b}$$

where (1.34b) is a **linear differential operator**, because it satisfies the **principle of superposition** (1.35b):

$$y_1,...,y_M \in \mathcal{D}^N(|C): \quad \left\{L\left(\frac{d}{dx}\right)\right\}\sum_{m=1}^{M} C_m y_m(x) = \sum_{m=1}^{M} C_m \left\{L\left(\frac{d}{dx}\right)\right\}y_m(x), \tag{1.35a, b}$$

for arbitrary constants $C_1,..., C_M$ and M functions that are and N-times differentiable (1.35a). The differential equation (1.33) is **unforced (forced)** if $B = 0\,(B \neq 0)$, in which case the zero function $y = 0$ is (is not) a solution. From (1.35b) it follows that if $y_1,..., y_M$ are solutions of the linear unforced equation (1.36a), then a linear combination of them (1.36b), with arbitrary constants $C_1,...,C_M$ is also a solution (1.36c):

$$\left\{L\left(\frac{d}{dx}\right)\right\}y_m(x)=0 \quad \wedge \quad y(x)\equiv\sum_{m=1}^{M}C_m y_m(x), \quad \Rightarrow \quad \left\{L\left(\frac{d}{dx}\right)\right\}y(x)=0. \qquad (1.36\text{a–c})$$

1.2.2 Superposition of Linearly Independent Solutions

If the number of terms M in (1.36b), is taken to be equal to the order N of the differential operator (1.34b), then the solution (1.36c) involves $N=M$ arbitrary constants of integration $C_1,...,C_N$, and is the general integral of the linear unforced differential equation. A necessary and sufficient condition is that the N functions $y_1,...,y_N$ be **linearly independent**, that a linear combination of the functions vanishes (1.37a) if and only if all coefficients are zero (1.37b):

$$\sum_{n=1}^{N}C_n y_n(x)=0 \qquad \Leftrightarrow \qquad C_1=C_2=...=C_N=0. \qquad (1.37\text{a, b})$$

If (1.37a) were met with at least one coefficient $C_n\neq 0$ being non-zero, then the function $y_n(x)$ would either be zero or a linear combination of the others; in both cases, substitution into (1.36b) would reduce the number of constants of integration below N, so that it could not be the general integral of a differential equation of order N. Thus, *the general integral of the linear (1.33) ≡ (1.34a, b) unforced differential equation (1.36c), is a linear combination (1.36b) of $M=N$ particular integrals (1.36a), which are linearly independent (1.37a, b).*

1.2.3 Wronskian (1812) and Linear Independence of Differentiable Functions

It is, thus, useful to have a criterion for the linear independence (1.37a, b) of a set of N functions $y_1,...,y_N$, that are $(N-1)$-times differentiable. Differentiating (1.37a) $m=0,...,N-1$ times (1.38a) leads to a linear homogeneous system of equations (1.38b):

$$m=0,...,N-1: \qquad \sum_{n=1}^{N}C_n y_n^{(m)}(x)=0 \quad \Leftrightarrow \quad C_1=C_2=...=C_n=0. \qquad (1.38\text{a–c})$$

The necessary condition that the linear homogeneous system of equations (1.38b) ≡ (1.39b):

$$y_n(x) \in \mathcal{D}^{N-1}(|C): \quad \begin{bmatrix} y_1(x) & y_2(x) & \cdots & y_N(x) \\ y_1'(x) & y_2'(x) & \ddots & y_N'(x) \\ \vdots & \vdots & \ddots & \vdots \\ y_1^{(N-1)}(x) & y_2^{(N-1)}(x) & \cdots & y_N^{(N-1)}(x) \end{bmatrix} \begin{bmatrix} C_1 \\ C_2 \\ \vdots \\ C_N \end{bmatrix} = 0, \tag{1.39a, b}$$

has only the trivial solution (1.38c), is that the determinant (1.40c) is non-zero:

$$n = 1, \ldots, N; m = 0, \ldots, N-1: \qquad 0 \neq W(y_1, \ldots, y_N) \equiv Det\left|y_n^{(m-1)}(x)\right|$$

$$= \begin{bmatrix} y_1(x) & y_2(x) & \cdots & y_N(x) \\ y_1'(x) & y_2'(x) & \ddots & y_N'(x) \\ \vdots & \vdots & \ddots & \vdots \\ y_1^{(N-1)}(x) & y_2^{(N-1)}(x) & \cdots & y_N^{(N-1)}(x) \end{bmatrix}. \tag{1.40a–c}$$

The determinant of a set of N functions (1.40a) that are (1.40b) differentiable ($N-1$)-times (1.39a) is called (1.40c) the **Wronskian** (1812). It has been shown that *a set N functions $y_1, \ldots, y_N$ that are $(N-1)$-times differentiable (1.39a) and has non-zero Wronskian (1.40c) is linearly independent (1.37a, b).*

1.2.4 General Integral of the Linear Unforced Differential Equation (Lagrange, 1765; Fuchs, 1866)

The preceding results provide *a method of solution of linear (1.33) ≡ (1.34a, b) unforced (1.36c) ordinary differential equations of order N: (i) N particular integrals $y_1, \ldots, y_N$ must be found that are N-times differentiable (1.41a); (ii) it should be checked that they are linearly independent (1.37a, b), that is have non-zero Wronskian (1.40a–c) and thus, form a* ***fundamental system (Fuchs, 1866)****; (iii) the general integral (1.41b) is* ***(Lagrange, 1765)*** *a linear combination of the N particular integrals, involving N arbitrary constants of integration $C_1, \ldots, C_N$:*

$$y_1,(x), \ldots, y_N(x) \in \mathcal{D}^N(|C): \qquad y(x) = \sum_{n=1}^{N} C_n \, y_n(x); \tag{1.41a, b}$$

(iv) the N constants of integration are determined from N independent and compatible boundary conditions, such as (1.5a, b) or (1.5a, c) or (1.6a, b). For example, the linear unforced second-order ordinary differential equation (1.42a):

$$(x-1)y'' - xy' + y = 0, \qquad y_1 = x, \qquad y_2 = e^x, \tag{1.42a, b, c}$$

has particular integrals (1.42b, c); their Wronskian (1.43a) is non-zero:

$$W(y_1) = \begin{vmatrix} y_1 & y_2 \\ y_1' & y_2' \end{vmatrix} = \begin{vmatrix} x & e^x \\ 1 & e^x \end{vmatrix} = (x-1)e^x = W\left(x, e^x\right) \neq 0, \; y(x) = C_1 x + C_2 e^x, \tag{1.43a, b}$$

implying that the particular integrals (1.42b, c) are linearly independent; hence, a linear combination (1.43b), with two arbitrary constants of integration C_1, C_2, is the general integral of the differential equation (1.42a).

1.2.5 A Particular Integral of the Linear Forced Equation

Consider now the general linear forced ordinary differential equation (1.33) ≡ (1.34a, b), and let $y_*(x)$ be any particular integral, the simpler the better, not involving any arbitrary constant:

$$B(x) = \left\{L\left(\frac{d}{dx}\right)\right\} y_*(x) = \sum_{n=0}^{N} A_n(x) \frac{d^n y_*}{dx^n}. \tag{1.44}$$

Since the operator (1.34b) is linear (1.35b), it follows from (1.34a; 1.44) that:

$$\left\{L\left(\frac{d}{dx}\right)\right\}\left[y(x) - y_*(x)\right] = \left\{L\left(\frac{d}{dx}\right)\right\} y(x) - \left\{L\left(\frac{d}{dx}\right)\right\} y_*(x) = B(x) - B(x) = 0, \tag{1.45}$$

the difference between the general y and a (1.44) particular y_* integral of the forced equation (1.33), is a solution (1.45) of the unforced equation, that is (1.36b) is replaced by (1.46):

$$y(x) - y_*(x) = \sum_{n=1}^{N} C_n y_n(x); \tag{1.46}$$

the r.h.s. of (1.46) is a linear combination of N linearly independent particular solutions of the homogeneous equation unforced differential equation.

Rewriting (1.46) in the form (1.47) specifies the complete integral of the forced differential equation:

$$y(x) = y_*(x) + \sum_{n=1}^{N} C_n y_n(x). \tag{1.47}$$

It can be checked that (1.47) satisfies the forced equation:

$$L\{y\} = L\{y_*\} + \sum_{n=1}^{N} C_N L\{y_n\} = L\{y_*\} = B; \tag{1.48}$$

also, it involves N arbitrary constants of integration $C_1,\ldots,C_N$, if the particular integrals $y_1,\ldots,y_N$ of the unforced equation (1.36a), are linearly independent (1.37a, b) or (1.40a–c).

1.2.6 Complete Integral of the Linear Forced Equation (D'Alembert, 1762)

It has been shown that: *the* ***complete integral*** *(1.47) of the linear forced* ***(D'Alembert, 1762)*** *differential equation (1.33) ≡ (1.34a, b), is the sum of: (i) the general integral (1.41b) of the unforced equation (1.36c), that is, a linear combination of N linearly independent (1.40a–c) particular integrals (1.36a) involving N arbitrary constants of integration* $C_1,\ldots,C_N$*; (ii) any particular integral* y_* *of the forced equation (1.44), involving no constants of integration, that is, the simpler the better.* For example, consider the linear, forced second-order differential equation:

$$(x-1)y'' - xy' + y = 2(1-x)\cos x + 2\sin x; \tag{1.49}$$

The linear differential operator is the same as in (1.42a), namely (1.50a):

$$\begin{aligned}
&\left\{(x-1)\frac{d^2}{dx^2} - x\frac{d}{dx} + 1\right\}(\cos x + \sin x) \\
&= (x-1)(-\sin x - \cos x) - x(\cos x - \sin x) + \cos x + \sin x \\
&= 2(1-x)\cos x + 2\sin x, \qquad y_*(x) = \cos x + \sin x,
\end{aligned} \tag{1.50a, b}$$

and (1.50a) shows that a particular integral of the forced equation is (1.50b). Since the general integral of the unforced equation (1.42a) has already been obtained (1.43b) the sum with (1.50b):

$$y(x) = C_1 x + C_2 e^x + \cos x + \sin x, \tag{1.51}$$

is the complete integral of the second-order linear forced differential equation (1.49). In the preceding examples, the solutions of differential equations were obtained by inspection. There are systematic methods to obtain solutions of certain classes of differential equations, such as the method of characteristic polynomials for linear differential equations with constant coefficients (sections 1.3–1.5).

1.3 Unforced Linear Equation with Constant Coefficients

A linear unforced differential equation with constant coefficient consists of a (subsection 1.3.1) characteristic polynomial of derivatives applied to the dependent variable. Two cases arise: depending on whether the roots of the characteristic polynomial are (*or* are not) all distinct [subsections 1.3.1–1.3.5 (1.3.6–1.3.12)]. The case of all roots distinct (subsection 1.3.1) leads to linearly independent (subsection 1.3.2) exponential solutions. In the case of a pair of complex conjugate (real distinct) roots, the exponentials may be replaced as particular integrals by circular (hyperbolic) cosines and sines [subsection 1.3.3 (1.3.4)]. In the case of multiple roots, the exponentials do not supply a sufficient number of linearly independent particular integrals (subsection 1.3.5). For each multiple root, additional particular integrals are obtained alternatively by the methods of variation of constants (parametric differentiation) in the subsection 1.3.6 (1.3.7). This is equivalent to multiplication by ascending powers (subsection 1.3.8) and ensures that the particular integrals are all linearly independent (subsection 1.3.9); this supplies a sufficient number of linearly independent particular integrals to form the general integral. Thus, the differential equations with constant real coefficients of order at least two (four) may have solutions involving products of powers by exponentials (circular or hyperbolic cosines and sines) corresponding (subsection 1.3.10) to multiple (multiple real distinct or complex conjugate roots), as shown in several examples (subsections 1.3.11–1.3.14).

1.3.1 Distinct Roots of the Characteristic Polynomial (Euler, 1743; Cauchy, 1827)

In the particular case of the linear equation (1.33), whose coefficients **(Euler, 1743)** are all constant (1.52a):

$$\sum_{n=0}^{N} A_n \frac{d^n y}{dx^n} = B(x), \qquad P_N(D) = \sum_{n=0}^{N} A_n D^n, \qquad (1.52a, b)$$

the linear operator (1.34b) is **(Cauchy, 1827)** a polynomial of derivatives (1.52b), where this notation is used:

$$D \equiv \frac{d}{dx}, \qquad D^n \equiv \frac{d^n}{dx^n}, \tag{1.53a, b}$$

respectively, for derivatives of first (1.53a) and n-th (1.53b) order. In the case of the **linear differential equation with constant coefficients** (1.52a), the particular integrals can be determined from the **characteristic polynomial** (1.52b). If the latter has simple roots $a_1,...,a_m$:

$$0 = \sum_{n=0}^{N} A_n \frac{d^n y}{dx^n} = \{P_N(D)\} y(x) = A_N \left\{ \prod_{m=1}^{N} (D - a_m) \right\} y(x), \tag{1.54}$$

then the unforced equation (1.54) is satisfied if any of the factors vanishes (1.55a):

$$0 = (D - a_m) y = \frac{dy}{dx} - a_m y, \qquad x = \int dx = a_m \int \frac{dy}{y} = a_m \log y. \tag{1.55a, b}$$

The solution of (1.55a) is (1.55b), which corresponds to the particular integral (1.56a):

$$y_m(x) = \exp(a_m x); \qquad y(x) = \sum_{m=1}^{N} C_m \exp(a_m x) = \sum_{n=1}^{N} C_m y_m(x). \tag{1.56a, b}$$

Thus, the general integral is given by (1.56b) as a linear combination of N particular integrals (1.56a) involving N arbitrary constants $C_1,...,C_N$ because the particular integrals (1.56a) are all linearly independent for distinct $(a_1,...,a_N)$, as proved in the sequel (subsection 1.3.2). It has been shown that *the linear unforced differential equation with constant coefficients (1.54), with characteristic polynomial (1.52b) having N simple roots $a_1,...,a_N$ all distinct (standard I), has N linearly independent particular integrals (1.56a), and general integral (1.56b), where $C_1,...,C_N$ are arbitrary constants of integration.*

1.3.2 Linear Independence of the Exponentials and Van der Monde Determinant

It has to be shown that the particular integrals (1.56a) are linearly independent for distinct $a_1,...,a_N$. In the case $N = 2$, the proof can be performed in three different ways: (i) two exponentials e^{ax}, e^{bx} are linearly dependent (1.57a) ≡ (1.57b):

$$e^{ax} + Ce^{bx} = 0 \Leftrightarrow e^{(a-b)x} = -C \Leftrightarrow (a-b)x = \log(-C) \Leftrightarrow (a = b, C = -1), \quad (1.57a–d)$$

only (1.57c) if the parameters coincide and the constant is unity (1.57d); (ii) the exponentials have a Wronskian (1.58a):

$$W\left(e^{ax}, e^{bx}\right) = \begin{vmatrix} e^{ax} & e^{bx} \\ \left(e^{ax}\right)' & \left(e^{bx}\right)' \end{vmatrix} = \begin{vmatrix} e^{ax} & e^{bx} \\ ae^{ax} & be^{bx} \end{vmatrix} = (b-a)e^{(a+b)x} \neq 0 \Rightarrow a \neq b,$$

(1.58a, b)

which is not zero (1.58a) if (1.58b) holds, that is, e^{ax} and e^{bx} are linearly independent if the coefficients are distinct; (iii) the exponentials (1.59b) are powers of the same variable (1.59a):

$$\xi = e^{x}, \qquad \exp(a_n x) = \xi^{a_n}, \quad (1.59a, b)$$

and if the exponents are distinct they are linearly independent. The proof (ii) extends readily from two (1.58a, b) to N exponentials (1.60a–c) as shown by the Wronskian of N exponentials:

$$W\left(\exp(a_1 x), \exp(a_2 x), \ldots, \exp(a_N x)\right) = Det\left\{\frac{d^m}{dx^m}\left[\exp(a_n x)\right]\right\}$$

$$\equiv \begin{vmatrix} \exp(a_1 x) & \exp(a_1 x) & \cdots & \exp(a_N x) \\ \left[\exp(a_1 x)\right]' & \left[\exp(a_1 x)\right]' & \cdots & \left[\exp(a_1 x)\right]' \\ \vdots & \vdots & \ddots & \vdots \\ \left[\exp(a_1 x)\right]^{(N-1)} & \left[\exp(a_2 x)\right]^{(N-1)} & \cdots & \left[\exp(a_2 x)\right]^{(N-1)} \end{vmatrix}$$

$$= \begin{vmatrix} \exp(a_1 x) & \exp(a_2 x) & \cdots & \exp(a_N x) \\ a_1 \exp(a_1 x) & a_2 \exp(a_2 x) & \cdots & a_N \exp(a_N x) \\ \vdots & \vdots & \ddots & \vdots \\ (a_1)^{N-1} \exp(a_1 x) & (a_2)^{N-1} \exp(a_1 x) & \cdots & (a_N)^{N-1} \exp(a_1 x) \end{vmatrix}$$

$$= V(a_1, a_2, \ldots, a_N) \exp\left[x\left(\sum_{n=1}^{N} a_n\right)\right],$$

(1.60a–c)

involves (1.60c) the **van der Monde determinant**:

$$V(a_1,\ldots,a_N) \equiv \begin{vmatrix} 1 & 1 & 1 & \cdots & 1 \\ a_1 & a_2 & a_3 & \cdots & a_2 \\ (a_1)^2 & (a_2)^2 & (a_3)^2 & \cdots & (a_N)^2 \\ \vdots & \vdots & \vdots & \ddots & \vdots \\ (a_1)^{N-1} & (a_1)^{N-1} & (a_1)^{N-1} & \cdots & (a_1)^{N-1} \end{vmatrix} \tag{1.61}$$

$$= \sum_{1 \le i < j \le N} (a_i - a_j),$$

which is evaluated as follows: (i) it vanishes when any two of the numbers $(a_1,\ldots,a_N)$ coincide, because the two columns are identical; (ii) thus all distinct factors $a_i - a_j$ must appear; (iii) they can appear only once with coefficient unity because the highest power of each a_n is $(a_n)^{N-1}$.

It has been shown that: (i) the van der Monde determinant (**van der Monde, 1771, 1772; Cauchy, 1815**) *is evaluated by (1.61) if all the N numbers $(a_1,\ldots,a_N)$ are distinct and vanishes if any two coincide; (ii) this proves that the exponentials with distinct factors $(a_1,\ldots,a_N)$ have non-zero Wronskian (1.60a–c), and hence are linearly independent; (iii) it follows that if the linear unforced ordinary differential equation with constant coefficients (1.54) has characteristic polynomial (1.52b) with all roots distinct, then the particular integrals (1.56a) are all linearly independent, and the general integral is their linear combination (1.56b) involving N arbitrary constants $(C_1,\ldots,C_N)$.*

1.3.3 Two Real Distinct Roots and Hyperbolic Functions

The case of two real distinct roots (1.62a) of the characteristic polynomial (1.62b):

$$a \neq b: \qquad P_2(D) = (D-a)(D-b) = D^2 - (a+b)D + ab, \tag{1.62a, b}$$

corresponds to the ordinary linear second-order differential equation with constant coefficients (1.63a):

$$y'' - (\mathrm{a}+\mathrm{b})y' + aby = 0, \qquad y(x) = C_1 e^{ax} + C_2 e^{bx}, \tag{1.63a, b}$$

whose general integral is (1.63b) where (C_1, C_2) are arbitrary constants. Using the sum (1.64a) and difference (1.63b) of roots leads to (1.64c, d):

$$\alpha = \frac{a+b}{2}, \qquad \beta = \frac{a-b}{2}: \qquad a = \alpha + \beta, \qquad b = \alpha - \beta. \tag{1.64a–d}$$

Substitution in (1.63b) specifies the general integral the form:

$$y(x) = e^{\alpha x}\left(C_1 e^{\beta x} + C_2\, e^{-\beta x}\right). \tag{1.65a–d}$$

Using the relation (II.5.1a) = (1.66) of the exponential with the hyperbolic cosine and sine:

$$\exp(\pm\beta x) = \cosh(\beta x) \pm \sinh(\beta x), \tag{1.66}$$

the general integral (1.63b) ≡ (1.65) is written in terms of hyperbolic functions:

$$y(x) = \exp\left(\frac{a+b}{2}x\right)\left[D_1 \cosh\left(\frac{a-b}{2}x\right) + D_2 \cosh\left(\frac{a-b}{2}x\right)\right], \tag{1.67}$$

where the pair of arbitrary constants of integration (1.68a, b):

$$D_1 = C_1 + C_2, \quad D_2 = C_1 - C_2: \quad 2C_1 = D_1 + D_2, \quad 2C_2 = D_1 - D_2, \tag{1.68a–d}$$

are related by (1.68c, d).

Another pair of arbitrary constants is (1.69a, b):

$$D_1 = E\cosh\gamma, \quad D_2 = E\sinh\gamma; \quad (D_1)^2 - (D_2)^2 = E^2, \quad \tanh\gamma = \frac{D_2}{D_1}, \tag{1.69a–d}$$

which are related to the preceding by (1.69c, d) and (1.70a–d):

$$E^2 = \left(\frac{C_1 + C_2}{2}\right)^2 - \left(\frac{C_1 - C_2}{2}\right)^2 = C_1 C_2, \quad \tanh\gamma = \frac{C_1 - C_2}{C_1 + C_2}, \tag{1.70a, b}$$

$$2C_1 = E(\cosh\gamma + \sinh\gamma), \quad 2C_2 = E(\cosh\gamma - \sinh\gamma). \tag{1.70c, d}$$

Substitution of (1.69a, b) and use of (II.5.49a):

$$\begin{aligned} D_1 \cosh(\beta x) + D_2 \cosh(\beta x) &= E\left[\cosh(\beta x)\cosh\gamma + \sinh(\beta x)\cosh\gamma\right] \\ &= E\cosh(\beta x + \gamma), \end{aligned} \tag{1.71}$$

specifies the general integral (1.67) in terms of a hyperbolic cosine with phase and amplitude:

$$y(x) = E\cosh\left(\frac{a+b}{2}x + \gamma\right). \tag{1.72}$$

It has been shown *that a pair of real distinct roots (1.62a) of the characteristic polynomial (1.62b) correspond (standard II) to a linear ordinary second-order differential equation with constant coefficients (1.63a). The general integral can be written in three equivalent forms: (i) a linear combination of exponentials (1.63b); (ii) a linear combination of hyperbolic cosine and sine (1.67); (iii) a hyperbolic cosine with amplitude and phase (1.72). The three pairs of arbitrary constants* $(C_1, C_2), (D_1, D_2)$ *and* (E, γ) *are related by (1.68a–d; 1.69a–d; 1.70a–d).*

1.3.4 Complex Conjugate Roots and Circular Functions

A polynomial with real coefficients can have complex conjugate pairs of roots (1.73):

$$\beta \neq 0: \qquad \begin{aligned} P_2(D) &= (D - \alpha - i\beta)(D - \alpha + i\beta) = (D-\alpha)^2 + \beta^2 \\ &= D^2 - 2\,\alpha\, D + \alpha^2 + \beta^2, \end{aligned} \tag{1.73a, b}$$

corresponding to the linear ordinary second-order differential equation with constant coefficients (1.74a).

$$0 = y'' - 2\,\alpha y' + \left(\alpha^2 + \beta^2\right)y; \qquad y(x) = e^{\alpha x}\left(C_1 e^{i\beta x} + C_2 e^{-i\beta x}\right), \tag{1.74a, b}$$

whose general integral (1.74b) is a linear combination of complex exponentials with (C_1, C_2) two arbitrary constants. If the coefficients (α, β) in the differential equations (1.74a) are real, the general integral (1.74b) must also be real; if the roots $\alpha \pm i\beta$ of the characteristic polynomial are complex conjugate, the particular integrals in (1.74b) are complex and the arbitrary constants (C_1, C_2) must also be complex. Using the relation between the exponential and the circular cosine and sine (II.5.1b) ≡ (1.75):

$$\exp(\pm i\beta x) = \cos(\beta x) \pm i\sin(\beta x), \tag{1.75}$$

the general integral (1.74b) becomes a linear combination of circular cosine and sine:

$$y(x) = e^{\alpha x}\left[D_1 \cos(\beta x) + D_1 \sin(\beta x)\right], \tag{1.76}$$

with arbitrary constants (1.77a, b).

$$D_1 = C_1 + C_2, \qquad D_2 = i(C_1 - C_2): \qquad 2C_1 = D_1 - iD_2, \qquad 2C_2 = D_1 + iD_2, \tag{1.77a–d}$$

related by (1.77c, d). Thus, replacing the exponentials with imaginary variables (1.74b) by their real and imaginary parts, which are respectively circular cosines and sines, the real general integral (1.76) is obtained involving real arbitrary constants (D_1, D_2).

Introducing as an amplitude and phase (1.78a, b) leads to (1.78c, d):

$$D_1 = E\cos\gamma, \quad D_2 = E\sin\gamma: \quad (D_1)^2 + (D_1)^2 = E^2, \quad \tan\gamma = \frac{D_2}{D_1}. \tag{1.78a–d}$$

Use of (II.5.47a) ≡ (1.79).

$$\begin{aligned} D_1 \cos(\beta x) + D_2 \sin(\beta x) &= E\left[\cos(\beta x)\cos\gamma + \sin(\beta x)\sin\gamma\right] \\ &= E\cos(\beta x - \gamma), \end{aligned} \tag{1.79}$$

specifies the general integral in terms of a circular cosine with amplitude and phase:

$$y(x) = Ee^{\alpha x}\cos(\beta x - \gamma), \tag{1.80}$$

related to the preceding constants by:

$$2C_1 = E(\cos\gamma - i\sin\gamma) = Ee^{-i\gamma}, \quad 2C_2 = E(\cos\gamma + i\sin\gamma) = Ee^{i\gamma}, \tag{1.81a, b}$$

$$E^2 = Ee^{i\gamma}Ee^{-i\gamma} = 4C_1C_2, \qquad i\tan\gamma = \frac{C_2 - C_1}{C_2 + C_1} = \tanh(i\gamma). \tag{1.82a, b}$$

It has been shown that *a pair of complex conjugate roots of the characteristic polynomial (1.73a, b) corresponds (standard III) to the ordinary linear second-order differential equation with constant coefficients (1.74a) whose general integral can be written in three equivalent forms: (i) as a linear combination of complex exponentials (1.74b); (ii) as a linear combination of circular cosine and sine (1.76); (iii) as a circular cosine with amplitude and phase (1.80). The three pairs of arbitrary constants are related by (1.77a–d; 1.78a–d; 1.81a, b; 1.82a, b).* Thus, have been covered *all cases of a linear ordinary differential equation with constant coefficients (1.54) for which the characteristic polynomial (1.52b) has all roots distinct: (standard I) an exponential (1.56a) for a single root (1.55a); (standard II) hyperbolic functions (1.63b) ≡ (1.67) ≡ (1.72) for (1.68a–d; 1.69a–d; 1.70a–d) real distinct roots (1.62a); (standard III) circular functions (1.74b) ≡ (1.76) ≡ (1.80) for (1.77a–d; 1.78a–d; 1.81a, b; 1.82a, b) a pair of complex conjugate roots (1.73).* All expressions apply real or complex quantities $\left(x, y, a, b, \alpha, \beta, \gamma, C_1, C_2, D_1, D_2, E\right)$. The remaining instances of repeated or multiple roots are considered after (subsection 1.3.6) a fourth-order case combining real and complex roots (subsection 1.3.5).

1.3.5 Circular and Hyperbolic Functions for Fourth-Order Equations

For example, the linear homogeneous fourth-order differential equation with constant coefficients:

$$y'''' - 2y''' + a^2 y'' + 2\,y' - \left(1 + a^2\right)y = 0, \tag{1.83}$$

has a characteristic polynomial:

$$\begin{aligned} P_4(D) &= D^4 - 2D^3 + a^2 D^2 + 2D - 1 - a^2 = a^2\left(D^2 - 1\right) + D^4 - 1 - 2D\left(D^2 - 1\right) \\ &= \left(D^2 - 1\right)\left(D^2 + 1 - 2D + a^2\right) = \left(D^2 - 1\right)\left[(D-1)^2 + a^2\right] \\ &= (D-1)(D+1)(D-1+ia)(D-1-ia), \end{aligned} \tag{1.84a–e}$$

with a pair of real and symmetric ± 1 and a pair of complex conjugate $1 \pm ia$ roots; hence, its general integral is (1.85b–d):

$$\begin{aligned} a \neq 0: \qquad y(x) &= C_1 e^{x} + C_2 e^{-x} + C_3 e^{x + iax} + C_4 e^{x - iax}, \\ &= D_1 \cosh x + D_2 \sinh x + e^{x}\left[D_3 \cos(ax) + D_4 \sin(ax)\right] \\ &= E_1\left(\cosh x + \gamma_1\right) + E_2 e^{x} \cos\left(ax - \gamma_2\right), \end{aligned} \tag{1.85a–d}$$

which holds for (1.85a). In the case $a = 0$, it is clear that (1.85b) cannot be the general integral because it involves only two constants of integration:

$$a = 0: \quad y(x) = (C_1 + C_2 + C_3)e^x + C_2 e^{-x} = C_0 e^x + C_2 e^{-x} \\ = D_1 \cosh x + D_2 \sinh x = E \cosh(x + \gamma); \tag{1.86a, b}$$

the reason is that for $a = 0$, three particular integrals in (1.86b) coincide because they correspond to the same triple root $D = 1$, of the characteristic polynomial. The case of multiple roots of the characteristic polynomial is considered next by two methods: (i) variation of constants (subsection 1.3.6); (ii) parametric differentiation (subsection 1.3.7).

1.3.6 *Root* of Multiplicity *M* and Variation of Constants

The preceding account leads to the problem of finding α linearly independent particular integrals, when the characteristic polynomial has (1.87b) a root a of multiplicity α:

$$Q_{N-\alpha}(a) \neq 0: \quad \{P_N(D)\}y(x) = \{(D-a)^\alpha Q_{N-\alpha}(D)\}y(x) = 0, \tag{1.87a, b}$$

where a is not (1.87a) a root of the polynomial $Q_{N-M}(D)$, that is, of degree $N - M$. The differential equation to be solved is (1.88a):

$$\{(D-a)^\alpha\}y(x) = 0, \qquad y(x) = C(x)e^{ax}, \tag{1.88a, b}$$

and the solution is sought in a form (1.88b), similar to the case (1.56a) of a single root e^{ax}, multiplied by a function $C(x)$, to be determined. This is an example of the **method of variation of constants** that will be applied again (section 3.3). Substituting (1.88b) into (1.88a), it is found that the operator $(D - a)$ applied to (1.88b) is equivalent to differentiating only C (1.89a):

$$(D-a)Ce^{ax} = \left(Ce^{ax}\right)' - aCe^{ax} = C'e^{ax}; \quad (D-a)^\alpha Ce^{ax} = C^{(\alpha)}e^{ax}; \tag{1.89a, b}$$

thus, the function $C(x)$ has (1.89b) zero α-th derivative (1.90a):

$$C^{(\alpha)}(x) = 0, \qquad C(x) = C_1 + C_2 x + \ldots + C_M x^{\alpha-1}, \tag{1.90a, b}$$

and hence is a polynomial (1.90b) of degree $\alpha - 1$. Substituting (1.90b) into (1.88b), follows (1.91b):

$$\beta = 1,\ldots,\alpha: \qquad y_\beta(x) = x^{\beta-1}e^{ax}, \qquad y(x) = \sum_{\beta=1}^{\alpha} C_\beta x^{\beta-1}e^{ax} = \sum_{\beta=1}^{\alpha} C_\beta y_\beta(x), \tag{1.91a–c}$$

Thus, *if the characteristic polynomial (1.52b), of the unforced linear differential equation with constant coefficients (1.54), has a root a of (1.87a, b) multiplicity α the corresponding (standard IV) part of the general integral is (1.91c), implying that the α linearly independent particular integrals are products of the exponential (1.56a) by powers (1.91b) with exponents (1.91a). In the case $\alpha = 1$ of a simple root (1.55a) of the characteristic polynomial (1.54) there are no powers (1.56a).*

1.3.7 Parametric Differentiation of Particular Integrals (D'Alembert, 1748)

The preceding result obtained by the method of variation of constants (subsection 1.3.6) can alternatively be obtained by a **method of parametric differentiation** (subsection 1.3.7). This method also starts from (1.88b) ≡ (1.92b) and uses the solution (1.92a) for a single root:

$$y_1(x) = e^{ax}: \qquad (D-a)^\alpha y_1 = (D-a)^\alpha e^{ax} = 0. \tag{1.92a–c}$$

Differentiating once with regard to parameter a gives (1.93a), which proves that (1.93b) is also a solution:

$$(D-a)^\alpha \frac{\partial y_1}{\partial \alpha} = \alpha(D-a)^{\alpha-1} y_1 = 0: \quad y_2(x) = \frac{\partial y_1}{\partial \alpha} = xe^{ax}. \tag{1.93a, b}$$

The process may be applied (1.94b):

$$\gamma = 1,\ldots,\alpha-1: \qquad (D-a)^\alpha \frac{\partial^\gamma y_1}{\partial a^\gamma} = \frac{\alpha!(-)^\gamma}{(\alpha-\gamma)!}(D-a)^{\alpha-\gamma} y_1 = 0, \tag{1.94a, b}$$

up to $(\alpha - 1)$ times, but not more, because $\gamma = \alpha, \alpha+1, \ldots$ no longer leads to a particular integral of the differential equation:

$$(D-a)^\alpha \frac{\partial^\alpha y_1}{\partial a^\alpha} = \alpha!(-)^\alpha y_1 \neq 0. \tag{1.95}$$

This proves *(D'Alembert, 1748) that if the characteristic polynomial (1.52b) of the unforced constant coefficients (1.54) has a root a of (1.87a, b) multiplicity* α*, then* α *linearly independent particular integrals are* obtained by **parametric differentiation** *(1.96b) up to* $(\alpha-1)$ *times (1.96a) of the particular integral (1.92a) for a simple root:*

$$\beta = 1,\ldots,\alpha: \qquad y_\beta(x) = \frac{\partial^{\beta-1}}{\partial a^{\beta-1}}\left(e^{ax}\right) = x^{\beta-1}e^{ax}. \tag{1.96a, b}$$

The results (1.96a, b) ≡ (1.91a–c) agree and are stated, in general, next (subsection 1.3.8) before confirming that the α particular integrals (1.91b) ≡ (1.96b) are linearly independent (subsection 1.3.9).

1.3.8 Multiple Roots of the Characteristic Polynomial

Combining the preceding results (subsections 1.3.8–1.3.9) it follows that *an ordinary linear unforced differential equation of order N with constant coefficients:*

$$0 = \sum_{n=1}^{N} A_n \frac{d^n y}{dx^x} = \left\{P_N\left(\frac{d}{dx}\right)\right\} y(x), \tag{1.97}$$

has a characteristic polynomial (1.98a) with M roots a_m *with multiplicities* α_n *adding (1.98a) to N:*

$$\sum_{m=1}^{M} \alpha_m = N: \qquad P_N(D) = A_N \prod_{m=1}^{M} (D - a_m)^{\alpha_m}. \tag{1.98a, b}$$

The corresponding general integral (standard IV) is:

$$y(x) = \sum_{m=1}^{M} \exp(a_m x) \prod_{\beta=1}^{\alpha_m} C_{m,\beta_m} x^{\beta_m - 1}, \tag{1.99}$$

given by a linear combination of exponentials, each multiplied by a polynomial of degree $\alpha_m - 1$*; the coefficients of the polynomials* C_{m,β_m} *are N arbitrary constants (1.98a). The general integral (1.99) ≡ (1.100a) is a linear combination of N particular integrals (1.100b):*

$$y(x) = \sum_{m=1}^{M} \sum_{\beta_m=1}^{\alpha_m} C_{m,\beta_m} y_{m,\beta_m}(x), \qquad y_{m,\beta_m}(x) = x^{\beta_m - 1} \exp(a_m x). \tag{1.100a, b}$$

For a given root α_m of multiplicity α_m of the characteristic polynomial (1.98a, b), the α_m particular integrals (1.101a) can be obtained from the first by parametric differentiation (1.101b):

$$\beta_m = 1,\ldots,\alpha_m: \qquad y_{m,\beta_m}(x) = \left(\frac{\partial}{\partial a_m}\right)^{\beta_m - 1}\left[\exp(a_m x)\right] = \left(\frac{\partial}{\partial a_m}\right)^{\beta_m - 1} y_{m,1}(x). \tag{1.101a, b}$$

The complete set of N particular integrals (1.100b) ≡ (1.101b) are all linearly independent because they differ either (i) in the exponential a_m or (ii) in the power β_m. The statement (i) has already been proved (1.60a–c) using the van der Monde determinant (1.61); the statement (ii) is considered next, omitting the common exponential factor e^{ax} in (1.99), so that only the linear independence of powers is to be proved.

1.3.9 Linear Independence of Powers with Fixed Base

In the case of powers with distinct exponents a, b, the Wronskian (1.102a):

$$W\left(x^a, x^b\right) \equiv \begin{vmatrix} x^a & x^b \\ \left(x^a\right)' & \left(x^b\right)' \end{vmatrix} = \begin{vmatrix} x^a & x^b \\ a x^{a-1} & b x^{b-1} \end{vmatrix} = (b-a)\, x^{a+b-1} \neq 0 \Leftrightarrow b \neq a, \tag{1.102a, b}$$

shows that they are linearly independent (1.102b). In the case of the first M powers, the Wronskian:

$$W\left(1, x, \ldots, x^M\right) \equiv Det\left\{\left(x^n\right)^{(m-1)}\right\} = \begin{vmatrix} 1 & x & x^2 & x^3 & \cdots & x^M \\ 0 & 1 & 2x & 3x^2 & \cdots & M x^{M-1} \\ 0 & 0 & 2 & 6x & \cdots & M(M-1)x^{M-2} \\ 0 & 0 & 0 & 6 & \cdots & M(M-1)(M-2)\, x^{M-3} \\ \vdots & \vdots & \vdots & \vdots & \ddots & \\ 0 & 0 & 0 & 0 & \cdots & M(M-1)\ldots. 2.1 \end{vmatrix}$$

$$= \prod_{m=2}^{M} m! = 2^{M-1}\, 3^{M-2} \ldots. (M-1)^2\, M = \prod_{m=2}^{M} m^{M-m+1} \neq 0, \tag{1.103}$$

shows that they are linearly independent. Note that the *Wronskian (1.103) [(1.60–1.61)] concerns the linear independence (1.59a, b) of powers with fixed (variable) base and variable (fixed) exponent.*

1.3.10 Multiple Pairs of Complex Conjugate or Real Roots

The solution just used (1.99) ≡ (1.100a, b), extends the result (1.56a–c) for a simple root $\alpha_m = 1$ to roots of any multiplicity $\alpha_m \geq 2$. In a similar way (1.56a) versus (1.96a, b) can be extended the results for two real (1.63b) ≡ (1.67) ≡ (1.72) [a complex conjugate pair (1.74b) ≡ (1.76) ≡ (1.81) of] roots to roots of multiplicity M in (1.104a, b) [(1.105a, b)]:

$$Q_{N-2M}(\alpha \pm i\beta) \neq 0: \quad P_N(D) = \left[(D-\alpha+i\beta)(D-\alpha-i\beta)\right]^M Q_{N-2M}(D) = \left[(D-\alpha)^2+\beta^2\right]^M Q_{N-2M}(D), \tag{1.104a, b}$$

$$Q_{N-2M}(\alpha \pm \beta) \neq 0: \quad P_N(D) = \left[(D-\alpha+\beta)(D-\alpha-\beta)\right]^M Q_{N-2M}(D) = \left[(D-\alpha)^2-\beta^2\right]^M Q_{N-2M}(D). \tag{1.105a, b}$$

If the characteristic polynomial (1.52b), of the unforced linear differential equation with constant coefficients (1.54), has a pair of complex conjugate (1.104a, b) [real and distinct (1.105a, b)] roots of multiplicity $M \leq N/2$, then [standard V (VI)] the corresponding part of the general integral is a product of circular (1.109a–c) [hyperbolic (1.110a–c)] functions, by polynomials of degree $M-1$ with constant coefficients, and by the exponential $e^{\alpha x}$:

$$y(x) = \sum_{m=0}^{M-1} x^m \left\{C_{1,m}\, e^{(\alpha+i\beta)}\, x + C_{2,m}\, e^{(\alpha-i\beta)x}\right\} = e^{\alpha x} \sum_{m=0}^{M-1} x^m \left\{D_{1,m} \cos(\beta x) + D_{2,m} \sin(\beta x)\right\} = e^{\alpha x} \sum_{m=0}^{M-1} x^m E_m \cos(\beta x - \gamma_m), \tag{1.106a–c}$$

$$y(x) = \sum_{m=0}^{M-1} x^m \left\{C_{1,m}\, e^{(\alpha+\beta)x} + C_{2,m}\, e^{(\alpha-\beta)x}\right\} = \sum_{m=0}^{M-1} x^n \left\{D_{1,m} \cosh(\beta x) + D_{2,m} \sinh(\beta x)\right\} = \sum_{m=0}^{M-1} x^m E_m \cosh(\beta x + \gamma_m), \tag{1.107a–c}$$

using different sets of 2M constants of integration $(C_{1,m}, C_{2,m}),(D_{1,m}, D_{2,m})$ and (E_m, γ_m) related by (1.77a–d; 1.78a–d; 1.82a–d) [(1.68a–d; 1.69a–d; 1.70a–d)].

1.3.11 Characteristic Polynomial with Single and Multiple Roots

The preceding theory covers the solution of the fourth-order ordinary differential equation (1.83) in the case (1.86a, b) of a triple root (1.108a, b):

$$a = 0: \qquad y'''' - 2y''' + 2y' - y = 0; \qquad P_4(D) = D^4 - 2D^3 + 2D - 1, \tag{1.108a–c}$$

the characteristic polynomial (1.108c) has with a single root –1 and a triple root +1:

$$P_4(D) = (D+1)(D^3 - 3D^2 + 3D - 1) = (D+1)(D-1)^3, \tag{1.109}$$

so that the general integral is:

$$\begin{aligned} a = 0: \qquad y(x) &= (C_1 + C_3 x + C_4 x^2)e^x + C_2 e^{-x} \\ &= D_1 \cosh x + D_2 \sinh x + x(C_3 + C_4 x)e^x, \\ &= E \cosh(x+\gamma) + x(C_3 + C_4 x)e^x, \end{aligned} \tag{1.110a–d}$$

using the change of arbitrary constants (1.68a–d). It has been shown *that the ordinary unforced differential equation with constant coefficients (1.83) has general integral (1.85b–d) [(1.110b–d)] in the case (1.85a) [(1.110a)] of four distinct (1.84a–d) [one triple and one single (1.108c) ≡ (1.109)] roots of the characteristic polynomial.*

1.3.12 Products of Powers and Circular or Hyperbolic Functions as Particular Integrals

An example of the fourth-order linear unforced differential equation with constant coefficients is (1.111):

$$y'''' + (a^2 + b^2)y'' + a^2 b^2 y = 0, \tag{1.111}$$

whose characteristic polynomial:

$$\begin{aligned} P_4(D) &= D^4 - (a^2 + b^2)D^2 + a^2 b^2 = (D + a^2)(D + b^2) \\ &= (D - ia)(D + ia)(D - ib)(D + ib), \end{aligned} \tag{1.112}$$

has roots $(\pm ia, \pm ib)$ leading to four cases for the general integral: (i) if neither parameter is zero and they do not coincide:

$$a \neq 0 \neq b \neq a: \quad y(x) = C_1\, e^{iax} + C_2\, e^{-iax} + C_3\, e^{ibx} + C_4\, e^{-ibx}$$
$$= D_1 \cos(ax) + D_2 \sin(ax) + D_3 \cos(bx) + D_4 \sin(bx)$$
$$= E_1 \cos(ax - \gamma_1) + E_2 \cos(bx - \gamma_2); \tag{1.113a–f}$$

(ii) if the parameters coincide and do not vanish:

$$a = b \neq 0; \quad y'''' + 2\, a^2\, y'' + a^4\, y = 0:$$
$$y(x) = \left(C_1 + C_3\, x\right) e^{iax} + \left(C_2 + C_4\, x\right) e^{-iax}$$
$$= D_1 \cos(ax) + D_2 \sin(ax) + x\left[D_3 \cos(ax) + D_4 \sin(ax)\right] \tag{1.114a–e}$$
$$= E_1 \cos\left(ax - \gamma_1\right) + E_2\, x \cos\left(ax - \gamma_2\right);$$

(iii) if one of the parameters is zero and the other is not:

$$a \neq 0 = b; \quad y'''' + a^2 y'' = 0:$$
$$y(x) = C_1 + C_2 x + C_3\, e^{iax} + C_4\, e^{-iax}$$
$$= C_1 + C_2\, x + D_3 \cos(ax) + D_4 \sin(ax) \tag{1.115a–e}$$
$$= C_1 + C_2 x + E \cos(ax - \gamma),$$

with another subcase for $a = 0 \neq b$; (iv) if both parameters are zero:

$$a = 0 = b: \quad y'''' = 0, \quad y(x) = C_1 + C_2\, x + C_3\, x^2 + C_4\, x^3, \tag{1.116a–d}$$

leading to a cubic polynomial.

1.3.13 Symmetric Real and Complex Conjugate Pairs of Roots of the Characteristic Polynomial

Changing b^2 to $-b^2$ in the fourth-order linear unforced ordinary differential equation with constant coefficients (1.111) leads to (1.117):

$$y'''' + \left(a^2 - b^2\right) y'' - a^2 b^2 y = 0; \tag{1.117}$$

the characteristic polynomial:

$$\begin{aligned} P_4(D) &= D^4 + \left(a^2 - b^2\right)D^2 - a^2b^2 \\ &= \left(D + a^2\right)\left(D - b^2\right) = (D - ia)(D + ia)(D - b)(D + b), \end{aligned} \tag{1.118}$$

has two real symmetric $\pm b$ and two imaginary conjugate $\pm ia$ roots. This leads to four cases for the general integrals: (i) both roots are non-zero:

$$a \neq 0 \neq b: \quad \begin{aligned} y(x) &= C_1 e^{iax} + C_2 e^{-iax} + C_3 e^{bx} + C_4 e^{-bx} \\ &= D_1 \cos(ax) + D_2 \sin(ax) + D_3 \cosh(bx) + D_4 \sinh(bx) \\ &= E_1 \cos(ax - \gamma_1) + E_2 \cosh(bx + \gamma_2); \end{aligned} \tag{1.119a–e}$$

(ii) only the real roots are non-zero:

$$a = 0 \neq b; \quad y'''' - b^2 y''' = 0: \quad \begin{aligned} y(x) &= C_1 + C_2 x + C_3 e^{bx} + C_4 e^{-bx} \\ &= C_1 + C_2 x + D_3 \cosh(bx) + D_4 \sinh(bx) \\ &= C_1 + C_2 x + E \cosh(bx + \gamma); \end{aligned} \tag{1.120a–e}$$

(iii) only the imaginary roots are non-zero:

$$a \neq 0 = b: \quad y'''' + a^2 y'' = 0: \quad \begin{aligned} y(x) &= C_1 + C_2 x + C_3 e^{iax} + C_4 e^{-iax} \\ &= C_1 + C_2 x + C_3 \cos(ax) + C_4 \sin(ax) \\ &= C_1 + C_2 x + E \cos(ax - \gamma); \end{aligned} \tag{1.121a–c}$$

(iv) all roots are zero (1.116a–d):

Following fourth-order unforced differential equations, whose characteristic polynomials have real symmetric and/or complex conjugate simple or double roots (subsections 1.3.12–1.3.13), the concluding example is of third-order (subsection 1.3.14).

1.3.14 Single and Multiple Roots of the Characteristic Polynomial

The third-order linear unforced differential equation with constant coefficients:

$$y''' - ay'' - y' + ay = 0, \tag{1.122}$$

has the characteristic polynomial:

$$P_3(D) = D^3 - aD^2 - D + a = (D^2 - 1)(D - a) = (D - 1)(D + 1)(D - a), \quad (1.123)$$

with roots $(\pm 1, a)$. This leads to three cases for the general integral: (i) all roots are distinct:

$$a \neq \pm 1: \quad \begin{aligned} y(x) &= C_1 e^x + C_2 e^{-x} + C_3 e^{ax} \\ &= D_1 \cosh x + D_2 \sinh x + C_3 e^{ax} \\ &= E \cosh(x + \gamma) + C_3 e^{ax}, \end{aligned} \quad (1.124a\text{–}d)$$

(ii) two coincident roots, with the two subcases:

$$a = \mp 1; \quad y''' \pm y'' - y' \mp y = 0: \quad \begin{aligned} y(x) &= C_1 e^{\pm x} + (C_2 + C_3 x) e^{\mp x} \\ &= D_1 \cosh x + D_2 \sinh x + C_3 e^{\mp x} x \\ &= E \cosh(x + \gamma) + C_3 e^{\mp x} x. \end{aligned} \quad (1.125a\text{–}d)$$

The preceding theory and examples cover all cases of solution of the unforced linear differential equation with constant coefficients (section 1.3). A variety of cases with forcing are considered next (sections 1.4–1.5).

1.4 General (Complete) Integral of the Unforced (Forced) Equation

Having solved the linear unforced ordinary differential equation with constant coefficients in all cases of simple or multiple roots (section 1.3) of the characteristic polynomial, the forced equation is considered next. To obtain the complete integral of the forced equation (subsection 1.2.6) it suffices to add: (i) general integral of the unforced equation already obtained (section 1.3); (ii) any particular integral of the forced equation (sections 1.4–1.5). The latter (ii) will be obtained by two methods, namely direct (inverse) use of the characteristic polynomial [sections 1.4 (1.5)]. The direct method is applied next (section 1.4) in the cases when the forcing term is: (a) an exponential (subsection 1.4.3); (b, c) hyperbolic (circular) cosine or sine [subsections 1.4.4 (1.4.5)]; (d, e) the product by an exponential of an hyperbolic (circular) cosine or sine [subsections 1.4.6 (1.4.7)]: (f) the triple product of an exponential by circular and hyperbolic cosines and sines (subsection 1.4.8). The particular integrals corresponding to these five cases (subsections 1.4.3–1.4.8) are: (α) of the same form as the forcing term in the non-resonant case; (β) have an extra power factor in the resonant case. The resonant (non-resonant) case corresponds to the coefficient in the exponential forcing term being (not being) a root of the characteristic polynomial and can be obtained by two alternative methods; (α) parametric differentiation (subsection 1.4.1); (β) use of L'Hôspital rule (subsection 1.4.2).

1.4.1 Parametric Differentiation of a Forced Solution (D'Alembert, 1762)

Next is considered a particular integral $y_*(x)$ of the linear forced (**D'Alembert, 1762**) differential equation with constant coefficients (1.52a, b):

$$B(x) = \sum_{n=0}^{N} A_n \frac{d^n y_*}{dx^n} = \left\{ P_N\left(\frac{d}{dx}\right) \right\} y_*(x), \tag{1.126}$$

when the **forcing term** $B(x)$ is an elementary function. For example, if the forcing term is an exponential (1.127a):

$$B(x) = Be^{bx}, \qquad y_*(x) = Ce^{bx}, \tag{1.127a, b}$$

the particular integral may be sought (1.127b) as a similar exponential, multiplied by a distinct coefficient C; the latter is determined by substitution into the differential equation (1.126):

$$Be^{bx} = \left\{ P_N\left(\frac{d}{dx}\right) \right\} Ce^{bx} = CP_N(b)e^{bx} = P_N(b)y_*(x). \tag{1.128}$$

If b is not a root of the characteristic polynomial (1.129a) then the particular integral, corresponding to the forcing term (1.127a), follows from (1.128), and is given by (1.129b):

$$P_N(b) \neq 0: \qquad y_*(x) = B\frac{e^{bx}}{P_N(b)}. \tag{1.129a, b}$$

The passage from (1.128) to (1.129b) cannot be made if b is a root of the characteristic polynomial (1.129a) since this would correspond to a division by zero.

In the sequel, it is convenient to use the short notation (I.19.27a) ≡ (1.130a), meaning that the function has (1.130b) a zero of order M at the point a:

$$f(D) \sim O\left((D-a)^M\right) \quad \Leftrightarrow \quad \lim_{D\to a}(D-a)^{-M} f(D) \neq 0, \infty. \qquad (1.130\text{a, b})$$

In the case of an M times differentiable function (1.131a), a zero of order at the point a is equivalent (1.131b) ≡ (1.131c) to a non-zero derivative of order M together with a zero value of the function and derivatives of lower order up to $M-1$:

$$f \in \mathcal{D}^M(|C): f(D) \sim O\left((D-a)^M\right) \Leftrightarrow f(a) = f'(a) = \ldots = f^{(M-1)}(a) = 0 \neq f^{(M)}(a). \qquad (1.131\text{a–c})$$

In the case of a polynomial P_N of degree N, a root of multiplicity M at a is equivalent (1.132a) to the factorization (1.132b), where the polynomial Q_{N-M} of degree $N-M$ has (1.132c) no root at a:

$$P_N(D) \sim O\left((D-a)^M\right) \quad \Leftrightarrow \quad P_N(D) = (D-a)^M Q_{N-M}(D), \quad Q_{N-M}(a) \neq 0. \qquad (1.132\text{a–c})$$

In this case, that is when b is a root of the characteristic polynomial, then (1.128) cannot be divided by $P_N(b)$ because it is zero; instead (1.128) is differentiated M times with regard to b, leading to (1.133a):

$$Bx^M e^{bx} = \frac{\partial^M}{\partial b^M}\left(Be^{bx}\right) = \frac{\partial^M}{\partial b^M}\left[Ce^{bx} P(b)\right] \qquad (1.133\text{a})$$

$$= C\sum_{m=0}^{M} \binom{M}{m} P_N^{(M-m)}(b) \frac{\partial^m}{\partial b^m}\left(e^{bx}\right) \qquad (1.133\text{b})$$

$$= CP_N^{(M)}(b) e^{bx}, \qquad (1.133\text{c})$$

where: (i) was used (1.133b) the Leibnitz chain rule for the derivative of order M of the product of two functions (I.13.31); (ii) by (1.131c) all the terms of the sum vanish (1.133c) except for $m = M$.

The result (1.133c) can be justified as follows: (i) if the differentiation with regard to b in (1.133a) is applied less than M-times to $P_N(b)$ the result is zero by (1.131c); (ii) in (1.133a) the differentiation with regard to b must be applied M-times to $P_N(b)$ leading to (1.133c).

Thus, the particular integral, corresponding to the forcing exponential term (1.127a) with b a root of multiplicity M of the characteristic polynomial (1.134a) is given by (1.134b):

$$P_N(D) \sim O\left((D-b)^M\right): \qquad y_*(x) = B\frac{x^M e^{bx}}{P_N^{(M)}(b)}. \tag{1.134a, b}$$

Setting $M = 0$ in (1.134a, b) leads back to (1.129a, b). Thus, *the particular integral (1.129b) [(1.134b)] of the linear differential equation with constant coefficients (1.126), with (standard VII) exponential forcing term (1.127a) has been obtained, where b is not a root (is a root of multiplicity M) of the characteristic polynomial (1.129a) [(1.134a)].*

The method of parametric differentiation has been applied to the linear differential equation with constant coefficients when the characteristic polynomial has multiple roots to: (i) find linearly independent particular integrals in the unforced case (subsection 1.3.7); (ii) obtain a resonant particular integral of the forced equation (subsection 1.4.1).

An alternative is to use: (i) the method of variation of constants for the unforced equation (subsection 1.3.6); (ii) the *L'Hôspital* rule for the forced equation (subsection 1.4.2). Thus, the resonant solution of linear differential equation with constant coefficients forced by an exponential can be obtained alternatively by: (i) the method of parametric differential (subsection 1.4.1); (ii) the *L'Hôspital* rule, as shown next (subsection 1.4.2).

1.4.2 Rule Applied to a Forced Solution (*L'Hôspital, 1696; Bernoulli, 1691*)

The result (1.134b) can be obtained alternatively by the method that follows. From the forced solution (1.129b) ≡ (1.135) of the linear differential equation with constant coefficients (1.126; 1.127a):

$$\bar{y}_*(x) = \lim_{a\to b} B\frac{e^{ax}}{P_N(a)}, \tag{1.135}$$

may be subtracted a particular integral of the unforced equation (1.136b):

$$C \equiv \frac{B}{P_N(a)}: \qquad \bar{y}_1(x) = Ce^{bx}, \tag{1.136a, b}$$

where the value (1.136a) is chosen for an arbitrary constant. Thus, a particular integral of the forced equation is the difference of (1.135) and (1.136b):

$$y_*(x) = \bar{y}_*(x) - \bar{y}_1(x) = \lim_{a\to b} B\frac{e^{ax} - e^{bx}}{P_N(a)}. \tag{1.137}$$

If b is a simple root of the characteristic polynomial (1.138a, b), then: (i) the denominator of (1.135) ≡ (1.129b) vanishes whereas the numerator is non-zero, and no solution of the forced differential equation is obtained; (ii) in contrast, as $a \to b$ in (1.137), both the denominator and numerator have a simple zero and the 0:0 indeterminacy is lifted using the *L'Hôspital* rule, (I.19.35) ≡ (1.138c), by differentiating separately the numerator and denominator before taking the limit $a \to b$:

$$P_N(b) = 0 \neq P_N'(b): y_*(x) = \lim_{a\to b} B\frac{(\partial/\partial a)\left(e^{ax} - e^{bx}\right)}{(\partial/\partial a)P_N(a)} = \lim_{a\to b} B\frac{xe^{ax}}{P_N'(a)} = B\frac{xe^{bx}}{P_N'(b)}. \tag{1.138a–c}$$

The result (1.138c) coincides with (1.134b) for a simple root $M = 1$ of the characteristic polynomial.

If b is a double root of the characteristic polynomial (1.138a–c), then xe^{bx} is a particular integral of the unforced equation, and a particular integral of the forced equation is given by (1.139):

$$y_*(x) = x\lim_{a\to b} B\frac{e^{ax} - e^{bx}}{P_N'(a)} = x\lim_{a\to b} B\frac{(\partial/\partial a)\left(e^{ax} - e^{bx}\right)}{(\partial/\partial a)P_N'(a)} = x^2\lim_{a\to b} B\frac{e^{ax}}{P_N''(a)} = B\frac{x^2e^{bx}}{P_N''(b)}. \tag{1.139}$$

This coincides with (1.134b) for $M = 2$ a double root of the characteristic polynomial. Applying the same method M times leads to (1.134b) for a root of multiplicity M of the characteristic polynomial. It has been shown that a *particular integral of the linear differential equation with constant coefficients (1.126) forced by an exponential (1.127a) where b is a root of multiplicity M of the characteristic polynomial (1.130a, b) ≡ (1.131a–c) ≡ (1.132a–c) can be obtained using l'Hôspital rule (I.19.35) ≡ (1.140) by differentiating M times numerator and denominator of (1.129b) with regard to b*:

$$\frac{(\partial/\partial b)^M\left(Be^{bx}\right)}{(\partial/\partial b)^M P_N(b)} = B\frac{x^M e^{bx}}{P_N^{(M)}(b)} = y_*(x). \tag{1.140}$$

In the case when b is (1.132a–c) ≡ (1.87a, b) a root of multiplicity M of the characteristic polynomial: (i) all the lower powers $x^m e^{bx}$ with $m = 0,\ldots, M-1$ satisfy (1.96a, b) the unforced equation (1.88a) and thus could not be a solution of the forced equation; (ii) the power $x^M e^{bx}$ satisfies (1.134b) the forced equation (1.126;1.127a) with coefficient given by (1.138); (iii) the differentiation of $e^{bx} = e^{ax}$ with regard to $a = b$ a number $m = 0,1,\ldots, M-1 (m = M)$ of times specifies the particular integrals of the *unforced (1.101b) [forced (1.140)] equation, that appear with arbitrary (1.91c) [fixed (1.134b)] coefficient in the complete integral.*

1.4.3 Resonant and Non-Resonant Forcing by an Exponential

As an example, for the equation (1.108b), with exponential forcing term:

$$y'''' - 2y''' + 2y' - y = 2e^{bx}, \tag{1.141}$$

the characteristic polynomial (1.108c) ≡ (1.109) ≡ (1.142a, b) has derivatives (1.142c–e):

$$P_4(D) = D^4 - 2D^3 + 2D - 1 = (D-1)^3(D+1), \tag{1.142a, b}$$

$$P_4'(D) = 4D^3 - 6D^2 + 2, \quad P_4''(D) = 12D^2 - 12D, \quad P_4'''(D) = 24D - 12, \tag{1.142c–e}$$

confirming that $-1(+1)$ is a simple (1.142f) [triple (1.142g) root:

$$P_4(-1) = 0 \neq -8 = P_4'(-1), \qquad P_4(1) = P_4'(1) = P_4''(1) = 0 \neq 12 = P_4'''(1). \tag{1.142f, g}$$

Thus, there are three cases for the particular integral of the forced differential equation (1.141): (i) if b is not a root of the characteristic polynomial (1.143a) the forced solution (1.129a, b) is non-resonant (1.143b):

$$b \neq \pm 1: \qquad y_*(x) = \frac{2e^{bx}}{P_4(b)} = \frac{2e^{bx}}{(b+1)(b-1)^3}. \tag{1.143a, b}$$

(ii, iii) The solution (1.143a, b) fails if b is a simple (1.144a) [triple (1.145a)] root of the characteristic polynomial (1.142f) [(1.142g)] in which case the forced solution (1.131a; 1.133c) is singly (1.144b) [triple (1.145b)] resonant:

$$b = -1: \qquad y_*(x) = \frac{2\,x\,e^{-x}}{P_4'(-1)} = -\frac{x}{4}e^{-x}, \tag{1.144a, b}$$

$$b = 1: \qquad y_*(x) = \frac{2x^3 e^x}{P_4'''(1)} = \frac{x^3}{6}e^x. \tag{1.145a, b}$$

The particular integral of the forced linear differential equation (1.141) could also be obtained by trial and error as follows: (i) substitution of (1.127b) yields

(1.143b) that fails for (1.144a) and (1.145a); (ii) for (1.144a) the solution Ce^{-x} fails because the left–hand side (LHS) of (1.141) yields zero but Cxe^{-x} gives $C = -1/4$ in agreement with (1.144b); (iii) for (1.145a) the solutions Ce^{x}, Cxe^{x} and Cx^2e^{x} all fail because the LHS yields zero and the Cx^3e^{x} gives $C = -1/6$ in agreement with (1.145b). The trial-and-error method may involve more calculation and risk of error than the method of the characteristic polynomial. In all cases, it is possible to substitute back the solution into the differential equation as a check.

1.4.4 Forcing by a Hyperbolic Cosine or Sine

A particular integral of the linear differential equation with constant coefficients (1.126) forced (standard VIII) by a hyperbolic cosine or sine:

$$B(x) = B\cosh,\sinh(cx) = B\frac{e^{cx} \pm e^{-cx}}{2}, \tag{1.146a, b}$$

is obtained: (i) by superposition (1.147b) of (1.129b) if $\pm c$ are not roots (1.129a) of the characteristic polynomial (1.147a):

$$P_N(\pm c) \neq 0: \qquad y_*(x) = \frac{B}{2}\left[\frac{e^{cx}}{P_N(c)} \pm \frac{e^{-cx}}{P_N(-c)}\right]$$

$$= \frac{B}{2}\left\{\cosh(cx)\left[\frac{1}{P_N(c)} + \frac{1}{P_N(-c)}\right] + \sinh(cx)\left[\frac{1}{P_N(c)} - \frac{1}{P_N(-c)}\right]\right\}, \tag{1.147a, b}$$

as a linear combination of hyperbolic sines and cosines; (ii) if $+c\,(-c)$ is a root of multiplicity M(S) of the characteristic polynomial (1.148a, b):

$$O\left((D-c)^M\right) \sim P_N(D) \sim O\left((D+c)^S\right): \qquad y_*(x) = \frac{B}{2}\left[\frac{x^M e^{cx}}{P_N^{(M)}(c)} \pm \frac{x^S e^{-cx}}{P_N^{(S)}(-c)}\right], \tag{1.148a–c}$$

the solution (1.148c) is the superposition of (1.134b).

As an example, consider the same differential operator (1.141;1.142a–g) with different forcing:

$$y'''' - 2y''' + 2y' - y = 2\cosh(cx) = e^{cx} + e^{-cx}. \tag{1.149}$$

The resonant solutions correspond to $c = \pm 1$, where the sign does not affect the right–hand side (RHS) of (1.149). Thus, there are two cases: (i) the non-resonant solution (1.150a, b); (ii) the resonant solution (1.151a, b):

$$c \neq \pm 1: \quad y_*(x) = \frac{e^{cx}}{P_4(c)} + \frac{e^{-cx}}{P_4(-c)} = \frac{1}{(c-1)(c+1)}\left[\frac{e^{cx}}{(c-1)^2} + \frac{e^{-cx}}{(c+1)^2}\right] \tag{1.150a, b}$$

$$= \frac{(c+1)^2 e^{cx} + (c-1)^2 e^{-cx}}{(c-1)^3 (c+1)^3} = \frac{2(c^2+1)\cosh(cx) + 4c\sinh(cx)}{(c^2-1)^3};$$

$$c = \pm 1: \quad y_*(x) = \frac{x^3 e^x}{P_4'''(1)} + \frac{xe^{-x}}{P_4'(-1)} = \frac{x^3 e^x}{12} - \frac{xe^{-x}}{8} \tag{1.151a, b}$$

$$= \frac{x}{4}\left[\left(\frac{x^2}{3} - \frac{1}{2}\right)\cosh x + \left(\frac{x^2}{3} + \frac{1}{2}\right)\sinh x\right].$$

In (1.150b) [(1.151b)] were used (1.142b) [(1.142f, g)].

1.4.5 Forcing by a Circular Sine or Cosine

A particular integral of the linear differential equation with constant coefficients (1.126) forced (standard IX) by a circular cosine or sine:

$$B(x) = B\cos,\sin(ax) = B\left\{\frac{e^{iax} + e^{-iax}}{2}, \frac{e^{iax} - e^{-iax}}{2i}\right\}, \tag{1.152}$$

is obtained: (i) by superposition (1.153b) of (1.129b) if $\pm ia$ *are not roots (1.129a) of the characteristic polynomial (1.153a):*

$$P_N(\pm ia) \neq 0: \qquad y_*(x) = \frac{B}{\{2, 2i\}}\left[\frac{e^{iax}}{P_N(ia)} \pm \frac{e^{-iax}}{P_N(-ia)}\right]; \tag{1.153a, b}$$

(ii) if $+ia(-ia)$ *is a root of multiplicity M(S) of the characteristic polynomial (1.154a) [(1.154b)] the resonant solution (1.154c) is the superposition of (1.134b):*

$$O\left((D-ia)^M\right) \sim P_N(D) \sim O\left((D+ia)^S\right): y_*(x) = \frac{B}{\{2, 2i\}}\left[\frac{x^M e^{iax}}{P_N^{(M)}(ia)} \pm \frac{x^S e^{-iax}}{P_N^{(S)}(-ia)}\right]. \tag{1.154a–c}$$

If the coefficient a in the forcing function (1.155c) is real (1.155b):

$$A_0,..,A_N,a\in|R: \qquad B(x)=B\cos,\sin(ax)=B\operatorname{Re},\operatorname{Im}\left(e^{iax}\right), \tag{1.155a–c}$$

and the coefficients of the differential equation are (1.126) real (1.155a) then: (i) either $\pm ia$ *are both not roots of the characteristic polynomial (1.156a) leading to a non-resonant solution (1.156b):*

$$P_N(ia)\neq 0: \qquad y_*(x)=B\operatorname{Re},\operatorname{Im}\left[\frac{e^{iax}}{P_N(ia)}\right]; \tag{1.156a, b}$$

$$P_N(D)\sim O\left((D-ia)^M\right): \qquad y_*(x)=Bx^M\operatorname{Re},\operatorname{Im}\left[\frac{e^{iax}}{P_N^{(M)}(ia)}\right], \tag{1.157a, b}$$

(ii) or $\pm ia$ *are both roots of multiplicity M of the characteristic polynomial (1.157a) leading to a resonant solution (1.157b).*

As an example, consider the linear differential equation with constant coefficients:

$$y'''-y''+y'-y=4\sin(ax)=4\operatorname{Im}\left(e^{iax}\right). \tag{1.158}$$

The characteristic polynomial is (1.159a–c):

$$P_3(D)=D^3-D^2+D-1=(D-1)\left(D^2+1\right)=(D-1)(D-i)(D+i), \tag{1.159a–c}$$

$$P_3'(D)=3D^2-2D+1: \quad P_3(1)=0\neq 2=P_3'(1), \quad P_3(\pm i)=0\neq -2\mp 2i=P_3'(\pm i), \tag{1.159d–f}$$

and its derivative (1.159d) confirms (1.159e, f) that $1,\pm i$ are single roots.

The general integral of the unforced equation is:

$$y(x)=C_1e^x+C_2e^{ix}+C_3e^{-ix}=C_1\,e^x+D_2\cos x+D_3\sin x. \tag{1.160a, b}$$

The forcing term on the RHS of (1.158) shows that resonant solutions occur when $\pm ia$ is a root of the characteristic polynomial (1.159a), which is possible (1.161a) only for two real values (1.161b) of a:

$$\pm ia=1,\pm i \quad\Rightarrow\quad a=\pm 1. \tag{1.161a, b}$$

Thus, there are two cases: (i) a non-resonant solution (1.162b) if a does not (1.162a) take the values (1.161b):

$$a \neq \pm 1: \quad y_*(x) = 4\,\mathrm{Im}\left[\frac{e^{iax}}{P_3(ia)}\right] = 4\,\mathrm{Im}\left[\frac{e^{iax}}{(a^2-1)(1-ia)}\right]$$
$$= \frac{4}{a^2-1}\mathrm{Im}\left[\frac{(1+ia)e^{iax}}{a^2+1}\right] = 4\frac{\sin(ax)+a\cos(ax)}{a^4-1}; \tag{1.162a, b}$$

(ii) the values (1.161b) ≡ (1.162a) correspond to the resonant solution (1.163b):

$$a = \pm 1: \quad y_*(x) = 4\,\mathrm{Im}\left[\frac{xe^{\pm ix}}{P_3'(\pm i)}\right] = 2x\,\mathrm{Im}\left(\frac{e^{\pm ix}}{-1 \mp i}\right)$$
$$= x\,\mathrm{Im}\left[(-1 \pm i)e^{\pm ix}\right] = \pm x(\cos x - \sin x). \tag{1.163a, b}$$

In (1.162b) [(1.163b)] was used (1.159b) [(1.159f)].

1.4.6 Product of an Exponential and a Hyperbolic Function

A particular integral of the linear differential equation with constant coefficients (1.126) forced (standard X) by the product (1.164) of an exponential (1.127a) and a hyperbolic cosine or sine (1.146b):

$$B(x) = Be^{bx}\cosh,\sinh(cx) = \frac{B}{2}\left[e^{(b+c)x} \pm e^{(b-c)x}\right], \tag{1.164}$$

is obtained: (i) by superposition (1.165b) of (1.129b) if $b \pm c$ are not (1.129a) roots of the characteristic polynomial (1.165a):

$$P_N(b \pm c) \neq 0: \qquad y_*(x) = \frac{B}{2}\left[\frac{e^{(b+c)x}}{P_N(b+c)} \pm \frac{e^{(b-c)x}}{P_N(b-c)}\right], \tag{1.165a, b}$$

that is, a linear combination of hyperbolic cosine and sines multiplied by the exponential:

$$y_*(x) = \frac{B}{2}e^{bx}\left\{\cosh(cx)\left[\frac{1}{P_N(b+c)} + \frac{1}{P_N(b-c)}\right] + \sinh(cx)\left[\frac{1}{P_N(b+c)} - \frac{1}{P_N(b-c)}\right]\right\}; \tag{1.165c}$$

(ii) if $b+c\left(b-c\right)$ is a root of multiplicity M(S) of the characteristic polynomial (1.166a) [(1.166b)] then, the resonant solution (1.166c) is the superposition of (1.134b):

$$O\left(\left(D-b-c\right)^M\right)\sim P_N\left(D\right)\sim O\left(\left(D-b+c\right)^S\right):\quad y_*\left(x\right)=\frac{B}{2}\left[\frac{x^M e^{(b+c)x}}{P_N^{(M)}\left(b+c\right)}\pm\frac{x^S e^{(b-c)x}}{P_N^{(S)}\left(b-c\right)}\right],$$
(1.165a–c)

As an example, consider the same fourth-order differential operator (1.141) with a forcing (1.167) different from (1.141):

$$y''''-2y'''+2y'-y=2e^{2x}\cosh\left(cx\right)=e^{(2+c)x}+e^{(2-c)x}. \tag{1.167}$$

The resonant solutions (1.168a) correspond:

$$2+c,\quad 2-c=\pm1\qquad\Rightarrow\qquad c=\pm1,\pm3, \tag{1.168a, b}$$

to (1.168b) where the signs do not affect (1.167). Thus, there are three cases: (i) the non-resonant (1.169a) solution (1.169b), where is used (1.142b):

$$c\neq\pm1,\pm3:\quad y_*(x)=\frac{e^{(2+c)x}}{P_4(2+c)}+\frac{e^{(2-c)x}}{P_4(2-c)}=\frac{e^{(2-c)x}}{(c+1)^3\,(c+3)}+\frac{e^{(2-c)x}}{(c-1)^3\,(c-3)}$$
$$=\frac{e^{2x}}{(c^2-1)^3(c^2-9)}[(c-1)^3(c-3)e^{cx}+(c+1)^3(c+3)e^{-cx}],$$
(1.169a, b)

(ii) the first resonant solution (1.170b) corresponds to (1.170a):

$$c=\pm1:\qquad y_*\left(x\right)=\frac{e^{3x}}{P_4\left(3\right)}+\frac{x^3e^x}{P_4'''\left(1\right)}=\frac{e^{3x}}{32}+\frac{x^3e^x}{12}; \tag{1.170a, b}$$

$$c=\pm3:\qquad y_*\left(x\right)=\frac{e^{5x}}{P_4\left(5\right)}+\frac{xe^{-x}}{P_4'(-1)}=\frac{e^{5x}}{384}-\frac{xe^{-x}}{8}, \tag{1.171a, b}$$

(iii) the second resonant solution (1.171b) corresponds to (1.171a). In (1.170b) [(1.171b)] are used (1.142a, g) [(1.142a, f)].

1.4.7 Product of an Exponential and a Circular Function

The determination of particular integrals of the linear ordinary differential equation with constant coefficients (1.126) can be extended from the case of exponential (subsection 1.4.3), not only to hyperbolic (circular) cosines and sines [subsections 1.4.4 (1.4.5)], but also to their product [subsections 1.4.6 (1.4.7)]. *The linear differential equation with constant coefficients (1.126), with (standard XI) forcing term specified by the product of an exponential and a circular cosine or sine:*

$$B(x) = Be^{\alpha x}\cos,\sin(ax) = \frac{B}{\{2,2i\}}\left[e^{(b+ia)x} \pm e^{(b-ia)x}\right], \tag{1.172}$$

has particular integrals given by: (i) the superposition of exponential solutions in the non-resonant case:

$$P_N(b \pm ia) \neq 0: \qquad y_*(x) = \frac{B}{\{2,2i\}}\left[\frac{e^{(b+ia)x}}{P_N(b+ia)} \pm \frac{e^{(b-ia)x}}{P_N(b-ia)}\right], \tag{1.173a, b}$$

and in the resonant case:

$$O\left((D-b-ia)^M\right) \sim P_N(D) \sim O\left((D-b+ia)^S\right):$$

$$y_*(x) = \frac{B}{\{2,2i\}}\left[\frac{x^M e^{(b+ia)x}}{P_N^{(M)}(b+ia)} \pm \frac{x^S e^{(b-ia)x}}{P_N^{(S)}(b-ia)}\right], \tag{1.174a–c}$$

that apply to a characteristic polynomial (1.52b) with complex coefficients $A_{1,\ldots,}A_N$ *and also complex (b, c); (ii) for real parameters (1.175b) and real characteristic polynomial (1.175a) the forcing term (1.175c):*

$$A_0,\ldots,A_N,a,b \in |R: \quad B(x) = Be^{bx}\cos,\sin(ax) = Be^{bx}\,\mathrm{Re},\mathrm{Im}\left(e^{iax}\right), \tag{1.175a–c}$$

leads to the non-resonant (1.176a, b):

$$P_N(b \pm ia) \neq 0: \qquad y_*(x) = B\,\mathrm{Re},\mathrm{Im}\left[\frac{e^{(b+ia)x}}{P_N(b+ia)}\right], \tag{1.176a, b}$$

$$P_N(D) \sim O\left((D-b \pm ia)^M\right): \qquad y_*(x) = Bx^M\,\mathrm{Re},\mathrm{Im}\left[\frac{e^{(b+ia)x}}{P_N^{(M)}(b+ia)}\right], \tag{1.177a, b}$$

and resonant (1.177a–c) solutions.

As an example, consider the second-order differential equation with constant coefficients:

$$y'' - 2y' + 2y = 2e^x \sin(ax) = 2\mathrm{Im}\left[e^{(1+ia)x}\right]; \tag{1.178}$$

the characteristic polynomial is (1.179a–c):

$$P_2(D) = D^2 - 2D + 2 = (D-1)^2 + 1 = (D-1-i)(D-1+i), \tag{1.179a–c}$$

$$P_2'(D) = 2D - 2, \qquad P_2(1 \pm i) = 0 \neq P_2'(1 \pm i) = \pm 2i, \tag{1.179d, e}$$

whose derivative (1.179d) confirms that $1 \pm i$ are simple roots (1.179e). The general integral of the unforced equation is:

$$y(x) = C_1 e^{(1+i)x} + C_2 e^{(1-i)x} = e^x (D_1 \cos x + D_2 \sin x) = E e^x \cos(x - \gamma). \tag{1.180a–c}$$

The forced solution of (1.178) is resonant (1.181a) for the values (1.181b) of a:

$$1 + ia = 1 \pm i \qquad \Rightarrow \qquad a = \pm 1. \tag{1.181a, b}$$

Thus, there are two cases: (i) the non-resonant solution (1.182a, b):

$$a \neq \pm 1: \qquad y_*(x) = 2\mathrm{Im}\left[\frac{e^{(1+ia)x}}{P_2(1+ia)}\right] = 2\, e^x \mathrm{Im}\left(\frac{e^{iax}}{1-a^2}\right) = \frac{2e^x \sin(ax)}{1-a^2}; \tag{1.182a, b}$$

and (ii) the resonant solution (1.183a, b):

$$a = \pm 1: \qquad y_*(x) = 2\mathrm{Im}\left[\frac{x e^{(1\pm i)x}}{P_2'(1 \pm i)}\right] = x e^x \mathrm{Im}\left(\frac{e^{\pm ix}}{\pm i}\right) = \mp x e^x \cos x. \tag{1.183a, b}$$

In (1.182b) [(1.183b)] was used (1.179b) [(1.179e)].

1.4.8 Product of an Exponential and a Circular and a Hyperbolic Function

All the preceding cases (subsections 1.4.3–1.4.7) are included in the *particular integral of a linear differential equation forced (1.126) forced (standard XII) by the product of an exponential by a hyperbolic cosine or sine by a circular cosine or sine:*

$$B(x) = Be^{bx} \cosh, \sinh(cx) \cos, \sin(ax) = Be^{bx} \frac{e^{cx} \pm e^{-cx}}{2} \frac{e^{iax} \pm e^{-iax}}{\{2, 2i\}}. \tag{1.184}$$

The non-resonant solution (1.185b) applies if $b \pm c \pm ia$ *are not roots of the characteristic polynomial (1.185a):*

$P_N(b \pm c \pm ia) \neq 0$:

$$y_*(x) = \frac{B}{\{4, 4i\}} \left[\frac{e^{(b+c+ia)x}}{P_N(b+c+ia)} \pm \frac{e^{(b-c+ia)x}}{P_N(b-c+ia)} \pm \frac{e^{(b+c-ia)x}}{P_N(b+c-ia)} + \frac{e^{(b-c-ia)x}}{P_N(b-c-ia)} \right]; \tag{1.185a, b}$$

the resonant solutions are modified as in (1.134b), and the results holds for complex (a, b, c) and complex characteristic polynomial (1.52b). In the case of real coefficients and parameters (1.186a) the forcing function (1.186b):

$$a, b, c, A_0, \ldots, A_N \in |R: \quad B(x) = Be^{bx} \cosh, \sinh(cx) \cos, \sin(ax) = \frac{B}{2} \operatorname{Re}, \operatorname{Im}\left[e^{(b+c+ia)x} \pm e^{(b-c+ia)x} \right], \tag{1.186a, b}$$

leads to the non-resonant integral (1.187a, b):

$$P_N(b \pm c + ia) \neq 0: \quad y_*(x) = Be^{bx} \operatorname{Re}, \operatorname{Im}\left[\frac{e^{(ia+c)x}}{P_N(b+c+ia)} \pm \frac{e^{(ia-c)x}}{P_N(b-c+ia)} \right], \tag{1.187a, b}$$

and the resonant cases are modified as in (1.134b).

As an example, the second-order differential equation (1.178) with a different forcing terms is considered (1.188):

$$y'' - 2y' + 2y = 2e^{2x} \sinh x \cos(ax) = \left(e^{3x} - e^{x}\right) \operatorname{Re}\left(e^{iax}\right). \tag{1.188}$$

The resonant solution occurs (1.189a) for the values (1.189b) of a:

$$3 + ia, 1 + ia = 1 \pm i \quad \Rightarrow \quad a = \pm 1, \tag{1.189a, b}$$

and only for the second term on the RHS of (1.188). Thus, there are three cases: (i) the non-resonant solution that fails for $a = \pm 1$:

$$\begin{aligned} a \neq \pm 1: \quad y_*(x) &= \operatorname{Re}\left[\frac{e^{(3+ia)x}}{P_2(3+ia)} - \frac{e^{(1+ia)x}}{P_2(1+ia)} \right] = \operatorname{Re}\left[\frac{e^{(3+ia)x}}{5 - a^2 + 4ia} - \frac{e^{(1+ia)x}}{1 - a^2} \right] \\ &= \frac{e^x}{a^2 - 1} \cos(ax) + \operatorname{Re}\left[\frac{5 - a^2 - 4ia}{(5 - a^2)^2 + 16a^2} e^{(3+ia)x} \right] \\ &= \frac{e^x}{a^2 - 1} \cos(ax) + \frac{e^{3x}}{a^4 + 6a^2 + 25} [(5 - a^2)\cos(ax) + 4a \sin(ax)], \end{aligned} \tag{1.190a, b}$$

(ii) in this case, it is replaced by the resonant solution (1.191a, b):

$$a = \pm 1: \quad y_*(x) = \mathrm{Re}\left[\frac{e^{(3\pm i)x}}{P_2(3\pm i)} - \frac{x\,e^{(1\pm i)x}}{P_2'(1\pm i)}\right] = \mathrm{Re}\left[\frac{e^{(3\pm i)x}}{4\pm 4i} - \frac{x\,e^{(1\pm i)x}}{\pm 2i}\right]$$

$$= \mathrm{Re}\left[\frac{1\mp i}{8}e^{(3\pm i)x} \pm i\frac{x}{2}e^{(1\pm i)x}\right] = \frac{e^{3x}}{8}(\cos x + \sin x) - \frac{x e^{x}}{2}\sin x. \tag{1.191a, b}$$

In (1.190b) [(1.191b)] were used (1.179a) [(1.179a, c)].

1.5 Polynomial of Derivatives and Inverse Operator

Two methods of obtaining a particular integral of a forced linear differential equation with constant coefficients are: (a) using the characteristic polynomial (section 1.4), for example, when the forcing term is a product of exponential and circular or hyperbolic cosines or sines; (b) using the algebraic inverse of the characteristic polynomial as an operator applied to the forcing term (section 1.5). In the latter method of (b) the algebraic inverse of the characteristic polynomial is interpreted as follows: (i) the inverse of the characteristic polynomial is a rational function that can be decomposed into partial fractions (subsections 1.5.3–1.5.4); (ii) each partial fraction is an inverse differential operator (subsection 1.5.1) corresponding to a geometric or binomial series of derivatives; (iii) the series of derivatives terminates when applied to a forcing function that is a polynomial (subsections 1.5.5–1.5.6); (iv) if the forcing function is a smooth function, it is infinitely differentiable and the resulting series must converge (subsection 1.5.7). The case (iv) applies to the forcing by the product of a smooth function by a polynomial (subsection 1.5.8) or other elementary functions (subsection 1.5.9); this includes the preceding cases (section 1.4) of resonant (subsection 1.5.11) and non-resonant (subsection 1.5.10) forcing, and zero or non-zero roots of the characteristic polynomial (subsection 1.5.12). The examples include the forcing of a linear differential equation with constant coefficients by the product of a power or polynomial by: (i) an exponential (subsection 1.5.13); (ii, iii) a hyperbolic (circular) cosine or sine [subsection 1.5.14 (1.5.15)]; (iv, v) an exponential times a hyperbolic (circular) cosine or sine [subsection 1.5.16 (1.5.17)]; (vi) an exponential times a hyperbolic times a circular cosine or sine (subsection 1.5.18). The examples of unforced and forced solutions can be superimposed (subsection 1.5.19). As a preliminary, the binomial series (subsection 1.5.1) is obtained.

1.5.1 Direct and Inverse Binomial Series

The Stirling-MacLaurin series (I.23.34b) ≡ (1.192b) for an analytic function (1.1921a):

$$f(z) \in \mathcal{A}(|C): \qquad f(x) = \sum_{n=0}^{\infty} \frac{x^n}{n!} f^{(n)}(0), \tag{1.192a, b}$$

applied to the function (1.193a) and its derivatives of all orders at the origin (1.193b):

$$f(x) = (x+a)^\nu: \quad f^{(n)}(0) = \lim_{x \to 0} \frac{d^n}{dx^n}\left[(x+a)^\nu\right]$$
$$= \nu(\nu-1)....(\nu-n+1)\lim_{x\to 0}(x+a)^{\nu-n} = \frac{\nu!}{(\nu-n)!}a^{\nu-n}, \tag{1.193a, b}$$

leads to the **binomial series** (1.194b) *involving the* **arrangements** (1.194c) *that converges for* (1.194a):

$$|x| < |a|: \qquad (x+a)^\nu = \sum_{n=0}^{\infty} \binom{\nu}{n} a^{\nu-n} x^n, \quad \binom{\nu}{n} \equiv \frac{\nu!}{n!(\nu-n)!}. \tag{1.194a–c}$$

The radius of convergence (1.194a) applies to all complex values of the exponent ν other than zero or a positive integer (section I.25.9). The expression (1.194b) coincides with (I.25.37b) apart from a misprint in the latter. The substitution (1.195a) in (1.194b) leads to (1.195b):

$$\nu = -\mu: \qquad (x+a)^{-\mu} = \sum_{n=0}^{\infty} \binom{-\mu}{n} a^{-\mu-n} x^n, \tag{1.195a, b}$$

where:

$$\binom{-\mu}{n}^n = \frac{(-\mu)(-\mu-1)....(-\mu-n+1)}{n!} = (-)^n \frac{\mu(\mu+1)....(\mu+n-1)}{n!} \equiv (-)^n \binom{\mu+n-1}{n}. \tag{1.195c}$$

Substitution of (1.195c) in (1.195b) specifies the inverse binomial series:

$$|x| < |a|: \qquad (x+a)^{-\mu} = \sum_{n=0}^{\infty} \binom{\mu+n-1}{n} a^{-\mu-n} (-x)^n; \tag{1.196a, b}$$

this coincides with (I.25.41b) apart from another misprint.

1.5.2 Interpretation of the Inverse Polynomial of Derivatives

A particular integral of the linear differential equation with constant coefficients (1.126) ≡ (1.197b) and forcing term is obtained by applying to the latter the inverse (1.197c) of a polynomial of derivatives (1.197a):

$$D \equiv \frac{d}{dx}: \qquad \{P_N(D)\} y_*(x) = B(x) \quad \Rightarrow \quad y_*(x) = \left\{\frac{1}{P_N(D)}\right\} B(x), \qquad (1.197a–c)$$

provided such an operator can be interpreted, for example, (i) the inverse of a derivative D is a primitive $1/D$:

$$D\{B(x)\} = \frac{dB}{dx}, \qquad \frac{1}{D}\{B(x)\} = \int^x B(\xi)\, d\xi; \qquad (1.198a, b)$$

(ii) the operator $(D-b)^{-1}$ can be expanded in an arithmetic series (I.21.62b):

$$\frac{1}{D-b} = \frac{-1/b}{1-D/b} = -\sum_{m=0}^{\infty} b^{-1-m} D^m; \qquad (1.199)$$

(iii) the operator $(D-b)^{-M}$ can be expanded in a binomial series (1.196b; 1.195c):

$$(D-b)^{-M} = \sum_{m=0}^{\infty} \frac{(M+n-1)!}{n!(M-1)!} (-b)^{-M-n} (-D)^n; \qquad (1.200)$$

(iv) a polynomial of derivatives (1.52b), for which zero is not a root (1.201a) has an inverse (1.201b), obtained using an arithmetic series (I.21.62c):

$$A_0 \neq 0: \qquad \frac{1}{P(D)} = \frac{1/A_0}{1 + \sum_{n=1}^{N} (A_n/A_0) D^n} = \sum_{m=0}^{\infty} (-)^m A_0^{-m-1} \left\{\sum_{n=1}^{N} A_n D^n\right\}^m, \qquad (1.201a, b)$$

(v) if zero is a root of multiplicity M of the polynomial of derivatives (1.132a) ≡ (1.132b, c) ≡ (1.202a, b), then it equals D^{-M} multiplied (1.202a) by a polynomial of degree $N-M$ for which zero is not a root (1.202b):

$$P_N(D) = D^M Q_{N-M}(D), \qquad Q_{N-M}(0) \neq 0: \qquad \frac{1}{P_N(D)} = D^{-M} \frac{1}{Q_{N-M}(D)}, \qquad (1.202a–c)$$

and the inverse of the latter polynomial is applied first (1.202c), followed by M primitives (1.198b). The series expansions (1.199; 1.200; 1.201b) in powers of (1.197a) are symbolic operators that if applied to a forcing term, that is: (i) a polynomial of degree S finish (subsections 1.5.5–1.5.6) at the derivative of order S; (ii) not a polynomial that requires the forcing function to be infinitely differentiable or smooth and that the resulting series must converge (subsections 1.5.7–1.5.10). The algebraic inverse of a polynomial of derivatives with simple (multiple) roots [subsection 1.5.3 (1.5.4)], via a partial fraction decomposition [section I.31.8 (I.31.9)] becomes a sum of terms of the form: (i) for zero roots (1.198b) and 1.202c); (ii) for non-zero roots can be decomposed into the sum of terms of the form (1.199) and (1.200) using [subsections 1.5.3 (1.5.4)] the partial fraction decomposition [subsection I.31.8 (I.31.9)].

1.5.3 Partial Fractions for the Inverse Characteristic Polynomial

If the characteristic polynomial (1.52b) ≡ (1.203a) has all roots distinct (1.54) ≡ (1.203b), its inverse can be decomposed into simple partial fractions (1.203c) with coefficients (1.203d):

$$P_N(D) = \sum_{n=0}^{N} A_n D^n = A_N \prod_{n=1}^{N} (D - a_n): \quad \frac{1}{P_N(D)} = \sum_{n=1}^{N} \frac{B_n}{D - a_n}, \quad B_n = \frac{1}{A_N} \prod_{\substack{m=1 \\ m \neq n}}^{N} \frac{1}{a_n - a_m}, \tag{1.203a–d}$$

corresponding to:

$$\frac{A_N}{P_N(D)} = \sum_{n=1}^{N} \frac{1}{(a_n - a_1)....(a_n - a_{n-1})(D - a_n)(a_n - a_{n+1})...(a_n - a_N)}. \tag{1.204}$$

The proof of (1.203a–c) uses the fact that a simple root $D = a_n$ of the characteristic polynomial (1.203b) is a simple pole of its inverse (1.203c); the coefficient B_n is the **residue at the simple pole** a_n, and is calculated by (1.205) ≡ (I.5.25a):

$$B_n = \lim_{D \to a_n} \frac{D - a_n}{P_N(D)}, \tag{1.205}$$

as follows from (1.203c):

$$\lim_{D \to a_n} \frac{D - a_n}{P_N(D)} = B_n + \lim_{D \to a_n} \prod_{\substack{m=1 \\ m \neq n}}^{N} B_m \frac{D - a_n}{D - a_m} = B_n, \tag{1.206}$$

since all terms with $m \neq n$ vanish when $D \to a_n$. In the case of the inverse of a polynomial with simple roots (1.203b), the residues (1.205) at the simple poles are given by:

$$B_n = \lim_{D \to a_n} \frac{D - a_n}{P_N(D)} = \lim_{D \to a_n} \frac{D - a_n}{A_N} \prod_{m=1}^{N} \frac{1}{D - a_m}$$
$$= \frac{1}{A_n} \lim_{D \to a_n} \prod_{\substack{m=1 \\ m \neq n}}^{N} \frac{1}{D - a_m} = \frac{1}{A_N} \prod_{\substack{m=1 \\ m \neq n}}^{N} \frac{1}{a_n - a_m}, \tag{1.207}$$

proving (1.203d). For example, the characteristic polynomial with two distinct roots (1.62a, b) has the inverse:

$$\frac{1}{P_2(b)} = \frac{1}{(D-a)(D-b)} = \frac{1}{b-a}\frac{1}{D-b} + \frac{1}{D-a}\frac{1}{a-b} = \frac{1}{a-b}\left(\frac{1}{D-a} - \frac{1}{D-b}\right); \tag{1.208}$$

thus *the partial fraction decomposition (1.204) of the inverse of the characteristic polynomial (1.62b) with two distinct roots (1.62a) is (1.208).*

1.5.4 Single and Multiple Poles of the Inverse Characteristic Polynomial

If the characteristic polynomial (1.52b) ≡ (1.209b) has multiple roots (1.98a, b) ≡ (1.209a, c), its algebraic inverse has the partial fraction decomposition (1.209d):

$$\sum_{m=1}^{M} \alpha_m = N, \qquad P_N(D) = \sum_{M=0}^{N} A_n D^n = A_N \prod_{m=1}^{N} (D - a_m)^{\alpha_m}: \tag{1.209a–c}$$

$$\frac{1}{P_N(D)} = \frac{1}{A_N} \sum_{m=1}^{M} \sum_{k=1}^{\alpha_m} B_{m,k} (D - a_m)^{-k}, \tag{1.209d}$$

with coefficients:

$$k = 1, 2, \ldots, \alpha_m: \quad B_{m,k} = \frac{(-)^{\alpha_m - k}}{(\alpha_m - k)!\, A_N} \prod_{\substack{n=1 \\ n \neq m}}^{M} \frac{(\alpha_m + \alpha_n - k)!}{(\alpha_n - 1)!} (a_m - a_n)^{k - \alpha_m - \alpha_n}. \tag{1.209e, f}$$

The proof of (1.209a–f) is made in two stages, first for the coefficients $B_{m,1}$ that are the residues, and then for the remaining coefficients $B_{m,k}$ with $k = 2, \ldots, \alpha_m$.

The root a_m of multiplicity α_m of the characteristic polynomial (1.209a-c) is a pole of order α_m of its inverse (1.209d); the **residue at a multiple pole** is the coefficient $B_{m,1}$ that is calculated by (1.210) ≡ (I.15.33b):

$$B_{m,1} = \frac{1}{(\alpha_m - 1)!} \lim_{D \to a_m} \left(\frac{d}{dD} \right)^{\alpha_m - 1} \left[\frac{(D - a_m)^{\alpha_m}}{P_N(D)} \right] \tag{1.210}$$

as follows from:

$$\begin{aligned} &\frac{1}{(\alpha_m - 1)!} \lim_{D \to a_m} \left(\frac{d}{dD} \right)^{\alpha_m - 1} \left[\frac{(D - a_m)^{\alpha_m}}{P_N(D)} \right] \\ &= \frac{1}{(\alpha_m - 1)!} \lim_{D \to a_m} \left(\frac{d}{dD} \right)^{\alpha_m - 1} \left[\sum_{k=1}^{\alpha_m} B_{m,k} (D - a_m)^{\alpha_m - k} \right] \\ &= \frac{1}{(\alpha_m - 1)!} \lim_{D \to a_m} \left(\frac{d}{dD} \right)^{\alpha_m - 1} \left[B_{m,1} (D - a_m)^{\alpha_m - 1} \right] \\ &= \frac{1}{(\alpha_m - 1)!} B_{m,1} (\alpha_m - 1)(\alpha_m - 2)....1 = B_{m,1}, \end{aligned} \tag{1.211a–d}$$

since: (i) all terms in (1.209d) vanish in the limit $D \to a_m$ except the m-th term in (1.211a); (ii) the m-th terms in (1.211a) also vanish unless $k = 1$ in (1.211b) that simplifies to (1.211c, d). In the case of the inverse of a polynomial with multiple roots (1.209c) the residues (1.210) at the poles of order α_m are given by:

$$\begin{aligned} B_{m,1} &= \frac{1}{(\alpha_m - 1)!} \lim_{D \to a_m} \left(\frac{d}{dD} \right)^{\alpha_m - 1} \left[\frac{(D - a_m)^{\alpha_m}}{P_N(D)} \right] \\ &= \frac{1}{(\alpha_m - 1)!} \lim_{D \to a_m} \left(\frac{d}{dD} \right)^{\alpha_m - 1} \left[\frac{1}{A_N} \prod_{\substack{n=1 \\ n \neq m}}^{M} (D - a_n)^{-\alpha_n} \right] \\ &= \frac{1}{(\alpha_m - 1)! A_N} \lim_{D \to a_m} \prod_{\substack{n=1 \\ n \neq m}}^{M} (D - a_n)^{-\alpha_n - \alpha_m + 1} \\ &\quad (-\alpha_n)(-\alpha_n - 1)...(-\alpha_n - \alpha_m + 1), \end{aligned} \tag{1.212}$$

that simplifies to:

$$B_{m,1} = \frac{(-)^{\alpha_m-1}}{(\alpha_m-1)!A_N} \prod_{\substack{n=1 \\ n\neq m}}^{M} \frac{(\alpha_m+\alpha_n-1)!}{(\alpha_n-1)!}(a_m-a_n)^{1-\alpha_m-\alpha_n}; \tag{1.213}$$

this proves (1.209f) for $k=1$.

The remaining coefficients (1.209e, f) at the pole a_m of order α_m in (1.209d) are obtained by the **extended residue rule** (1.214) ≡ (I.31.85a, b):

$$B_{m,k} = \frac{1}{(\alpha_m-k)!} \lim_{D\to a_m} \left(\frac{d}{dD}\right)^{\alpha_m-k} \left[\frac{(D-a_m)^{\alpha_m}}{P_N(D)}\right], \tag{1.214}$$

which includes (1.210) for $k=1$. The residue for simple (1.205) ≡ (1.206) and multiple (1.210) ≡ (1.211) pole are included in the **extended residue rule** (1.214) ≡ (1.215) that follows from (1.209d):

$$\begin{aligned}
&\frac{1}{(\alpha_m-k)!} \lim_{D\to \alpha_m} \left(\frac{d}{dD}\right)^{\alpha_m-k} \left[\frac{(D-a_m)^{\alpha_m}}{P_N(D)}\right] \\
&= \frac{1}{(\alpha_m-k)!} \lim_{D\to \alpha_m} \left(\frac{d}{dD}\right)^{\alpha_m-k} \left[\sum_{\ell=1}^{\alpha_m} B_{m,\ell}(D-a_m)^{\alpha_m-\ell}\right] \\
&= \frac{1}{(\alpha_m-k)!} \lim_{D\to \alpha_m} \left(\frac{d}{dD}\right)^{\alpha_m-k} \left[B_{m,k}(D-a_m)^{\alpha_m-k}\right] \\
&= \frac{1}{(\alpha_m-k)!} B_{m,k}(\alpha_m-k)(\alpha_m-k-1)....1 = B_{m,k},
\end{aligned} \tag{1.215a–d}$$

since: (i) all terms in (1.209d) vanish in the limit $D \to a_m$ except the m-th term in (1.215a); (ii) all the terms in (1.215a) vanish except for $\ell = k$ in (1.215b) simplifying to (1.215c, d). In the case of a the inverse of a polynomial with multiple roots (1.209c) the coefficients of its partial fraction decomposition (1.209g) are given by:

$$\begin{aligned}
B_{m,k} &= \frac{1}{(\alpha_m-k)!} \lim_{D\to a_m} \left(\frac{d}{dD}\right)^{\alpha_m-k} \left[\frac{(D-a_m)^{\alpha_m}}{P_N(D)}\right] \\
&= \frac{1}{(\alpha_m-k)!} \lim_{D\to a_m} \left(\frac{d}{dD}\right)^{\alpha_m-k} \left[\frac{1}{A_N} \prod_{\substack{n=1 \\ n\neq m}}^{M} (D-a_n)^{-\alpha_n}\right] \\
&= \frac{1}{(\alpha_m-k)!A_N} \lim_{D\to a_m} (D-a_n)^{-\alpha_n-\alpha_m+k} \\
&= (-\alpha_n)(-\alpha_n-1)...(-\alpha_n-\alpha_m+k),
\end{aligned} \tag{1.216}$$

that simplifies to:

$$B_{m,k} = \frac{(-)^{\alpha_m - k}}{(\alpha_m - k)!A_N} \prod_{\substack{n=1 \\ n \neq m}}^{M} \frac{(\alpha_n + \alpha_n - k)!}{(\alpha_m - 1)!} (a_m - a_n)^{k - \alpha_m - \alpha_n}. \tag{1.217}$$

The coefficient (1.217) with $k = 1$ coincides with the residue (1.213) at the pole of order α_m, and for other values (1.209e) of k proves the coefficients (1.209f).

As an example, consider the cubic characteristic polynomial (1.218b) with a single and a double root (1.218a):

$$a \neq b: \qquad P_3(D) = (D-a)(D-b)^2: \qquad \frac{1}{P_3(D)} = \frac{B_1}{D-a} + \frac{B_{2,1}}{D-b} + \frac{B_{2,2}}{(D-b)^2}. \tag{1.218a–c}$$

The inverse of the characteristic polynomial (1.218b) has partial fraction decomposition (1.218c) with coefficients: (i) the residue (1.219a) at the simple pole at a:

$$B_1 = \lim_{D \to a} \frac{D-a}{P_3(D)} = \lim_{D \to a} \frac{1}{(D-b)^2} = \frac{1}{(a-b)^2}; \tag{1.219a}$$

$$B_{2,1} = \lim_{D \to a} \frac{d}{dD} \left[\frac{(D-b)^2}{P_3(D)} \right] = \lim_{D \to b} \frac{d}{dD} \frac{1}{(D-a)} = -\frac{1}{(b-a)^2}, \tag{1.219b}$$

$$B_{2,2} = \lim_{D \to a} \frac{(D-b)^2}{P_3(D)} = \lim_{D \to b} \frac{1}{D-a} = \frac{1}{b-a}, \tag{1.219c}$$

(ii, iii) the residue (1.219b) and other coefficient (1.219c) at the double pole b. Substitution of (1.219a–c) in (1.218c) leads to:

$$\frac{1}{(D-a)(D-b)^2} = \frac{1}{b-a} \left[\frac{1}{b-a} \left(\frac{1}{D-a} - \frac{1}{D-b} \right) + \frac{1}{(D-b)^2} \right]. \tag{1.220}$$

This specifies *the partial fraction decomposition (1.220) of the inverse of a cubic characteristic polynomial (1.218b) with a single and a double root (1.218a), and corresponds to the identity:*

$$(b-a)^2 = (D-b)^2 - (D-a)(D-b) + (b-a)(D-a), \tag{1.221}$$

obtained multiplying by the denominators in (1.220).

1.5.5 Particular Integral for Polynomial Forcing

As an alternative to the partial fraction decompositions (subsections 1.5.3–1.5.4) the inverse of a characteristic polynomial can be expanded by (1.201a, b), for example, to second-order:

$$\begin{aligned}\frac{1}{P_N(D)} &= \frac{1}{A_0 + A_1 D + A_2 D^2 + O(D^3)} \\ &= \frac{1}{A_0}\left[1 + \frac{A_1}{A_0}D + \frac{A_2}{A_0}D^2 + O(D^3)\right]^{-1} \\ &= \frac{1}{A_0}\left[1 - \frac{A_1}{A_0}D - \frac{A_2}{A_0}D^2 + \left(\frac{A_1}{A_0}D + \frac{A_2}{A_0}D^2\right)^2 + O(D^3)\right] \\ &= \frac{1}{A_0}\left[1 - \frac{A_1}{A_0}D - \frac{A_2 A_0 - (A_1)^2}{(A_0)^2}D^2 + O(D^3)\right].\end{aligned} \tag{1.222}$$

Thus, *the inverse of the characteristic polynomial (1.52b) can be expanded to order zero (1.223a), one (1.223b), and two (1.223c):*

$$\frac{1}{P_N(D)} = \frac{1}{A_0} + O(D) = \frac{1}{A_0} - \frac{A_1}{(A_0)^2}D + O\left(D^2\right), \tag{1.223a, b}$$

$$= \frac{1}{A_0} - \frac{A_1}{(A_0)^2}D - \left[\frac{A_2}{(A_0)^2} - \frac{(A_1)^2}{(A_0)^3}\right]D^2 + O\left(D^3\right); \tag{1.223c}$$

(1.223c) is sufficient to obtain the particular integral due to forcing by a polynomial of degree two, because the derivatives of order three and higher vanish. As an example, the same polynomial forcing term is applied to the three linear differential equations with constant coefficients (1.178) ≡ (1.224a), (1.158) ≡ (1.224b) and (1.141) ≡ (1.224c):

$$x^2 - x + 1 = y'' - 2y' + 2y, \quad y''' - y'' + y' - y, \quad y'''' - 2y''' + 2y' - y. \tag{1.224a–c}$$

The corresponding particular integrals are respectively:

$$\begin{aligned}y_*(x) &= \frac{1}{2}\frac{1}{1 - D + D^2/2}\left(x^2 - x + 1\right) \\ &= \frac{1}{2}\left[1 + D - \frac{D^2}{2} + \left(D - \frac{D^2}{2}\right)^2 + O\left(D^3\right)\right]\left(x^2 - x + 1\right) \\ &= \frac{1}{2}\left[1 + D + \frac{D^2}{2} + O\left(D^3\right)\right]\left(x^2 - x + 1\right) = \frac{x^2 + x + 1}{2},\end{aligned} \tag{1.225a}$$

$$y_*(x) = -\frac{1}{1 - D + D^2 - D^3}\left(x^2 - x + 1\right)$$

$$= -\left[1 + D - D^2 + \left(D - D^2\right)^2 + O\left(D^3\right)\right]\left(x^2 - x + 1\right) \tag{1.225b}$$

$$= -\left[1 + D + O\left(D^3\right)\right]\left(x^2 - x + 1\right) = -x^2 - x.$$

$$y_*(x) = -\frac{1}{1 - 2D + 2D^3 - D^4}\left(x^2 - x + 1\right)$$

$$= -\left[1 + 2D + 4D^2 + O\left(D^3\right)\right]\left(x^2 - x + 1\right) = -x^2 - 3x - 7. \tag{1.225c}$$

In (1.225a–c), the expansion was made explicitly only to $O\left(D^2\right)$, since all derivatives of higher order give zero when applied to the quadratic polynomial on the LHS of (1.224a–c).

1.5.6 Trial Solution and Determination of Coefficients

An alternative to the use of the characteristic polynomial is to substitute in the differential equation a trial solution with some coefficients to be determined. For example, the solution of (1.224a–c) must be a polynomial of the second degree (1.226a):

$$y_*(x) = ax^2 + bx + c, \qquad y_*' = 2ax + b, \qquad y_*'' = 2a, \qquad y_*''' = 0 = y_*'''', \tag{1.226a–e}$$

with coefficients (a, b, c) to be determined by substitution, together with all the derivatives (1.226b–e) appearing in the differential equation. Substitution of (1.226a–e) in (1.224a–c) gives, respectively, (1.227a–c):

$$x^2 - x + 1 = 2ax^2 + 2(b - 2a)x + 2(a + c - b), \tag{1.227a}$$

$$= -ax^2 + (2a - b)x + b - c - 2a, \tag{1.227b}$$

$$= -ax^2 + (4a - b)x + 2b - c. \tag{1.227c}$$

Equating the coefficients of equal powers leads respectively to the linear systems (1.228a–c), (1.229a–c), and (1.230a–c):

$$2a = 1, \qquad b - 2a = -\frac{1}{2}, \qquad a + c - b = \frac{1}{2}, \tag{1.228a–c}$$

$$-a = 1, \qquad b - 2a = 1, \qquad b - 2a - c = 1. \tag{1.229a–c}$$

$$-a = 1, \qquad b - 4a = 1, \qquad 2b - c = 1. \tag{1.230a–c}$$

These can be solved for the coefficients:

$$\{a\,,\,b\,,\,c\}=\left\{\frac{1}{2}\,,\,\frac{1}{2}\,,\,\frac{1}{2}\right\},\{-1\,,\,-1\,,\,0\},\{-1\,,\,-3\,,\,-7\}. \tag{1.231a–c}$$

Substituting the coefficients (1.231a–c) in (1.226a) confirms the particular integrals (1.225a–c). Thus, *a particular integral of a linear differential equation with constant coefficients (1.126) forced (standard XIII) by a polynomial of degree M in (1.232a) is a polynomial of at most the same degree (1.232b):*

$$\sum_{m=0}^{N} A_n \frac{d^n y_*}{dx^n} = \sum_{m=1}^{M} B_m x^m, \qquad y(x)=\sum_{m=1}^{M} C_m x^m, \tag{1.232a, b}$$

whose coefficients C_m may be obtained in terms of (A_n, B_m) substituting (1.232b) in (1.232a) and equating to zero the coefficients of all powers of x. An alternative method, that is not restricted to forcing by polynomials, is to use (1.197a–c) the inverse of the polynomial of derivatives: (i) by performing a partial fraction decomposition in the case of simple (1.203a–d; 1.204) [multiple (1.209a–f)] roots leading to a sum of terms (1.199) [(1.200)]; (ii) in the case of forcing (1.232a) by a polynomial (1.232b) of degree M, the derivatives terminate at order M; (iii) in the case of a smooth or infinitely differentiable function the series must converge (chapter I.21). The method of the characteristic polynomial (1.197a–c) [trial solution (1.232a, b)]: (i) is general, that is, it specifies the form of the solution (requires an 'a priori' guess of the form of the solution); (ii) is direct, in the sense that the calculations are usually minimized (may lead to more extensive computations). For these reasons, the method of the characteristic polynomial has been preferred before and will continue to be used in the sequel. The inverse of the characteristic polynomial is a series (1.201b) that: (i) terminates when applied to a polynomial (subsection 1.5.5); (ii) does not terminate and must converge when applied to a non-algebraic function, that must be smooth, that is infinitely differentiable (subsection 1.5.7).

1.5.7 Series of Derivatives Applied to a Smooth Function

The application of a series of derivatives to a smooth function $B(x)$, terminates on the p-th term, if it is a polynomial of degree p, for example, from (1.199):

$$\frac{1}{D-b}x^p = -\sum_{n=0}^{\infty} b^{-1-n} D^n x^p = -\sum_{n=0}^{p} b^{-1-n} \frac{p!}{(p-n)!} x^{p-n}; \tag{1.233a}$$

this formula (1.233a) can be confirmed taking the inverse operator (1.233c):

$$m = n+1: \qquad (D-b)\left\{\sum_{n=0}^{p} b^{-1-n}\frac{p!}{(p-n)!}x^{p-n}\right\}$$

$$= \sum_{n=0}^{p-1} b^{-1-n}\frac{p!}{(p-n-1)!}x^{p-n-1} - \sum_{n=0}^{p} b^{-n}\frac{p!}{(p-n)!}x^{p-n} \quad (1.233\text{b, c})$$

$$= \sum_{m=1}^{p} b^{-m}\frac{p!}{(p-m)!}x^{p-m} - \sum_{n=0}^{p} b^{-n}\frac{p!}{(p-n)!}x^{p-n} = -x^{p},$$

where: (i) was made change of dummy variable of summation (1.233b); (ii) all terms in (1.233b) cancel except $n = 0$. If the function $B(x)$ is not a polynomial, the series of derivatives applied to it should lead to a convergent expansion, for example, from (1.199):

$$\frac{1}{D-b}e^{ax} = -\sum_{n=0}^{\infty} b^{-1-n}D^{n}e^{ax}$$

$$= -\frac{e^{ax}}{b}\sum_{n=0}^{\infty}\left(\frac{a}{b}\right)^{n} = -\frac{e^{ax}}{b}\left(1-\frac{a}{b}\right)^{-1} = \frac{e^{ax}}{a-b}. \quad (1.234\text{a})$$

The formula (1.234a) can be confirmed taking the inverse operator:

$$(D-b)\frac{e^{ax}}{a-b} = (a-b)\frac{e^{ax}}{a-b} = e^{ax}. \quad (1.234\text{b})$$

It has been shown that *a forced linear differential equation with constant coefficients (1.197a, b) and has particular integral (1.197c), where the inverse of a polynomial of derivatives is interpreted according to: (i) the expansions in series of derivatives (1.199; 1.200; 1.201a, b; 1.202a–c); (ii) the decompositions in partial fractions (1.203a–d) ≡ (1.204) and (1.209a–f); (iii) the latter are sums of terms of the form of the form (1.199; 1.200). It is assumed that the forcing function is smooth (1.237a) that is infinitely differentiable and the application of the series of derivatives is: (i) a finite expansion if the forcing function is a polynomial, for example, (1.232a); (ii) a converging series, for example, (1.234a). The latter (1.234a) may be extended to (1.235a):*

$$(D-b)^{-M}e^{ax} = (a-b)^{-M}e^{ax}, \qquad \frac{1}{P_N(D)}e^{ax} = \frac{e^{ax}}{P_N(a)}, \quad (1.235\text{a, b})$$

that implies (1.235b) using the partial fraction decompositions (1.203a–d) ≡ (1.204) or (1.209a–f). The property (1.235b) is generalized next (subsection 1.5.8) to the product of the exponential by a smooth function.

1.5.8 Forcing by the Product of a Smooth Function and an Exponential

The preceding method is applied next to a forcing term, consisting of the product of an exponential and a smooth function (1.236a), which is infinitely differentiable:

$$D^{\infty}(|C) \equiv \left\{I(x): \forall_{x \in |C, n \in |N} \ \exists f^{(n)}(x)\right\}: \quad D\left\{e^{bx} I(x)\right\} = e^{bx}(I' + bI) = e^{bx}(D+b)I(x); \tag{1.236a, b}$$

the differentiation property (1.236b) extends to a polynomial (1.52b) of derivatives (1.237):

$$\{P(D)\} e^{bx} I(x) = e^{bx} \{P(D+b)\} I(x). \tag{1.237}$$

The inverse of (1.237) is (1.238a):

$$e^{bx} I(x) = \frac{1}{P(D)} \left\{e^{bx} P(D+b) I(x)\right\}; \qquad J(x) \equiv \{P(D+b)\} I(x), \tag{1.238a, b}$$

defining the smooth (1.239a) function $J(x)$ by (1.238b) and substituting in (1.238a) yields (1.239b):

$$J \in D^{\infty}(|C): \qquad \left\{\frac{1}{P(D)}\right\} e^{bx} J(x) = e^{bx} \left\{\frac{1}{P(D+b)}\right\} J(x). \tag{1.239a, b}$$

Thus, *an inverse polynomial of derivatives applied to the product of an exponential and a smooth function (1.239a) is equivalent (1.239b) to: (i) taking the exponential e^{bx} 'out' of the operator; (ii) replacing in the operator D by D + b. Thus, a particular integral of a linear differential equation with constant coefficients (1.126) forced (standard XIV) by the product (1.240a) of an exponential by a smooth function (1.239a):*

$$\{P_N(D)\} y_*(x) = e^{bx} J(x): \qquad y_*(x) = e^{bx} \left\{\frac{1}{P_N(D+b)}\right\} J(x), \tag{1.240a, b}$$

is given by (1.240b) using the inverse of the characteristic polynomial of D + b. Even if b is a root of the characteristic polynomial $P_N(b) = 0$ generally $P_N(D+b) \neq 0$ is not zero and (1.240b) applies in all cases either non-resonant (subsection 1.5.10) or resonant (subsection 1.5.11).

1.5.9 Products of Smooth and Elementary Functions

Applying to the linear differential equation with constant coefficients (1.197a–c) forced by (standard XIV – XV) an exponential (1.241a), a (standard XVI) hyperbolic cosine or sine (1.241b, c), or (standard XVII) their product (1.241d, e), with a smooth function (1.239a) as a further factor, the particular integrals are respectively (1.242a–e):

$$\left\{P_N\left(\frac{d}{dx}\right)\right\}y(x)=\left\{e^{bx};\cosh,\sinh(cx);e^{bx}\cosh,\sinh(cx)\right\}J(x), \tag{1.241a–e}$$

$$y_*(x)=\left\{\frac{e^{bx}}{P_N(D+b)},\frac{1}{2}\left[\frac{e^{cx}}{P_N(D+c)}\pm\frac{e^{-cx}}{P_N(D-c)}\right],\right.$$

$$\left.\frac{e^{bx}}{2}\left[\frac{e^{cx}}{P_N(D+b+c)}\pm\frac{e^{cx}}{P_N(D+b-c)}\right]\right\}J(x). \tag{1.242a–e}$$

If the forcing term involves (standard XVIII) circular cosines or sines (1.243a, b) or (standard XIX) their product by an exponential (1.243c, d) besides a smooth function (1.239a) the particular integrals are, respectively, (1.244a–d) valid for complex parameters and coefficients:

$$\left\{P_N\left(\frac{d}{dx}\right)\right\}y(x)=\left\{\cos,\sin(ax),2e^{bx}\cos,\sin(ax)\right\}J(x), \tag{1.243a–d}$$

$$y_*(x)=\frac{1}{\{2,2i\}}\left\{\frac{e^{iax}}{P_N(D+ia)}\pm\frac{e^{-iax}}{P_N(D-ia)},\frac{e^{(b+ia)x}}{P_N(D+b+ia)}\pm\frac{e^{(b-ia)x}}{P_N(D+b-ia)}\right\}J(x). \tag{1.244a–d}$$

If the parameters and coefficients are real (1.245a) the forcing by the product of a smooth function (1.239a) and a circular cosine or sine (1.245b, c), multiplied by (standard XIX) an exponential (1.245d, c) and an (standard XX) hyperbolic cosine or sine (1.245f, g) leads respectively to the particular integrals (1.246b–g):

$$a,b,c,A_0,\ldots,A_N\in|R:$$

$$\left\{P_N\left(\frac{d}{dx}\right)\right\}y(x)=\cos,\sin(ax)\left\{1;e^{bx};2e^{bx}\cosh,\sinh(cx)\right\}J(x)$$

$$=\operatorname{Re},\operatorname{Im}\left\{e^{iax};e^{(b+ia)x};e^{(b+ia+c)x}\pm e^{(b+ia-c)x}\right\}J(x), \tag{1.245a–g}$$

$$J\in D^{\infty}(|R):\quad y_*(x)=\text{Re},\text{Im}\left\{\frac{e^{iax}}{P_N(D+ia)};\frac{e^{(b+ia)x}}{P_N(D+b+ia)};\right.$$

$$\left.\frac{e^{(b+ia+c)x}}{P_N(D+b+ia+c)}\pm\frac{e^{(b+ia-c)x}}{P_N(D+b+ia-c)}\right\}J(x);\tag{1.246a–g}$$

thus, (1.245b–d; 1.246b–d) simplify (1.243a–d; 1.244a–d) for real coefficients.

1.5.10 Forcing by Products of Elementary Functions

A polynomial (1.52b) ≡ (1.247a) is an analytic function that coincides with its MacLaurin series (I.23.34b) = (1.247b) that has $N+1$ terms:

$$P_N(D)=\sum_{n=0}^{N}A_nD^n,\qquad A_n=\frac{1}{n!}P_N^{(n)}(0).\tag{1.247a, b}$$

The inverse polynomial of derivatives applied to a constant (1.248a) is equivalent to dividing by the value of the polynomial at the origin (1.248b):

$$I(x)=C=const:\quad \frac{1}{P_N(D)}C=\frac{1}{A_0+O(D)}C=\frac{1}{A_0}\left[1+O(D)\right]C=\frac{C}{A_0}=\frac{C}{P_N(0)}.\tag{1.248a, b}$$

Applying (1.248a, b) to (1.239a, b) leads to:

$$\frac{1}{P_N(D)}Ce^{ax}=e^{ax}\frac{1}{P_N(D+a)}C=\frac{Ce^{ax}}{P_N(a)},\tag{1.249}$$

in agreement with (1.235b) for $C=1$. Thus, *if the smooth function (1.239a) is unity $J=1$ the particular integrals (1.241a–c, 1.242a–e; 1.243a–d, 1.244a–d; 1.245a–g, 1.246a–g) hold with $D=0$.* The particular integrals with $D=0$ agree with previous results for forcing by: (i) exponentials (1.241a, 1.242a) ≡ (1.126; 1.127a; 1.129a, b); (ii) hyperbolic cosines or sines (1.241b, c; 1.242b, c) ≡ (1.126; 1.146a, b; 1.147a, b); (iii) circular cosines and sines (1.243a, b; 1.244a, b) ≡ (1.126; 1.152; 1.153a, b) for complex and (1.245a, b; 1.246a, b) ≡ (1.126; 1.155b, c; 1.156a, b) for real coefficients and parameters; (iii) product of exponentials and hyperbolic cosines and sines, for example, with real coefficients and parameters (1.245a, f, g; 1.246f, g) ≡ (1.126; 1.185a, b; 1.186a, b). The preceding cases (i–v) concern non-resonant particular integrals; the resonant particular integrals were considered before (subsections 1.4.1–1.4.6) and can also be obtained by the method of the inverse characteristic polynomial (subsection 1.5.11).

1.5.11 Distinction between Resonant and Non-Resonant Cases

As a simple example of how the method of the inverse polynomial of derivatives distinguishes resonant from non-resonant cases, consider the linear second-order differential equation with constant coefficients forced by a sinusoid:

$$y'' + a^2 y = B\cos(bx) = \mathrm{Re}\left(Be^{ibx}\right). \tag{1.250}$$

The characteristic polynomial (1.251a) has simple roots $\pm ia$ in (1.251b):

$$P_2(D) = D^2 + a^2 = (D - ia)(D + ia), \quad P_2'(\pm ia) = \pm 2ia. \tag{1.251a, b}$$

The particular solution in the non-resonant case (1.252a) is (1.252b):

$$b \neq a: \qquad y_*(x) = \mathrm{Re}\left\{\frac{B}{P_2(D)} e^{ibx}\right\} = \mathrm{Re}\left\{\frac{e^{ibx}}{P_2(D+ib)} B\right\} = \mathrm{Re}\left\{\frac{e^{ibx}}{(D+ib)^2 + a^2} B\right\}$$

$$= \mathrm{Re}\left\{\frac{e^{ibx}}{a^2 - b^2 + 2ibD + D^2} B\right\} = \mathrm{Re}\left\{\left[\frac{e^{ibx}}{a^2 - b^2} + O(D)\right] B\right\}$$

$$= \mathrm{Re}\left\{\frac{Be^{ibx}}{a^2 - b^2}\right\} = \frac{B}{a^2 - b^2}\cos(bx), \tag{1.252a, b}$$

where since B is a constant it vanishes under differentiation.

The solution (1.252a, b) coincides (1.129a, b) with (1.253a, b):

$$b \neq a: \qquad y_*(x) = \mathrm{Re}\left\{\frac{B}{P_2(ib)} e^{ibx}\right\} = \mathrm{Re}\left\{\frac{Be^{ibx}}{a^2 - b^2}\right\} = \frac{B}{a^2 - b^2}\cos(bx). \tag{1.253a, b}$$

In the resonant case (1.254a) do not hold (1.252b) ≡ (1.253b), and the forced solution is given by (1.254b), using the method of the inverse characteristic polynomial of derivatives:

$$b = a: \qquad y_*(x) = \mathrm{Re}\left\{\frac{e^{ibx}}{D\,(2ib + D)} B\right\} = \mathrm{Re}\left\{\frac{e^{iax}}{2ia}\frac{1}{D}\left(1 + \frac{D}{2ia}\right)^{-1} B\right\}$$

$$= \mathrm{Re}\left\{\frac{e^{iax}}{2ia}\frac{1}{D}[1 + O(D)]B\right\} = \mathrm{Re}\left\{-\frac{iB}{2a} e^{iax} x\right\} = \frac{Bx}{2a}\sin(ax). \tag{1.254a, b}$$

The same result is obtained using (1.134a, b):

$$b \neq a: \qquad y_*(x) = \operatorname{Re}\left\{\frac{Bxe^{iax}}{P_2'(ia)}\right\} = Bx\operatorname{Re}\left\{\frac{e^{iax}}{2ia}\right\} = \frac{Bx}{2a}\sin(ax). \qquad (1.255\text{a, b})$$

It has been shown that *the solution of the linear second-order differential equation (1.250) with constant coefficients forced by a sinusoid can be obtained equivalently using the inverse (direct) characteristic polynomial both in the non-resonant (1.252a, b) [(1.253a, b)] and resonant (1.254a, b) [(1.255a, b)] cases.*

1.5.12 Zero as a Root of the Characteristic Polynomial

A power or polynomial forcing function does not lead to a resonant particular integral unless the characteristic polynomial has a root zero. The case of a characteristic polynomial with root zero can be simplified as follows: (i) if zero is a root of multiplicity M of the characteristic polynomial it must be of the form (1.256a, b) leading to the unforced differential equation (1.256c):

$$A_{N-M} \neq 0: \quad P_N(D) = D^M \sum_{n=0}^{N-M} A_n D^n, \quad \sum_{n=0}^{N-M} A_n \frac{d^{M+n}y}{dx^{M+n}} = 0; \qquad (1.256\text{a–c})$$

(ii) the change of dependent variable (1.257a) leads to a differential equation (1.257b) of order $N - M$:

$$z \equiv \frac{d^M y}{dx^M}: \qquad \sum_{n=0}^{N-M} A_n \frac{d^n z}{dx^n} = 0. \qquad (1.257\text{a, b})$$

Thus, an unforced linear differential equation with constant coefficients for which the characteristic polynomial (1.256a, b) has zero as a root of order M is the form (1.256c) reducible to a differential equation (1.257b) of degree N – M, whose N – M + 1 coefficients are arbitrary constants of integration. From the new dependent variable (1.257a), the original dependent variable is recovered by M integrations:

$$y(x) = \sum_{m=0}^{M-1} C_m x^m + \int^{x} d\xi_1 \int^{\xi_1} d\xi_2 \ldots \int^{\xi_{M-1}} z(\xi_M)\, d\xi_M, \qquad (1.257\text{c})$$

thus, adding a polynomial of degree M – 1. In the case of a forced equation, the additional M integrations specify the resonant terms (subsection 1.5.11).

For example, the linear differential equation with constant coefficients of order five (1.258a) has characteristic polynomial (1.258b) with zero as a triple root:

$$y^{\mathrm{v}} + a^2 y''' = 0: \qquad P_5(D) = D^3\left(D^2 + a^2\right) = D^3(D - ia)(D + ia). \tag{1.258a, b}$$

This implies that it is equivalent to a second-order differential equation (1.259b) for the variable (1.259a), whose general integral is (1.259c) where (C_1, C_2) are arbitrary constants:

$$z \equiv y''': \qquad z'' + a^2\, z = 0, \qquad z(x) = C_1 \cos(ax) + C_2 \sin(ax). \tag{1.259a–c}$$

Integrating (1.259c) three times leads to (1.260), where D_{1-5} are arbitrary constants, that is, the general integral of (1.258a):

$$y(x) = D_1 \cos(ax) + D_2 \sin(ax) + D_3 + D_4 x + D_5 x^2; \tag{1.260}$$

the general integral (1.260) of the differential equation (1.258a) can also be obtained from the characteristic polynomial (1.258b). Next is considered the case when the smooth function (1.240a) is a polynomial of degree S so that the series of derivatives terminates with the derivative of order S. This specifies particular integrals for a linear differential equation with constant coefficients forced by: (i) a power or polynomial (subsection 1.5.5); (ii) its product by an exponential (subsection 1.5.13); (iii) its product by a hyperbolic (circular) cosine or sine [subsection 1.5.14 (1.5.15)]; (iv) the product of a power by an exponential by a hyperbolic (circular) cosine or sine [subsection 1.5.16 (1.5.17)]; (v) the product of all four, that is power, exponential and hyperbolic, and circular cosines or sines (subsection 1.5.18).

1.5.13 Forcing by the Product of a Polynomial and Exponential

Since the principle of superposition holds for linear differential equations, it is sufficient to consider forcing by a term of the polynomial, that is, a power multiplied by an exponential, for example, (standard XV) forcing the differential equation (1.224c):

$$y'''' - 2y''' + 2y' - y = xe^x. \tag{1.261}$$

A corresponding (1.241a; 1.242a) particular integral is:

$$y_*(x) = \frac{1}{D^4 - 2D^3 + 2D - 1} x e^x = \frac{1}{(D-1)^3 (D+1)} x e^x$$

$$= e^x \frac{1}{D^3 (D+2)} x = \frac{e^x}{2} \frac{1}{D^3} \left(1 + \frac{D}{2}\right)^{-1} x = \frac{e^x}{2} \frac{1}{D^3} \left(1 - \frac{D}{2}\right) x \tag{1.262}$$

$$= \frac{e^x}{2} \frac{1}{D^3} \left(x - \frac{1}{2}\right) = \frac{e^x}{48} x^3 (x-2),$$

where it is sufficient to expand to $O(D)$ since higher-order derivatives vanish. The triple resonance is due to the characteristic polynomial having the triple root unity. The unforced differential equation (1.108b) has general integral (1.110b), including the linearly independent particular integrals $e^{\pm x}, xe^x$, and $x^2 e^x$. Thus, the forced equation (1.261) can have particular integrals involving higher powers of x, namely, the resonant solution:

$$y_*(x) = x^3 (\alpha + \beta x) e^x, \tag{1.263}$$

where the lowest power is $x^3 e^x$, corresponds to forcing by e^x, and the linear function $\alpha + \beta x$ corresponds to the factor x. Substitution of (1.263) in (1.261) determines the constants (α, β). The method of the inverse characteristic polynomial (1.262) yields the same result more simply.

1.5.14 Product of a Power by a Hyperbolic Cosine or Sine

The third-order differential equation (1.224b) is taken as example (standard XVI):

$$y''' - y'' + y' - y = 2x \sinh x = x\left(e^x - e^{-x}\right). \tag{1.264}$$

A particular integral (1.241c; 1.242c) is given by:

$$y_*(x) = \frac{1}{D^3 - D^2 + D - 1} \left[x\left(e^x - e^{-x}\right) \right]$$

$$= e^x \frac{1}{(D+1)^3 - (D+1)^2 + (D+1) - 1} x - e^{-x} \frac{1}{(D-1)^3 - (D-1)^2 + (D-1) - 1} x$$

$$= e^x \frac{1}{2D + 2D^2 + D^3} x - e^{-x} \frac{1}{-4 + 6D - 4D^2 + D^3} x$$

$$= \frac{e^x}{2D}\left[1 - D + O\left(D^2\right)\right]x + \frac{e^{-x}}{4}\left[1 + \frac{3D}{2} + O\left(D^2\right)\right]x$$

$$= \frac{e^x}{2}\left(\frac{x^2}{2} - x\right) + \frac{e^{-x}}{4}\left(x + \frac{3}{2}\right) \tag{1.265}$$

$$= \frac{1}{4}\left[\left(x^2 - x + \frac{3}{2}\right)\cosh x + \left(x^2 - 3x - \frac{3}{2}\right)\sinh x\right],$$

where $1/D$ corresponds to an integration (1.197b) and to a resonant term. The unforced differential equation (1.158) has (1.160a) linearly independent particular integrals e^{-x} and $e^{\pm ix}$; thus, the equation (1.264) forced by $xe^{\pm x}$ has for particular integral the solution (1.266):

$$y_*(x) = e^x\left(\alpha_1 + \alpha_2 x + \alpha_3 x^2\right) + e^{-x}\left(\beta_1 + \beta_2 x + \beta_3 x^2\right), \tag{1.266}$$

where the constants $\left(\alpha_1, \alpha_2, \alpha_3, \beta_1, \beta_2, \beta_3\right)$ may be determined substituting (1.266) in (1.264). The result (1.265) is obtained more simply using the inverse characteristic polynomial.

1.5.15 Product of a Power by a Circular Cosine or Sine

The forcing is applied (standard XVIII) to the second-order differential equation (1.224a):

$$y'' - 2y' + 2y = x\cos x = \operatorname{Re}\left(xe^{ix}\right), \tag{1.267}$$

a particular integral (1.243a; 1.244a) is:

$$y_*(x) = \operatorname{Re}\left(\frac{1}{D^2 - 2D + 2}xe^{ix}\right) = \operatorname{Re}\left(e^{ix}\frac{1}{(D+i)^2 - 2(D+i) + 2}x\right)$$

$$= \operatorname{Re}\left(e^{ix}\frac{1}{1 - 2i - 2(1-i)D + D^2}x\right) = \operatorname{Re}\left\{\frac{e^{ix}}{1-2i}\left[1 + \frac{2(1-i)}{1-2i}D + O\left(D^2\right)\right]x\right\}$$

$$= \operatorname{Re}\left\{\frac{1+2i}{5}e^{ix}\left[x + \frac{2(1-i)(1+2i)}{5}\right]\right\} = \frac{x}{5}(\cos x - 2\sin x) + \operatorname{Re}\left[\frac{2(1+7i)}{25}e^{ix}\right]$$

$$= x\frac{\cos x - 2\sin x}{5} + \frac{2\cos x - 14\sin x}{25}. \tag{1.268}$$

The unforced differential equation (1.178) has general integral (1.180c) with linearly independent particular integrals $e^x(\cos x, \sin x)$; these do not include the forcing term in (1.267), and thus, a particular integral is the non-resonant solution:

$$y_*(x) = (\alpha_1 + \beta_1 x)\cos x + (\alpha_2 + \beta_2 x)\sin x; \tag{1.269}$$

substitution of (1.269) in (1.267) specifies the constants $(\alpha_1, \alpha_2; \beta_1, \beta_2)$. The same result (1.268) is obtained more simply using the inverse characteristic polynomial.

1.5.16 Product of a Power by an Exponential and a Hyperbolic Function

The forcing (standard XVII) is applied to the same fourth-order differential equation (1.224c):

$$y'''' - 2y''' + 2y' - y = 2x^2 e^x \cosh x = x^2\left(e^{2x} - 1\right). \tag{1.270}$$

A particular integral (1.241d; 1.242d) is:

$$\begin{aligned}
y_*(x) &= \frac{1}{D^4 - 2D^3 + 2D - 1} x^2 \left(e^{2x} - 1\right) \\
&= e^{2x} \frac{1}{(D+2)^4 - 2(D+2)^3 + 2(D+2) - 1} x^2 - \frac{1}{D^4 - 2D^3 + 2D - 1} x^2 \\
&= e^{2x} \frac{1}{3 + 10D + 12D^2 + O\left(D^3\right)} x^2 + \frac{1}{1 - 2D + O\left(D^3\right)} x^2 \\
&= \frac{e^{2x}}{3} \frac{1}{1 + 10D/3 + 4D^2 + O\left(D^3\right)} x^2 + \left[1 + 2D + O\left(D^3\right)\right] x^2 \\
&= \frac{e^{2x}}{3}\left[1 - \left(\frac{10D}{3} + 4D^2\right) + \left(\frac{10D}{3} + 4D^2\right)^2 + O\left(D^3\right)\right] x^2 + x^2 + 4x \\
&= \frac{e^{2x}}{3}\left[1 - \frac{10}{3} D + \frac{64}{9} D^2 + O\left(D^3\right)\right] x^2 + x^2 + 4x \\
&= \frac{e^{2x}}{3}\left(x^2 - \frac{20}{3} x + \frac{128}{9}\right) + x(x+4),
\end{aligned} \tag{1.271}$$

where the expansions in powers of derivatives are quite different for the two terms on the RHS of (1.271). The unforced differential equation (1.108b) has general integral (1.110b), involving the linearly independent particular integrals e^{-x}, e^x, xe^x, and x^2e^x that do not appear in the forcing term in (1.270); thus, a particular integral of the forced equation (1.270) is the non-resonant solution:

$$y_*(x) = \alpha_1 x^2 + \beta_1 x + \gamma_1 + e^{2x}\left(\alpha_2 x^2 + \beta_2 x + \gamma_2\right); \tag{1.272}$$

the constants $(\alpha_1, \alpha_2, \beta_1, \beta_2, \gamma_1, \gamma_2)$ can be determined substituting (1.272) in (1.270). The same result is obtained more simply using the inverse characteristic polynomial (1.271).

1.5.17 Product of a Power by an Exponential by a Circular Function

The forcing (standard XIX) is applied to the third-order differential equation (1.224b):

$$y''' - y'' + y' - y = xe^x \cos x = \operatorname{Re}\left[xe^{(1+i)x}\right]. \tag{1.273}$$

A particular integral (1.245c; 1.246c) is:

$$\begin{aligned} y_*(x) &= \operatorname{Re}\left[\frac{1}{D^3 - D^2 + D - 1} xe^{(1+i)x}\right] \\ &= \operatorname{Re}\left[e^{(1+i)x} \frac{1}{(D+1+i)^3 - (D+1+i)^2 + D + i} x\right] \\ &= \operatorname{Re}\left[e^{(1+i)x} \frac{1}{i - 2 + (4i-1)D + O(D^2)} x\right] \\ &= -\operatorname{Re}\left\{\frac{e^{(1+i)x}}{2-i}\left[1 - \frac{1-4i}{2-i} D + O\left(D^2\right)\right] x\right\} \\ &= -\frac{e^x}{5} \operatorname{Re}\left\{\left[(2+i)\, x - \frac{19-8i}{5}\right] e^{ix}\right\} \\ &= \frac{e^x}{5}\left[x(\sin x - 2\cos x) + \frac{19\cos x + 8\sin x}{5}\right]. \end{aligned} \tag{1.274}$$

The unforced differential equation (1.158) has general integral (1.160b) involving the linearly independent particular integrals e^x, $\cos x$, and $\sin x$ that do not appear in the forcing term in (1.273). Thus, the forced differential equation has a particular integral in the non-resonant form (1.275):

$$y_*(x) = e^x\left[(\alpha_1 + \beta_1 x)\cos x + (\alpha_2 + \beta_2 x)\sin x\right]; \tag{1.275}$$

the constants $(\alpha_1, \alpha_2, \beta_1, \beta_2)$ can be determined substituting (1.275) in (1.273). The same solution (1.274) is obtained more simply using the inverse characteristic polynomial.

1.5.18 Product of a Power by an Exponential and Circular and Hyperbolic Functions

This forcing (standard XX) is applied to the second-order differential equation (1.224a):

$$y'' - 2y' + 2y = 2xe^{-x}\cos x \sinh(2x) = \text{Re}\left\{x\left[e^{(1+i)x} - e^{(i-3)x}\right]\right\}. \tag{1.276}$$

A particular integral (1.245f; 1.246f) is:

$$y_*(x) = \text{Re}\left\{\frac{1}{D^2 - 2D + 2}x\left[e^{(1+i)x} - e^{(i-3)x}\right]\right\}$$

$$= \text{Re}\left\{e^{(1+i)x}\frac{1}{(D+1+i)^2 - 2(D+1+i) + 2}x - e^{(i-3)x}\frac{1}{(D+i-3)^2 - 2(D+i-3) + 2}x\right\}$$

$$= \text{Re}\left\{e^{(1+i)x}\frac{1}{2iD + D^2}x - e^{(i-3)x}\frac{1}{16 - 8i + (2i-8)D + D^2}x\right\}$$

$$= \text{Re}\left\{\frac{e^{(1+i)x}}{2iD}\left(1 + \frac{D}{2i}\right)^{-1}x - \frac{e^{(i-3)x}}{8(2-i)}\left[1 - \frac{i-4}{4(2-i)}D + O\left(D^2\right)\right]x\right\}^{-1}$$

$$= \text{Re}\left\{\frac{e^{(1+i)x}}{2iD}\left[1 - \frac{D}{2i} + O\left(D^2\right)\right]x - \frac{e^{(i-3)x}}{40}(2+i)\left[1 + \frac{9+2i}{20}D + O\left(D^2\right)\right]x\right\}$$

$$= \text{Re}\left\{\frac{e^{(1+i)x}}{2i}\left(\frac{x^2}{2} - \frac{x}{2i}\right) - \frac{e^{(i-3)x}}{40}\left[(2+i)\,x + \frac{16+13i}{20}\right]\right\}$$

$$= \frac{xe^x}{4}(\cos x + x\sin x) - \frac{e^{-3x}}{40}\left[x(2\cos x - \sin x) + \frac{16\cos x - 13\sin x}{20}\right], \tag{1.277}$$

where the first (second) term on the RHS of (1.277) is resonant (non-resonant) because $1+i$ $(i-3)$ is (is not) a root of the characteristic polynomial (1.179c) of the differential operator in (1.178) and (1.276). The general integral (1.180c) of the unforced differential equation (1.178) involves the linearly independent particular integrals $e^{(1\pm i)x}$ of which one appears in the forcing term in (1.276). Thus, a particular integral of the forced differential equation (1.276) consists of a resonant (non-resonant) solution for the first (second) term:

$$\begin{aligned} y_*(x) = e^x x\left[\alpha_1 \cos x + \beta_1 \sin x + x(\alpha_2 \cos x + \beta_1 \sin x)\right] \\ + e^{-3x}\left[\alpha_3 \cos x + \beta_3 \sin x + x(\alpha_4 \cos x + \beta_4 \sin x)\right]; \end{aligned} \tag{1.278}$$

the constants $(\alpha_{1-4}, \beta_{1-4})$ may be determined by substitution of (1.278) in (1.276). The same solution (1.277) is obtained more simply using the inverse characteristic polynomial. In (1.252b; 1.254b; 1.262; 1.265; 1.268; 1.271; 1.274; 1.277) the inverse of the characteristic polynomial was expanded in powers of derivatives as in (1.222; 1.225a–c). As alternative procedure is: (i) to factorize the characteristic polynomial, leading to simple (1.54) [or multiple (1.98a, b) roots]; (ii) to decompose the inverse of the characteristic polynomial into partial fractions (1.203a–d) ≡ (1.204) [(1.209a–f)]; (iii) to use the inverse operators (1.199; 1.200), for example, (1.233a; 1.234a; 1.235a, b). The preceding examples (sections 1.3–1.5) are partially summarized next.

1.5.19 Forced Differential Equation with Constant Coefficients

The complete integral of a forced linear differential equation is (subsection 1.2.6), the sum of: (i) the general integral of the unforced equation; (ii) the sum of particular integrals for each forcing term. As examples are considered with parameters $(a=1, b=2, c=3)$ the following three linear differential equations with constant coefficients: (i) second-order (1.178; 1.180c) with forcings (1.178, 1.183b; 1.188, 1.191b; 1.224a, 1.225a; 1.267, 1.268; 1.276, 1.277):

$$\begin{aligned} y'' - 2y' + 2y = 2e^x \sin x + 2e^{2x} \sinh x \cos x + x^2 - x + 1 + x\cos x \\ + 2xe^{-x} \cos x \sinh(2x), \end{aligned} \tag{1.279}$$

$$\begin{aligned} y(x) = E e^x \cos(x-\gamma) - xe^x\left(\cos x + \frac{\sin x}{2}\right) \\ + \frac{e^{3x}}{8}(\sin x + \cos x) + \frac{x^2+x+1}{2} + x\frac{\cos x - 2\sin x}{5} + \frac{2\cos x - 14\sin x}{25} \\ + \frac{xe^x}{4}(\cos x + x\sin x) - \frac{e^{-3x}}{40}\left[x(2\cos x - \sin x) + \frac{16\cos x - 13\sin x}{20}\right], \end{aligned} \tag{1.280}$$

where (E, γ) are arbitrary constants; (ii) third-order (1.158; 1.160b) with forcings (1.158, 1.163b; 1.224b, 1.225b; 1.264, 1.265; 1.273, 1.274):

$$y''' - y'' + y' - y = 4\sin x + x^2 - x + 1 + 2x\sinh x + xe^x \cos x, \tag{1.281}$$

$$\begin{aligned} y(x) = {} & C_1 e^x + D_2 \cos x + D_3 \sin x + x(\cos x - \sin x) - x(1+x) \\ & + \frac{1}{4}\left[\left(x^2 - x + \frac{3}{2}\right)\cosh x + \left(x^2 - 3x - \frac{3}{2}\right)\sinh x\right] \\ & + \frac{e^x}{5}\left[x(\sin x - 2\cos x) + \frac{19\cos x + 8\sin x}{5}\right], \end{aligned} \tag{1.282}$$

where (C_1, D_2, D_3) are arbitrary constants; (iii) fourth-order (1.108b; 1.110c) with forcings (1.141, 1.143b; 1.149, 1.150b; 1.167, 1.171b; 1.224c, 1.225c; 1.261, 1.262; 1.270, 1.271):

$$\begin{aligned} y'''' - 2y''' + 2y' - y = {} & 2e^{2x} + 2\cosh(3x) + 2e^{2x}\cosh(3x) \\ & + x^2 - x + 1 + xe^x + 2x^2 e^x \cosh x, \end{aligned} \tag{1.283}$$

$$\begin{aligned} y(x) = {} & D_1 \cosh x + D_2 \sinh x + xe^x (C_3 + C_4 x) + \frac{2}{3}e^{2x} \\ & + \frac{5\cosh(3x) + 3\sinh(3x)}{128} + \frac{e^{5x}}{384} - \frac{xe^{-x}}{8} - x^2 - 3x - 7 \\ & + \frac{x^3 e^x}{48}(x-2) + \frac{e^{2x}}{3}\left(x^2 - \frac{20}{3}x + \frac{128}{9}\right) + x(x+4), \end{aligned} \tag{1.284}$$

where $(D_1, D_2 C_3, C_4)$ are arbitrary constants. The examples (1.279, 1.280; 1.281, 1.282; 1.283, 1.284) provide a sample of the methods used to solve forced linear differential equations with constant coefficients (sections 1.3–1.5) that have a characteristic polynomial. Additional cases are considered in the example 10.1. Similar methods apply to two other types of equations with a characteristic polynomial: (i) homogeneous linear differential equations (sections 1.6–1.8) where each derivative is multiplied by a power with the same exponent as the order of derivation; (ii) linear finite difference equations with constant coefficients (section 1.9).

1.6 Homogenous Linear Differential Equation with Power Coefficients (Euler, 1769)

A particular class of linear ordinary differential equations with variable coefficients (section 1.2) is the **Euler (1769)** type for which the n-th derivative of the dependent variable is multiplied by the n-th power of the independent variable; this may be designated the homogeneous linear differential equation (subsection 1.6.1) because it is unchanged when the independent variable is multiplied by a constant. The homogeneous can be transformed to a linear differential equation with constant coefficients via change of independent variable (subsection 1.6.2); the relation between the characteristic polynomial of the linear differential equations with constant (homogeneous) coefficients leads to a relation between ordinary (homogeneous) derivatives (subsection 1.6.5). Both for the linear differential equation with constant (homogeneous) coefficients the general integral in the unforced case is specified by the roots of the characteristic polynomial [section 1.4 (1.6)]; in the general integral are distinguished the cases of simple (multiple) roots [subsection 1.6.2 (1.6.3)]. The general integral of an unforced linear differential equation with homogeneous coefficients of arbitrary order (subsection 1.6.6) is illustrated by: (i) solutions of the centrally symmetric Laplace equation in N dimensions (subsection 1.6.7), including in particular the linear, logarithmic, and power-law potentials (subsection 1.6.8); (ii) examples of second (third) order equations [subsection 1.6.9 (1.6.10)].

1.6.1 Transformation into a Linear Equation with Constant Coefficients

The method of the characteristic polynomial can be used to solve not only (sections 1.3–1.5) the linear differential equation with constant coefficients (1.52a), but also an equation with power-type coefficients, namely the **Euler (1769) homogeneous linear equation**:

$$\sum_{n=0}^{N} A_n x^n \frac{d^n y}{dx^n} = B(x), \tag{1.285}$$

where the coefficient of the n-th order derivative is a power of exponent n multiplied by a constant. Thus, the linear homogeneous differential operator (1.286c) is unchanged by multiplication of the independent variable (1.286b) by a constant (1.286a):

$$\lambda \in |C: \qquad z = \lambda x: \qquad \sum_{n=0}^{N} A_n x^n \frac{d^n}{dx^n} = \sum_{n=0}^{N} A_n z^n \frac{d}{dz^n}. \tag{1.286a–c}$$

The homogeneous differential operator is linear (1.287a) ≡ (1.34b):

$$\sum_{n=0}^{N} A_n x^n \frac{d^n}{dy^n} = \sum_{n=0}^{N} A_n(x) \frac{d^n}{dy^n}, \qquad A_n(x) = A_n x^n, \qquad (1.287\text{a, b})$$

and has variable coefficients (1.287b) such that the operator is homogeneous (1.286a–c). Hence, it is distinct from the linear differential equation with constant coefficients (1.52a) that involves a polynomial of derivatives (1.52b). *Performing the change of variable:*

$$x = e^t, \qquad t = \log x, \qquad dx = e^t\, dt = x dt, \qquad \frac{d}{dx} = e^{-t} \frac{d}{dt}, \qquad (1.288\text{a–d})$$

the coefficients of (1.285) become constants:

$$\left\{ \sum_{n=0}^{N} A_n e^{nt} \left(e^{-t} \frac{d}{dt} \right)^n \right\} y\left(e^t\right) = B\left(e^t\right), \qquad (1.289)$$

and the Euler or homogeneous differential equation (1.285) transforms to a linear type with constant coefficients (1.289). The unforced linear differential equation with constant coefficients has particular integrals of the form (1.96a, b) ≡ (1.290a):

$$m = 1,\ldots,M: \qquad y_m\left(e^t\right) = t^{m-1} e^{at} = x^a \log^{m-1} x = y_m(x), \qquad (1.290\text{a, b})$$

that are exponentials (multiplied by powers) for simple $M = 1$ (multiple $M \geq 2$) roots of the characteristic polynomial; hence the unforced Euler or homogeneous equation has particular integrals (1.290a, b) that are powers (multiplied by logarithms). It is simpler to solve the linear differential equation with homogeneous coefficients (1.285) directly (subsection 1.6.2) rather than transforming (1.288a–d; 1.289) to constant coefficients; the transformation can be used to relate the ordinary and homogeneous derivatives (subsection 1.6.5).

1.6.2 Simple Roots of the Characteristic Polynomial

Considering the unforced Euler a homogeneous linear differential equation (1.285) ≡ (1.291a), it has power solutions (1.248b):

$$\sum_{n=0}^{N} A_n x^n \frac{d^n y}{dx^n} = 0, \qquad y(x) = x^a, \qquad (1.291\text{a, b})$$

whose exponent satisfy:

$$0 = x^a \left\{ \sum_{n=0}^{N} A_n a(a-1)...(a-n+1) \right\} \equiv x^a P_N(a), \qquad (1.292a)$$

where (2.192b) is the **characteristic polynomial** of degree N:

$$P_N(\delta) \equiv \sum_{n=0}^{N} A_n \delta(\delta-1)....(\delta-n+1) = \sum_{n=0}^{N} A_n \frac{\delta!}{(\delta-n)!}. \qquad (1.292b, c)$$

The factorials (2.292c) can be replaced by the **Pochhammer symbol** (I.29.79a, b) ≡ (2.293a) and the characteristic polynomial (1.292b), and becomes (2.293b):

$$(b)_n \equiv b(b+1)...(b+n-1): \qquad P_N(\delta) = \sum_{n=0}^{N} A_n (\delta-n+1)_n. \qquad (1.293a, b)$$

The (standard XXI) simple roots (1.294a) of the characteristic polynomial (1.282a):

$$P_N(\delta) = A_N \prod_{m=1}^{N} (\delta - a_m), \quad P_N(a_m) = 0 \neq P_N'(a_m), y_m(x) = x^{a_m}, \quad y(x) = \sum_{m=1}^{N} C_m x^{a_m}, \qquad (1.294a\text{–}d)$$

specify the particular integrals (1.294c); these are linearly independent (1.58a, b) because the roots that appear as exponents are distinct and their linear combination specifies the general integral (1.294d) of the homogeneous equation, involving N arbitrary constants of integration $C_1,...,C_N$.

1.6.3 Multiple Roots of the Characteristic Polynomial

If a is a root of multiplicity M (1.130a, b) ≡ (1.131a–c) ≡ (1.132a–c) if any of the three equivalent conditions (1.295a) ≡ (1.295b, c) ≡ (1.295d, e) hold:

$$P_N(\delta) \sim O\left((\delta-a)^M\right) \iff P_N(\delta) = (\delta-a) Q_{N-M}(\delta), \qquad Q_{N-M}(a) \neq 0$$
$$\iff P_N(a) = P_N'(a) = ... = P_N^{(M-1)}(a) = 0 \neq P_N^{(M)}(a). \qquad (1.295a\text{–}e)$$

In this case, the M particular integrals x^a would coincide in (1.294c), and the corresponding constants of integration would coalesce to one; thus, it is necessary to obtain new particular integrals as for the linear differential equation with constant coefficients. For the latter, the particular integrals (1.96a, b) for a root a of multiplicity M are obtained by parametric differentiation with regard to a up to $(M-1)-$ times of the integral for a single root; applying the same type of parametric differentiation to the particular integral x^a, leads to:

$$m = 1,\ldots,M: \qquad y_m(x) = \left(\frac{\partial}{\partial a}\right)^{m-1} x^a = x^a \log^{m-1} x, \tag{1.296a, b}$$

as particular integrals for roots of multiplicity M in agreement with (1.290a, b). In (1.296b), the definition of power with non-integral exponential (II.3.76a, b) ≡ (1.297a) was used:

$$x^a \equiv \exp\left[\log\left(x^a\right)\right] = \exp\left(a \log x\right), \tag{1.297a}$$

$$\frac{\partial}{\partial a}\left(x^a\right) = \left[\exp\left(a \log x\right)\right] \log x = x^a \log x, \tag{1.297b}$$

from which follows its derivative of first-order (1.297b) ≡ (II.3.79) and (1.296b) of higher order $n = m - 1$.

1.6.4 General Integral of the Homogenous Differential Equation

To a root a of multiplicity M of the homogeneous differential equation (1.291a) corresponds a set of terms:

$$y(x) = x^a \sum_{m=1}^{M} C_m \log^{m-1} x, \tag{1.298}$$

where $C_1,\ldots,C_M$ are arbitrary constants. It has been shown that *the unforced linear equation with power coefficients of Euler or homogeneous type (1.291a) has the characteristic polynomial (1.292a–c) ≡ (1.293a, b). If (standard XXI) all its roots are distinct (1.294a, b), they specify the exponents of the particular N linearly independent powers-type integrals (1.294c), and the general integral (1.294d) is a linear combination involving N arbitrary constants of integration* $C_1,\ldots,C_N$. *If (standard XXII)* a_m *is a root of multiplicity* α_m *of the characteristic polynomial (1.299a, b), the corresponding particular integrals (1.296a, b) lead to the terms (1.298) in the general integral (1.299c):*

$$\sum_{m=1}^{M} \alpha_m = M; \quad P_N(\delta) = A_N \prod_{m=1}^{N} (\delta - a_m)^{\alpha_m}: \quad y(x) = \sum_{m=1}^{M} x^{a_m} \sum_{\beta_m=1}^{\alpha_m} C_{m,\beta_m} \log^{\beta_m - 1} x. \tag{1.299a–c}$$

The general case (1.299a–c) includes (1.294a–c) for simple roots $\alpha_m = 1$ and $M = N$.

1.6.5 Relation between Ordinary and Homogenous Derivatives

The **homogeneous derivative** is defined by (1.300c), which is unchanged multiplying the variable (1.300b) by a constant (1.300a):

$$\lambda \in |R: \qquad z = \lambda x: \qquad \delta \equiv x\frac{d}{dz} = z\frac{d}{dz}. \tag{1.300a–c}$$

An ordinary (homogeneous) derivative applied to an exponential (power) is equivalent to multiplication by the coefficient (1.301a) [exponent (1.301b)]:

$$D\{e^{ax}\} \equiv \frac{d}{dx}(e^{ax}) = ae^{ax}, \qquad \delta(x^a) = x\frac{d}{dx}(x^a) = ax^a. \tag{1.301a, b}$$

A linear differential operator with constant (1.52a) [homogeneous (1.285)] coefficients involves a characteristic polynomial (1.52b) ≡ (1.302b) [(1.292b) ≡ (1.303b)] consisting of ordinary (1.53a) ≡ (1.302a) [homogeneous (1.300c) ≡ (1.303a)] derivatives:

$$D \equiv \frac{d}{dx}: \quad B(x) = \{P_N(D)\}y(x) = \sum_{n=0}^{N} A_n D^n y = \sum_{n=0}^{N} A_n \frac{d^n y}{dx^n}, \tag{1.302a, b}$$

$$\delta \equiv x\frac{d}{dx}: \quad B(x) = \{P_N(\delta)\}y(x) = \sum_{n=0}^{N} A_n x^n \frac{d^n y}{dx^n} = \sum_{n=0}^{N} A_n \delta(\delta - 1)\dots(\delta - n + 1)y. \tag{1.303a, b}$$

In (1.303b) appears the relation between ordinary and homogeneous derivatives of order M:

$$x^M \frac{d^M}{dx^M} = x\frac{d}{dx}\left(x\frac{d}{dx}-1\right)....\left(x\frac{d}{dx}-M+1\right), \tag{1.304}$$

that is proved next.

The proof of (1.304) is made by induction showing that: (i) it holds for $M = 2$; (ii) if it holds for M it also holds for $M+1$. Concerning (i) the identity (1.305a):

$$\delta^2 = xD(xD) = x^2D^2 + xD = x^2D^2 + \delta, \quad x^2D^2 = \delta^2 - \delta = \delta(\delta-1), \tag{1.305a, b}$$

corresponds (1.305b) to (1.304) with $M = 2$. Concerning (ii) consider:

$$\delta\left(x^M D^M\right) = xD\left(x^M D^M\right) = x^{M+1}D^{M+1} + Mx^M D^M; \tag{1.306a}$$

assuming that (1.304) holds it can be substituted in (1.306a) leading to:

$$x^{M+1}D^{M+1} = (\delta - M)\left(x^M D^M\right) = (\delta-M)(\delta-M+1)(\delta-M+2)...(\delta-2)(\delta-1)\delta, \tag{1.306b}$$

which coincides with (1.304) for $M+1$. QED. The solution (1.299a–c) of unforced linear homogeneous differential equation (1.291a) of arbitrary order N, with multiple roots (1.299a, b) is illustrated next by examples of the second (third) order [subsection 1.6.9 (1.6.10)] after considering pairs of real and distinct or complex conjugate roots of the characteristic polynomial (subsection 1.6.6) and solutions of the centrally symmetric Laplace equation (subsections 1.6.7–1.6.8).

1.6.6 Real Distinct and Complex Conjugate Roots

If the characteristic polynomial (1.292b, c) ≡ (1.293a, b) of the unforced linear homogeneous differential equation (1.291a) has two real distinct roots (1.307a), then the corresponding part of the general integral is (1.307b, c):

$$a_1 \equiv a \neq b \equiv a_2: \qquad y(x) = C_1 x^a + C_2^b = x^\alpha\left(C_1 x^\beta + C_2 x^{-\beta}\right), \tag{1.307a–c}$$

using (1.64a–d). The definition of power with arbitrary exponent is (I.5.28) ≡ (1.297a) leads to:

$$x^{\pm\beta} \equiv \exp\left[\log\left(x^{\pm\beta}\right)\right] = \exp(\pm\beta\log x) = \cosh(\beta\log x) \pm \sinh(\beta\log x). \tag{1.308}$$

Substituting (1.308) in (1.307b) gives the alternative forms:

$$y(x) = x^{(a+b)/2}\left[D_1\cosh\left(\frac{a-b}{2}\log x\right) + D_2\sinh\left(\frac{a-b}{2}\log x\right)\right]$$
$$= x^{(a+b)/2}E\cosh\left(\frac{a-b}{2}\log x + \gamma\right), \tag{1.309a, b}$$

using (1.68a–d; 1.69a–d). Thus, *a pair of real distinct roots (1.307a) of the characteristic polynomial (1.293a, b) ≡ (1.292b, c) of the linear homogenous differential equation (1.291a) corresponds (standard XXIII) in the general integral to (1.307c) ≡ (1.309a) ≡ (1.309b) with the pairs of arbitrary constants* $(C_1, C_2), (D_1, D_2)$ *and* (E, γ) *related by (1.68a–d;1.69a–d;1.70a–d).*

If the unforced linear homogeneous differential equation (1.291a) has real coefficients, so does its characteristic polynomial (1.293a, b), and any complex roots must appear as complex conjugate pairs (1.310a) leading to the contribution (1.310b) to the general integral:

$$a_{1,2} = \alpha \pm i\beta: \qquad y(x) = C_1 x^{\alpha_1} + C_2 x^{a_2} = x^{\alpha}\left(C_1 x^{i\beta} + C_2 x^{-i\beta}\right). \tag{1.310a, b}$$

Using (I.1.24) ≡ (1.311):

$$x^{\pm i\beta} \equiv \exp\left[\log\left(x^{\pm i\beta}\right)\right] = \exp(\pm i\beta\log x) = \cos(\beta\log x) \pm i\sin(\beta\log x), \tag{1.311}$$

in (1.310b) leads to:

$$y(x) = x^{\alpha}\left[D_1\cos(\beta\log x) + D_2\sin(\beta\log x)\right] = x^{\alpha}E\cos(\beta\log x - \gamma), \tag{1.312a, b}$$

using (1.77a–d; 1.78a–d). Thus, *a pair of complex conjugate roots (1.310a) of the characteristic polynomial (1.292b, c) ≡ (1.293a, b) of the unforced linear homogeneous differential equation (1.291a) corresponds (standard XXIV) in the general integral specified by (1.310b) ≡ (1.312a) ≡ (1.312b) where the three pairs of arbitrary constants of integration are related by (1.77a–d; 1.78a–d; 1.81a, b; 1.82a, b).* The isotropic Laplace equation in any dimension (section III.9.2) and the multi-harmonic operators (section III.4.6) lead to linear homogeneous differential equations, as shown next (subsections 1.6.7–1.6.8).

1.6.7 Isotropic Multidimensional Laplace Equation

The hyperspherical Laplace equation (III.9.35b) ≡ (1.313b) depending only on the radial distance in N-dimensions is (III.9.35a) ≡ (I.313a):

$$R \equiv \left| \sum_{n=1}^{N} (x_n)^2 \right|^{1/2} : \quad 0 = \nabla^2 \Phi_N = \frac{1}{R^{N-1}} \frac{d}{dR}\left(R^{N-1} \frac{d\Phi_N}{dR} \right) = \frac{d\Phi_N}{dR} + \frac{N-1}{R} \frac{d\Phi_N}{dR}, \tag{1.313a, b}$$

and the general case in hyperspherical coordinates (8.375b) will be considered subsequently (notes 8.6–8.17). The radially symmetric (1.313a) case (1.313b) leads to a linear homogeneous differential equation of the second-order (1.314a) with characteristic polynomial (1.314b) of the second degree:

$$0 = R^2 \Phi_N'' + (N-1) R \Phi_N' : \quad P_2(\delta) = \delta(\delta - 1) + (N-1)\delta = \delta(\delta + N - 2). \tag{1.314a, b}$$

It has a double root zero (1.315b) in the plane case (1.315a) leading to the **logarithmic potential** (1.315d) ≡ (I.18.25c) for the two-dimensional Laplace equation (1.315c):

$$N = 2: \quad P_2(\delta) = \delta^2, 0 = \frac{1}{R} \frac{d}{dR}\left(R \frac{d\Phi_2}{dR} \right) = \frac{d^2\Phi_2}{dR^2} + \frac{1}{R} \frac{d\Phi_2}{dR}, \Phi_2(R) = C_- + C_+ \log R; \tag{1.315a–d}$$

in all other dimensions (1.316a) the roots are distinct (1.316b, c) and the **hyperspherical potential** (1.316d) ≡ (III.9.43c):

$$N \neq 2: \quad \delta_1 = 0, \quad \delta_2 = 2 - N: \qquad \Phi_N(R) = C_- + C_+ R^{2-N}, \tag{1.316a–d}$$

involves besides a constant and inverse power of the radius with exponent $N - 2$.

1.6.8 Linear, Logarithmic, and Power-Law Potentials

The general case (1.316a–d) includes the cases (1.317a) [(1.318a)] specifying the **linear (spherical) potential** (1.317a) ≡ (III.9.85b) [(1.318c) ≡ (III.9.101b), which satisfies the one (three)-dimensional Laplace equation (1.317b) [(1.318b)]:

$$N = 1: \qquad 0 = \frac{d^2\Phi_1}{dR^2}, \qquad \Phi_1(R) = C_- + C_+ R, \tag{1.317a–c}$$

$$N = 3: \quad 0 = \frac{1}{R^2}\frac{d}{dR}\left(R^2\frac{d\Phi_3}{dR^2}\right) = \frac{d^2\Phi_3}{dR^2} + \frac{2}{R}\frac{d\Phi_3}{dR}, \qquad \Phi_3(R) = C_- + \frac{C_+}{R}. \tag{1.318a–c}$$

The general (1.316a–d) [two-dimensional (1.315a–d)] case can be obtained from (1.313b) by direct integration (1.319a–c) [(1.320a–c)]:

$$N \neq 2: \quad R^{N-1}\frac{d\Phi_N}{dR} = (2-N)C_+, \qquad \Phi_N(R) = C_- + C_+R^{2-N}, \tag{1.319a–c}$$

$$N = 2: \quad R\frac{d\Phi_2}{dR} = C_+, \qquad \Phi_2(R) = C_- + C_+\log R. \tag{1.320a–c}$$

It has been shown that *the multidimensional Laplace equation (1.313b) has for isotropic solution (1.313a) the hyperspherical potential (1.316d) ≡ (1.319c), except in two dimensions (1.315a) ≡ (1.320a) when the logarithmic potential (1.315c) ≡ (1.320c) is the solution of the cylindrical Laplace equation (1.315c). The particular cases include the linear (1.317c) [spherical (1.318c)] potential for the Laplace equation in one (1.317b) [three 1.318b)] dimension(s).*

1.6.9 A Second-Order Linear Homogeneous Differential Equation

Considering, for example, (1.321a):

$$x^2y'' \pm xy' + y = 0, \qquad P_2^{\pm}(\delta) = \delta(\delta-1) \pm \delta + 1, \tag{1.321a, b}$$

which has characteristic polynomial (1.321b). In the case of the lower sign, there is a double root $a = 1$ in (1.322a):

$$P_2^{-}(\delta) = \delta^2 - 2\delta + 1 = (\delta-1)^2: \qquad y_+(x) = x(C_1 + C_2\log x), \tag{1.322a, b}$$

and the general integral is (1.322b); in the case of the upper sign, there are a pair of complex conjugate roots $\pm i$ in (1.323a):

$$P_2^{+}(\delta) = \delta^2 + 1 = (\delta - i)(\delta + i): \qquad y_+(x) = C_1x^i + C_2x^{-i}, \tag{1.323a, b}$$

and the general integral is (1.323b), which can be written in the alternative forms:

$$y_-(x) = D_1\cos(\log x) + D_2\sin(\log x) = E\cos(\log x - \gamma), \tag{1.323c, d}$$

with the arbitrary constants of integration related by (1.77a–d; 1.78a–d; 1.81a, b; 1.82a, b)).

1.6.10 Third-Order Linear Homogeneous Differential Equation

Considering, for example:

$$x^3y''' + 2x^2y'' \pm xy' \mp y = 0, \tag{1.324}$$

the corresponding characteristic polynomial is:

$$P_3^{\pm}(\delta) = \delta(\delta-1)(\delta-2) + 2\delta(\delta-1) \pm \delta \mp 1 = \delta^2(\delta-1) \pm (\delta-1) = (\delta-1)(\delta^2 \pm 1). \tag{1.325}$$

The lower sign leads to a single plus a double root of the characteristic polynomial (1.326a), corresponding to the general integral (1.326b):

$$P_3^{-}(\delta) = (\delta-1)^2(\delta+1): \qquad y_-(x) = x(C_1 + C_2 \log x) + \frac{C_3}{x}; \tag{1.326a, b}$$

the upper sign leads to one real and two complex imaginary roots of the characteristic polynomial (1.327a):

$$P_3^{+}(\delta) = (\delta-1)(\delta-i)(\delta+i): \qquad y_+(x) = Cx + E\cos(\log x - \gamma), \tag{1.327a, b}$$

and the general integral (1.327b) where (C, E, γ) are arbitrary constants.

1.7 Homogeneous Derivatives and Characteristic Polynomial

Similar methods apply to the solution of the linear ordinary differential equation with constant (homogeneous) coefficients, both for: (i) the general integral in the unforced case [section 1.3 (1.6)]; (ii) the complete integral in the forced case using either the characteristic polynomial [section 1.4 (1.7)] or its inverse [section 1.5 (1.8)]. The ordinary (homogeneous) derivatives lead to a general integral of the unforced equation involving exponentials/powers/circular-hyperbolic cosines-sines (powers/logarithms/circular-hyperbolic cosines-sines of logarithms). This applies also to the particular integral of the linear ordinary differential equation with homogeneous coefficients when the forcing term (section 1.7) is: (i) a power (subsection 1.7.1); (ii, iii) the hyperbolic (circular) cosine or sine of a logarithm [subsection 1.7.2 (1.7.3)]; (iv, v) the product of a power by a hyperbolic (circular) cosine or sine of a logarithm [subsection 1.7.4 (1.7.5)]; (v, vi) the triple product of a power times a hyperbolic times a circular cosine or sine of a logarithm (subsection 1.7.6).

1.7.1 Homogeneous Differential Equation Forced by a Power

The methods of solution are similar for the linear differential equation with constant (1.52a) [homogeneous (1.285)] coefficients replacing (1.288a–d) exponential (powers) and powers (logarithms) as in (1.290a, b) for particular integrals of the unforced equation, and also for particular integrals of the forced equation. For example, the analogues of (1.126; 1.127a; 1.129a, b; 1.134a, b) are: *a particular integral of the homogeneous linear differential equation (1.285), with (standard XXV) power-type forcing term (1.328b):*

$$P_N(b) \neq 0: \qquad B(x) = Bx^b, \qquad y_*(x) = B\frac{x^b}{P_N(b)}, \tag{1.328a–c}$$

is the same power (1.328c) divided by the characteristic polynomial (1.293a, b), if b is not a root (1.328a); if b is a root of multiplicity M in (1.329a) the particular integral (1.329b) involves the M-th power of the logarithm:

$$P_N(\delta) \sim O\left((\delta - b)^M\right): \qquad y_*(x) = B\frac{x^b \log^M x}{P_N^{(M)}(b)}. \tag{1.329a, b}$$

The proof of the preceding results follows by substitution of (1.330b) in (1.285; 1.328b) ≡ (1.330a) leading to (1.330c):

$$\{P_N(\delta)\}y(x) = Be^b, \quad y(x) = Cx^b: \quad Cx^b = \{P_N(\delta)\}Be^b = BP_N(b)x^b, \tag{1.330a–c}$$

to two cases: (i) if b is not a root of the characteristic polynomial (1.328a), then division by the characteristic polynomial in (1.330c) is permissible leading to (1.328c); (ii) if b is a root of multiplicity M of the characteristic polynomial (1.329a), then the *L'Hospital* rule (as in subsection 1.4.2) of differentiation M times with regard to b in the numerator and denominator of (1.328c) leads to:

$$y_*(x) = \frac{(\partial/\partial b)^M x^b}{(\partial/\partial b)^M P_N(b)} = \frac{x^b \log^M x}{P_N^{(M)}(b)}, \tag{1.331}$$

that coincides with (1.329b) ≡ (1.331).

Considering, for example, the linear second-order homogeneous differential equation (1.321a) ≡ (1.332a) with upper sign (1.321b) ≡ (1.332b) forced by a power:

$$x^2y'' + xy' + y = 2x^b, \quad P_2(\delta) = \delta^2 + 1, \quad P_2(\pm i) = 0 \neq \pm 2i = P_2'(\pm i), \tag{1.332a–c}$$

the characteristic polynomial (1.332b) has two single roots (1.332c). The particular integral of (1.332a) is (1.333b) in the non-resonant case (1.333a):

$$b \neq \pm i: \qquad y_*(x) = \frac{2x^b}{P_2(b)} = \frac{2x^b}{1+b^2}; \tag{1.333a, b}$$

$$b = \pm i: \quad y_*(x) = \frac{2x^{\pm i}\log x}{P_2'(\pm i)} = \mp i x^{\pm i}\log x = \log x\left\{\sin(\log x) \mp i\cos(\log x)\right\}. \tag{1.334a, b}$$

in the resonant case (1.334a) the particular integral is (1.334b).

1.7.2 Forcing by a Hyperbolic Cosine or Sine of a Logarithm

The principle of superposition applied to (1.328a–c; 1.329a, b) specifies *a particular integral of a linear homogeneous differential equation (1.285) forced (standard XXVI) by the hyperbolic cosine or sine of a logarithm*:

$$B(x) = B\cosh,\sinh(c\log x) = \frac{B}{2}\left(x^c \pm x^{-c}\right), \tag{1.335}$$

(i) in the non-resonant case (1.336b) when $\pm c$ *is not a root of the characteristic polynomial (1.336a)*:

$$P_N(\pm c) \neq 0: \qquad y_*(x) = \frac{B}{2}\left[\frac{x^c}{P_N(c)} \pm \frac{x^{-c}}{P_N(-c)}\right]; \tag{1.336a, b}$$

(ii) in the resonant case (1.337c) when $+c(-c)$ *is a root of multiplicity* $M(S)$ *of the characteristic polynomial (1.337a) [(1.337b)]*:

$$O\left((\delta-c)^M\right) \sim P_N(\delta) \sim O\left((\delta+c)^S\right): \quad y_*(x) = \frac{B}{2}\left[\frac{x^c \log^M x}{P_N^{(M)}(c)} \pm \frac{x^{-c}\log^S x}{P_N^{(S)}(-c)}\right]. \tag{1.337a–c}$$

For $M = 0 = S$ then (1.337a–c) simplifies to (1.336a, b).

As an example, consider the third-order linear homogeneous differential equation (1.324) ≡ (1.338) with the lower sign (1.326a) forced by the hyperbolic sine of a logarithm:

$$x^3y''' + 2\,x^2y'' - xy' + y = 2\sinh(c\log x) = x^c - x^{-c}; \tag{1.338}$$

the resonant case (1.326a) is $c = \pm 1$. Excluding this (1.339a), a non-resonant particular integral is (1.339b):

$$c \neq \pm 1: \qquad y_*(x) = \frac{x^c}{P_3(c)} - \frac{x^{-c}}{P_3(-c)} = \frac{1}{c^2-1}\left(\frac{x^c}{c-1} + \frac{x^{-c}}{c+1}\right)$$

$$= \frac{(c+1)x^c + (c-1)x^{-c}}{(c^2-1)^2} = \frac{2c\cosh(c\log x) + 2\sinh(c\log x)}{(c^2-1)^2}; \qquad \text{(1.339a, b)}$$

the resonant case (1.340a) involves a single and a double root of the characteristic polynomial:

$$c = \pm 1: \qquad y_*(x) = \pm\left[\frac{x\log^2 x}{P_3''(1)} - \frac{x^{-1}\log x}{P_3'(-1)}\right] = \pm\frac{\log x}{4}\left(x\log x - \frac{1}{x}\right), \qquad \text{(1.340a, b)}$$

leading to the particular integral (1.340b), since $-1(+1)$ is a simple (1.341d) [double (1.341e)] root:

$$P_3(\delta) = \delta^3 - \delta^2 - \delta + 1: \qquad P_3'(\delta) = 3\delta^2 - 2\delta - 1, \qquad P_3''(\delta) = 6\delta - 2, \qquad \text{(1.341a–c)}$$

$$P_3(-1) = 0 \neq 4 = P_3'(-1), \qquad P_3(1) = P_3'(1) = 0 \neq 4 = P_3''(1), \qquad \text{(1.341d, e)}$$

of the characteristic polynomial (1.326a) ≡ (1.341a), which has first (second) order derivative (1.341b) [(1.341c)].

1.7.3 Forcing by the Circular Cosine or Sine of a Logarithm

The forcing (standard XXVII) by a circular cosine or sine of a logarithm (1.342) of a linear homogeneous differential equation (1.285):

$$B(x) = B\cos,\sin(a\log x) = \frac{B}{\{2, 2i\}}\left(x^{ia} \pm x^{-ia}\right), \qquad \text{(1.342)}$$

leads to the particular integral; (i) in the non-resonant case:

$$P_N(\pm ia) \neq 0: \qquad y_*(x) = \frac{B}{\{2, 2i\}}\left[\frac{x^{ia}}{P_N(ia)} \pm \frac{x^{-ia}}{P_N(-ia)}\right]; \qquad \text{(1.343a, b)}$$

(ii) in the resonant case:

$$O\left(\left(\delta - ia\right)^M\right) \sim P_N(\delta) \sim O\left(\left(\delta + ia\right)^S\right): \quad y_*(x) = \frac{B}{\{2, 2i\}}\left[\frac{x^{ia}\log^M x}{P_N^{(M)}(ia)} \pm \frac{x^{-ia}\log^S x}{P_N^{(S)}(-ia)}\right]. \tag{1.344a–c}$$

In (1.343a, b; 1.344a–c) the parameter c and the coefficients $(A_1,\ldots,A_N)$ *of the linear homogeneous differential operator (1.293a, b) may be complex.*

If they are real (1.345a):

$$a, A_0,\ldots,A_N \in |R: \qquad B(x) = B\,\mathrm{Re},\mathrm{Im}\left(x^{ia}\right), \tag{1.346a, b}$$

then the forcing term simplifies to (1.345b) and a particular integral is:

$$P_N(ia) \neq 0: \qquad y_*(x) = \frac{B}{2}\mathrm{Re},\mathrm{Im}\left[\frac{x^{ia}}{P_N(ia)}\right], \tag{1.346a, b}$$

(i) in the non-resonant case (1.346a, b), and:

$$P_N(\delta) \sim O\left(\left(\delta - ia\right)^M\right): \qquad y_*(x) = \frac{B}{2}\log^M x\,\mathrm{Re},\mathrm{Im}\left[\frac{x^{ia}}{P_N^{(M)}(ia)}\right], \tag{1.347a, b}$$

(ii) in the resonant case (1.347a, b).

As an example, consider the linear homogeneous third-order differential equation (1.324) ≡ (1.348) with the upper sign (1.327a) forced by the circular cosine of a logarithm:

$$x^3 y''' + 2x^2 y'' + xy' - y = 2\cos\left(a\log x\right) = 2\,\mathrm{Re}\left(x^{ia}\right), \tag{1.348}$$

whose characteristic polynomial (1.327a) ≡ (1.349a) has derivative (1.349b) confirming (1.349c, d) that all roots are simple:

$$P_3(\delta) = (\delta - 1)\left(\delta^2 + 1\right) = \delta^3 - \delta^2 + \delta - 1, \qquad P_3'(\delta) = 3\delta^2 - 2\delta + 1, \tag{1.349a, b}$$

$$P_3(1) = 0 \neq 2 = P_3'(1), \qquad P_3(\pm i) = 0 \neq -2 \mp 2i = P_3'(\pm i). \tag{1.349c, d}$$

For real a, the possible (1.349e) resonant cases are (1.349f) corresponding to the forcing (1.349g):

$$ia = 1, \pm i \;\Rightarrow\; a = \pm 1: \qquad \mathrm{Re}\left(x^{\pm i}\right) = \cos\left(\log x\right). \tag{1.349e–g}$$

There are two possible cases: (i) non-resonant (1.350 a, b) leading to (1.350c):

$$a \neq \pm 1, \quad ia \neq \pm i: \quad y_*(x) = 2\,\mathrm{Re}\left\{\frac{x^{ia}}{P_3(ia)}\right\} = \frac{2}{a^2-1}\mathrm{Re}\left(\frac{x^{ia}}{1-ia}\right)$$

$$= \frac{2}{a^2-1}\mathrm{Re}\left(\frac{1+ia}{a^2+1}x^{ia}\right) = \frac{2}{a^4-1}[\cos(a\log x) - a\sin(a\log x)]; \tag{1.350a–c}$$

(ii) the single resonant cases (1.351a, b) leading to (1.351c):

$$a = \pm 1, \quad ia = \pm i: \quad y_*(x) = 2\log x\,\mathrm{Re}\left\{\frac{x^{\pm i}}{P_3'(\pm i)}\right\} = -\log x\,\mathrm{Re}\left(\frac{x^{\pm i}}{1\pm i}\right)$$

$$= -\log x\,\mathrm{Re}\left(\frac{1\mp i}{2}x^{\pm i}\right) = -\frac{\log x}{2}\left[\cos(\log x) + \sin(\log x)\right], \tag{1.351a–c}$$

corresponding to the forcing (1.349g).

1.7.4 Product of a Power and a Hyperbolic Function of a Logarithm

A particular integral of the linear homogeneous differential equation (1.285) forced (standard XXVIII) by the product of a power by the hyperbolic cosine or sine of a logarithm:

$$B(x) = Bx^b \cosh,\sinh\left(c\log x\right) = \frac{B}{2}\frac{x^{b+c} \pm x^{b-c}}{2}, \tag{1.352}$$

is given by:

$$P_N(b\pm c) \neq 0: \qquad y_*(x) = \frac{B}{2}\left[\frac{x^{b+c}}{P_N(b+c)} \pm \frac{x^{b-c}}{P_N(b-c)}\right], \tag{1.353a, b}$$

(i) in the non-resonant case (1.353a, b), and:

$$O\left((\delta-b-c)^M\right) \sim P_N(\delta) \sim O\left((\delta-b+c)^S\right): \quad y_*(x) = \frac{B}{2}\left[\frac{x^{b+c}\log^M x}{P_N^{(M)}(b+c)} \pm \frac{x^{b-c}\log^S x}{P_N^{(S)}(b-c)}\right], \tag{1.354a, b}$$

(ii) in the resonant case (1.354a, b).

As an example is the linear second-order homogeneous differential equation (1.321a) ≡ (1.355) with the lower sign (1.322a) forced by the product of a power by a hyperbolic cosine of a logarithm:

$$x^3 y'' - x\, y' + y = 2x^2 \cosh\left(c \log x\right) = x^{2+c} + x^{2-c}. \tag{1.355}$$

The roots of the characteristic polynomial (1.322a) are (1.356a) and lead to the resonant case (1.356b):

$$2 \pm c = 1 \qquad \Rightarrow \qquad c = \pm 1. \tag{1.356a, b}$$

The particular integral is (1.357b):

$$\begin{aligned} c \neq \pm 1: \qquad y_*(x) &= \frac{x^{2+c}}{P_2(2+c)} + \frac{x^{2-c}}{P_2(2-c)} \\ &= \frac{x^{2+c}}{(c+1)^2} + \frac{x^{2-c}}{(c-1)^2} \\ &= x^2 \frac{(c-1)^2 x^c + (c+1)^2 x^{-c}}{(c^2-1)^2} \\ &= \frac{2\, x^2}{(c^2-1)^2}\left[\left(c^2+1\right)\cosh(c \log x) - 2c \sinh(c \log x)\right], \end{aligned} \tag{1.357a, b}$$

(i) in the non-resonant case (1.357a), and (1.358b):

$$c = \pm 1: \qquad y_*(x) = \frac{x^3}{P_2(3)} + \frac{x \log^2 x}{P_2''(1)} = \frac{x}{2}\left(\frac{x^2}{2} + \log^2 x\right), \tag{1.358a, b}$$

(ii) in the resonant case (1.358a), since 3(1) is not a root (1.359d) [is a double root (1.358e)]:

$$\begin{gathered} P_2(\delta) = \delta^2 - 2\delta + 1, \quad P_2'(\delta) = 2\delta - 2, \quad P_2''(\delta) = 2: \\ P_2(3) = 4, P_2(1) = P_2'(1) = 0 \neq 2 = P_2''(1), \end{gathered} \tag{1.359a–e}$$

of the characteristic polynomial (1.322a) ≡ (1.359a) with first (second) derivative (1.359b) [(1.359c)].

1.7.5 Product of a Power and Circular Functions of a Logarithm

Applying (1.328a–c; 1.329a–c) to:

$$B(x) = Bx^b \cos, \sin(a \log x) = \frac{B}{\{2, 2i\}}\left(x^{b+ia} \pm x^{b-ia}\right), \tag{1.360}$$

it follows that *a particular integral of the linear homogeneous differential equation (1.285) forced (standard XXIX) by the product of a power by a circular cosine or sine of a logarithm has a particular integral specified: (i) by (1.361b) in the non-resonant case (1.361a):*

$$P_N(b \pm ia) \neq 0: \qquad y_*(x) = \frac{B}{\{2, 2i\}}\left[\frac{x^{b+ia}}{P_N(b+ia)} \pm \frac{x^{b-ia}}{P_N(b-ia)}\right]; \tag{1.361a, b}$$

(ii) by (1.362c) in the resonant case (1.360a, b):

$$O\left((\delta - b - ia)^M\right) \sim P_N(\delta) \sim O\left((\delta - b + ia)^S\right):$$

$$y_*(x) = \frac{B}{\{2, 2i\}}\left[\frac{x^{b+ia} \log^M x}{P_N^{(M)}(b+ia)} \pm \frac{x^{b-ia} \log^S x}{P_N^{(S)}(b-ia)}\right]. \tag{1.362a–c}$$

In (1.360; 1.361a, b; 1.362a–c), the parameters (a, b) and the coefficients $(A_1, \ldots, A_N)$ of the linear homogeneous differential operator (1.293a, b) may be complex.

If they are all real (1.363a) the forcing term (1.363b):

$$a, b, A_0, \ldots, A_N: \ \in |R: \quad B(x) = Bx^b \cos, \sin(a \log x) = B \operatorname{Re}, \operatorname{Im}\left(x^{b+ia}\right), \tag{1.363a, b}$$

simplifies the particular integral: (i) to (1.364b) in the non-resonant case (1.364a):

$$P_N(b+ia) \neq 0: \qquad y_*(x) = B \operatorname{Re}, \operatorname{Im}\left[\frac{x^{b+ia}}{P_N(b+ia)}\right]; \tag{1.364a, b}$$

(ii) to (1.365b) in the resonant case (1.365a):

$$P_N(\delta) \sim O\left((\delta - b - ia)^M\right): \qquad y_*(x) = B \log^M x \operatorname{Re}, \operatorname{Im}\left[\frac{x^{b+ia}}{P_N^{(M)}(b+ia)}\right]. \tag{1.365a, b}$$

The particular integral (1.361a, b) [(1.362a–c)] for general, complex characteristic polynomial and coefficients, is a superposition of power solutions (1.328a–c) [(1.329a–c)] in the non-resonant (resonant) case; in the case of real characteristic polynomial and coefficients the complex roots always appear as conjugate pairs $b \pm ia$, and using $P(a - ia) = P^*(b + ia)$, where * denotes complex conjugate, the particular integral (1.361a, b) [(1.362a–c)] simplifies to (1.364a, b) [(1.365a, b)].

As an example, consider the linear second-order homogeneous differential equation (1.366) forced by the product of a power and the sine of a logarithm:

$$x^2 y'' - xy' + 2y = 2x \sin(a \log x) = 2\operatorname{Im}\left(x^{1+ia}\right). \tag{1.366}$$

The characteristic polynomial is (1.367):

$$P_2(\delta) = \delta(\delta - 1) - \delta + 2 = \delta^2 - 2\delta + 2 = (\delta - 1)^2 + 1 = (\delta - 1 - i)(\delta - 1 + i), \tag{1.367}$$

and has (1.368a–c) simple roots $1 \pm i$:

$$P_2'(\delta) = 2\delta - 2: \qquad P_2(1 \pm i) = 0 \neq \pm 2i = P_2'(1 \pm i). \tag{1.368a–c}$$

The general integral of the unforced equation is:

$$y(x) = x\left[C_1 \cos(\log x) + C_2 \sin(\log x)\right], \tag{1.369}$$

where C_1, C_2 are arbitrary constants.

A resonance can occur if the exponent in (1.366) equals one of the roots of the characteristic polynomial (1.368a, b), corresponding (1.370a) to the values (1.370b) of a:

$$1 + ia = 1 \pm i \qquad \Rightarrow \qquad a = \pm 1. \tag{1.370a, b}$$

(i) in the non-resonant case (1.371a), the particular integral is (1.371b):

$$a \neq \pm 1: \quad y_*(x) = 2\operatorname{Im}\left[\frac{x^{1+ia}}{P_2(1+ia)}\right] = 2x \operatorname{Im}\left[\frac{x^{ia}}{i(a-1)i(a+1)}\right] = \frac{2x}{1-a^2}\sin(a \log x); \tag{1.371a, b}$$

(ii) in the resonant case (1.372a), the particular integral is (1.372b):

$$a = \pm 1: \qquad y_*(x) = 2\,\mathrm{Im}\left[\frac{x^{1\pm i}\log x}{P_2'(1\pm i)}\right] = 2x\log x\,\mathrm{Im}\left(\frac{x^{\pm i}}{\pm 2i}\right)$$
$$= x\log x\,\mathrm{Im}\left(\mp i x^{\pm i}\right) = \mp x\log x\cos(\log x). \tag{1.372a, b}$$

Next (subsection 1.7.6) is considered forcing by the product of all three factors, namely the power (1.328b), the hyperbolic (1.352), and the circular (1.360) cosine or sine of a logarithm.

1.7.6 Product of a Power by Hyperbolic and Circular Functions of a Logarithm

The forcing by the product of a power by a hyperbolic and a circular cosine or sine of a logarithm (1.373b):

$$a, b, c, A_0, \ldots, A_N \in |R: \qquad B(x) = Bx^b \cosh, \sinh(c\log x)\cos, \sin(a\log x)$$
$$= \frac{B}{2}\mathrm{Re}, \mathrm{Im}\left(x^{(b+c+ia)x} \pm x^{b-c+ia}\right), \tag{1.373a–c}$$

is considered in the case of real parameters (1.373a) and coefficients of the homogeneous characteristic polynomial (1.293a, b) to simplify the explicit expressions (1.373c). The forcing (standard XXX) of a linear homogeneous differential equation (1.285) leads to a particular integral, specified by (1.374b):

$$P_N(b\pm c + ia) \neq 0: \qquad y_*(x) = \frac{B}{2}\mathrm{Re}, \mathrm{Im}\left[\frac{x^{b+c+ia}}{P_N(b+c+ia)} \pm \frac{x^{b-c+ia}}{P_N(b-c+ia)}\right], \tag{1.374a, b}$$

(i) in the non-resonant case (1.374a) and by (1.375c):

$$O\left((\delta - b - c - ia)^M\right) \sim P_N(\delta) \sim O\left((\delta - b + c + ia)^S\right):$$

$$y_*(x) = \frac{B}{2}\mathrm{Re}, \mathrm{Im}\left[\frac{x^{b+c+ia}\log^M x}{P_N^{(M)}(b+c+ia)} \pm \frac{x^{b-c+ia}\log^S x}{P_N^{(S)}(b-c+ia)}\right], \tag{1.375a–c}$$

(ii) and in the resonant case (1.375a, b).

An example is the linear homogeneous second-order differential equation (1.366) ≡ (1.376) forced by a product of a power and a hyperbolic sine and a circular cosine of a logarithm:

$$x^2y'' - xy' + 2y = x\cos(\log x)\cosh(c\log x) = \frac{1}{2}\mathrm{Re}\left(x^{1+i+c} - x^{1+i-c}\right). \tag{1.376}$$

The resonant condition is that at least one of the exponents of the powers on the RHS of (1.376) equals one root of the characteristic polynomial (1.367) and this is possible (1.377a) only for (1.377b) and (1.377c) the root $1 + i$:

$$1+i\pm c = 1\pm i: \qquad c = 0, \qquad 1+i\pm c = 1+i. \tag{1.377a–c}$$

Thus, the non-resonant (1.378a) particular integral is (1.378b):

$$\begin{aligned}
c \neq 0: \quad y_*(x) &= \frac{1}{2}\mathrm{Re}\left[\frac{x^{1+i+c}}{P_2(1+i+c)} + \frac{x^{1+i-c}}{P_2(1+i-c)}\right] \\
&= \frac{x}{2c}\mathrm{Re}\left(\frac{x^{i+c}}{c+2i} + \frac{x^{i-c}}{c-2i}\right) = \frac{x}{2c\,(c^2+4)}\mathrm{Re}[x^{i+c}(c-2i) + x^{i-c}(c+2i)] \\
&= \frac{x}{2c\,(c^2+4)}\left\{x^c\,[c\cos(\log x) + 2\sin(\log x)] + x^{-c}[c\cos(\log x) - 2\sin(\log x)]\right\} \\
&= \frac{x}{c\,(c^2+4)}[c\cos(\log x)\cosh(c\log x) + 2\sin(\log x)\sinh(c\log x)];
\end{aligned} \tag{1.378a, b}$$

(ii) in the remaining case (1.379a) the resonance occurs (1.379b) only in the first root $1 + i$:

$$c = 0: \qquad y_*(x) = \mathrm{Re}\left[\frac{x^{1+i}\log x}{P_2'(1+i)}\right] = x\log x\,\mathrm{Re}\left(\frac{x^i}{2i}\right) = \frac{x}{2}\log x\sin(\log x). \tag{1.379a, b}$$

1.8 Inverse Polynomial of Homogeneous Derivatives

The linear differential equation with constant (homogeneous) coefficients [sections 1.3–1.5 (1.6–1.8)] corresponds to: (i) a characteristic polynomial of ordinary (homogeneous) derivatives of the independent variable;

(ii) applied to the dependent variable [section 1.3 (1.6)]; (iii) equated to a forcing function of the independent variable [section 1.4 (1.7)]. A formal particular integral is obtained applying to the forcing function an inverse polynomial of ordinary (homogeneous) derivatives [section 1.5 (1.8)]. Decomposing the algebraic inverse of the characteristic polynomial in partial fractions (subsections 1.5.3–1.5.4), or otherwise, leads to a series expansion of ordinary (homogeneous) derivatives [subsection 1.5.2 (1.8.1)] that: (i) terminates if applied [subsection 1.5.5 (1.8.2)] to a polynomial (a polynomial of logarithms); (ii) if it is applied to another type of smooth forcing function results in a series that should converge [subsections 1.5.6–1.5.18 (1.8.6–1.8.13). The method of the inverse characteristic polynomial of homogeneous derivatives can be used as an alternative to the method of substitution (subsection 1.8.3), for example, to determine the particular integral of a linear homogeneous differential equation forced by a polynomial of logarithms (subsection 1.8.4).

Using the analogy between linear differential equations with constant (homogeneous) coefficients (subsection 1.8.5), it is shown that the inverse characteristic polynomial of ordinary (homogeneous) derivatives applied to an exponential (power) times a smooth function [subsection 1.5.8 (1.8.6)] is equivalent to applying a modified characteristic polynomial only to the smooth function. This specifies a particular integral of the linear homogeneous differential equation forced by a power multiplied by: (i) a polynomial of logarithms (subsection 1.8.7); (ii, iii) a hyperbolic (circular) cosine or sine of a logarithm [subsection 1.8.8 (1.8.9); (iv, v) the polynomial logarithms times a hyperbolic (circular) cosine or sine of a logarithm [subsection 1.8.10 (1.8.11)]; (vi) the power of a logarithm times a hyperbolic and a circular cosine or sine of a logarithm for a total of four factors in the forcing function (subsection 1.8.12). The principle of superposition allows addition (subsection 1.8.13) of the particular integrals of the unforced (forced) linear homogeneous differential equation [section(s) 1.6 (1.7–1.8)].

1.8.1 Series Expansion for the Inverse of a Polynomial

A particular integral of the forced linear differential equation with constant (1.52b) ≡ (1.126) [homogeneous (1.285) ≡ (1.380b)] coefficients is obtained applying to the forcing function the inverse characteristic polynomial (1.197c) [(1.380c)] of ordinary (1.197a) [homogeneous (1.380a)] derivatives:

$$\delta \equiv x\frac{d}{dx}: \qquad \{P_N(\delta)\}\, y_*(x) = B(x) \Rightarrow y_*(x) = \left\{\frac{1}{P_N(\delta)}\right\} y(x). \qquad (1.380a\text{–}c)$$

The algebraic inverse of the characteristic polynomial is a rational function that can be expanded in partial fractions: (i) consisting (1.203a–d) ≡ (1.204) of a sum of terms of the form (1.199):

$$\frac{1}{\delta - b} = \frac{-1/b}{1-\delta/b} = \sum_{n=0}^{\infty} b^{-1-n}\delta^n, \tag{1.381}$$

if all roots of the characteristic polynomial are simple (1.294a): (ii) if the characteristic polynomial has multiple roots (1.299a, b) the partial fraction decomposition (1.209a–g) involves terms of the form (1.200):

$$(\delta - b)^{-M} = \sum_{n=0}^{\infty} \frac{(M+n-1)!}{(M-1)!n!}(-b)^{-M-m}\delta^n. \tag{1.382}$$

The series of ordinary (1.199; 1.200) [homogeneous (1.381; 1.382)] derivatives: (i) terminate at order N when applied to a polynomial (polynomial of logarithms) of degree N; (ii) must lead to a convergent series when applied to a smooth, that is, an infinitely differentiable function (1.237a). The aspects (i) [(ii)] are addressed in the sequel [subsections 1.8.2–1.8.4 (1.8.5–1.8.12)].

1.8.2 Homogeneous Derivatives of a Polynomial of Logarithms

The ordinary (homogeneous) derivative of the variable (logarithm of the variable) is unity (1.383a) [(1.383b)]:

$$Dx = \frac{d}{dx}(x) = 1 = x\frac{d}{dx}(\log x) = \delta \log x. \tag{1.383a, b}$$

From (1.383a) [(1.383b)] follows the *ordinary (homogeneous) derivative applied to a power (1.384a, b) [power of a logarithm (1.385a, b)]:*

$$D^n x^p \equiv \frac{d^n}{dx^n}\left(x^p\right) = \begin{cases} \dfrac{p!}{(p-n)!}x^{p-n} & \text{if} \quad n \le p, & (1.384a) \\ 0 & \text{if} \quad n > p. & (1.384b) \end{cases}$$

$$\delta^n \log^p x = \left(x\frac{d}{dx}\right)^n \log p = \begin{cases} \dfrac{p!}{(p-n)!}\log^{p-n} x & \text{if} \quad n \le p, & (1.385a) \\ 0 & \text{if} \quad n > p, & (1.385b) \end{cases}$$

and their inverse (1.386b) [(1.386c)]:

$$q = p - n: \qquad \frac{1}{D^n} x^q = \frac{q!}{(q+n)!} x^{q+n}, \qquad \frac{1}{\delta^n} \log^q x = \frac{q!}{(q+n)!} \log^{q+n} x, \tag{1.386a–c}$$

obtained setting (1.386a). The proof of (1.385a) follows from:

$$p \ge n: \qquad \delta^n \left\{ \log^p x \right\} = \left(x \frac{d}{dx} \right)^n \log^p x = p \left(\frac{d}{dx} \right)^{n-1} \log^{p-1} x$$
$$= p(p-1)\ldots(p-n+1)\log^{p-1} x = \frac{p!}{(p-n)!} \log^{p-n} x. \tag{1.387}$$

If $p = n$ this reduces to a constant:

$$\delta^p \left\{ \log^p x \right\} = p! = D^p \left(x^p \right), \tag{1.388a, b}$$

and higher-order derivatives are zero (1.385b). The consistency of the direct (1.385a) and inverse (1.386a) homogeneous derivatives follows from the identity (1.389b):

$$q = p - n: \qquad \log^p x = \frac{1}{\delta^n} \delta^n \log^p x = \frac{1}{\delta^n} \frac{p!}{(p-n)!} \log^{p-n} x; \tag{1.389a, b}$$

the substitution (1.389a) leads from (1.389b) to (1.386c). Thus, *there is an analogy between the ordinary (homogeneous) derivative of a power (1.384a, b) [power of a logarithm (1.385a, b)] that extends to the inverse operators (1.386b) [(1.386c)]*. The relations (1.385a, b; 1.388a) specify the particular integral of a linear homogeneous differential equation forced by a polynomial of logarithms (subsections 1.8.3–1.8.4).

1.8.3 Solution by Substitution by the Inverse Characteristic Polynomial

From (1.380b, c), it follows that *a particular integral of the linear homogeneous differential equation (1.285) forced (standard XXXI) by a polynomial of derivatives (1.390a)*:

$$\left\{ P_N\left(x \frac{d}{dx} \right) \right\} y(x) = \sum_{m=0}^{M} B_p \log^m x, \quad y(x) = \frac{1}{P_N\left(x \frac{d}{dx} \right)} \left\{ \sum_{m=1}^{M} B_m \log^m x \right\}, \tag{1.390a, b}$$

is obtained by applying the inverse polynomial of homogeneous derivatives to the forcing term (1.390b):

$$\frac{1}{P_N(\delta)} = \frac{1}{A_0}\left(1+\sum_{n=1}^{N}\frac{A_n}{A_0}\delta^n\right)^{-1} = \sum_{p=1}^{\infty} A_0^{-1-p}(-)^p\left(\sum_{n=1}^{N}A_n\delta^n\right)^p, \tag{1.391}$$

implying that the expansion terminates (1.385a, b) at order $p = M$ equal to the degree of forcing polynomial. As five examples, the same polynomial of logarithms of degree two is used as a forcing term in the five linear homogeneous differential equations (1.321a) ≡ (1.392a, b), (1.324) ≡ (1.392c, d) and (1.366) ≡ (1.392e):

$$\log^2 x + 2\log x - 1 = x^2y'' \pm xy' + y,\quad x^3y''' + 2x^2y'' \pm xy' \mp y,\quad x^2y'' - xy' + 2y. \tag{1.392a–e}$$

The solution is a polynomial of logarithms of the second degree:

$$y_*(x) = \alpha\log^2 x + \beta\log x - \gamma, \tag{1.393}$$

where the coefficients (α, β, γ) are determined by substitution in (1.392a–e). An alternative is to use the inverse polynomial of homogeneous derivatives (subsection 1.8.4).

1.8.4 Homogeneous Equation Forced by a Polynomial of Logarithms

The second-order linear homogeneous differential equations (1.392a, b) have particular integrals:

$$y_*(x) = \frac{1}{1 \pm \delta + \delta\,(\delta - 1)}\left(\log^2 x + 2\,\log x - 1\right), \tag{1.394}$$

corresponding to (1.395a) [(1.395b)] for the upper (lower) sign:

$$\begin{aligned} y_*^+(x) &= \frac{1}{1+\delta^2}\left(\log^2 x + 2\,\log x - 1\right) \\ &= \left[1 - \delta^2 + O(\delta^4)\right]\left(\log^2 x + 2\,\log x - 1\right) \\ &= \log^2 x + 2\,\log x - 3, \end{aligned} \tag{1.395a}$$

$$\begin{aligned} y_*^+(x) &= \frac{1}{1 - 2\delta + \delta^2}\left(\log^2 x + 2\,\log^2 x - 1\right) \\ &= \left[1 + 2\delta - \delta^2 + \left(2\delta - \delta^2\right)^2 + O(\delta^3)\right]\left(\log^2 x + 2\,\log x - 1\right) \\ &= \left[1 + 2\delta + 3\delta^2 + O(\delta^3)\right]\left(\log^2 x + 2\,\log x - 1\right) \\ &= \log^2 x + 6\,\log x + 9, \end{aligned} \tag{1.395b}$$

where terms $O(\delta^3)$ can be omitted.

The third-order linear homogeneous differential equations (1.392c, d) have particular integrals:

$$\begin{aligned} y_*^{\pm}(x) &= \mp\frac{1}{1-\delta\mp 2\delta(\delta-1)\mp\delta(\delta-1)(\delta-2)}\left(\log^2 x+2\log x-1\right) \\ &= \mp\frac{1}{1-\delta\pm\delta^2+O\left(\delta^3\right)}\left(\log^2 x+2\log x-1\right) \\ &= \mp\left[1+\delta\mp\delta^2+\left(\delta\mp\delta^2\right)^2+O\left(\delta^3\right)\right]\left(\log^2 x+2\log x-1\right), \end{aligned} \tag{1.396}$$

corresponding to (1.397a) [(1.397b)]:

$$y_*^{+}(x) = -\left[1+\delta+O\left(\delta^3\right)\right]\left(\log^2 x+2\log x-1\right) = -\log^2 x-4\log x-1, \tag{1.397a}$$

$$y_*^{-}(x) = \left[1+\delta+2\delta^2+O\left(\delta^3\right)\right]\left(\log^2 x+2\log x-1\right) = \log^2 x+4\log x+5, \tag{1.397b}$$

for the upper (lower) sign.

The second-order linear homogeneous differential equation (1.392e) has a particular integral:

$$\begin{aligned} y_*(x) &= \frac{1}{2}\frac{1}{1-\delta/2+\delta(\delta-1)/2}\left(\log^2 x+2\log x-1\right) \\ &= \frac{1}{2}\frac{1}{1-\delta+\delta^2/2}\left(\log^2 x+2\log x-1\right) \\ &= \frac{1}{2}\left[1+\delta-\frac{\delta^2}{2}+\left(\delta-\frac{\delta^2}{2}\right)^2+O\left(\delta^3\right)\right]\left(\log^2 x+2\log x-1\right) \\ &= \frac{1}{2}\left[1+\delta+\frac{\delta^2}{2}+O\left(\delta^3\right)\right]\left(\log^2 x+2\log x-1\right) \\ &= \frac{1}{2}\log^2 x+2\log x+1. \end{aligned} \tag{1.398}$$

Next, products of polynomials of logarithms by smooth functions are considered, and smooth means infinitely differentiable functions.

1.8.5 Linear Differential Equations with Constant/Homogeneous Coefficients

The relation between linear differential equations with constant (1.197a–c) [homogeneous (1.380a–c)] coefficients corresponds to the substitution of: (i) ordinary (homogeneous) derivatives (1.399a) in the characteristic polynomial:

$$d \equiv \frac{d}{dx} \quad \leftrightarrow \quad \delta \equiv x\frac{d}{dx}; \qquad e^{ax} \quad \leftrightarrow \quad x^a, \qquad x^m \quad \leftrightarrow \quad \log^m x, \tag{1.399a–c}$$

and (ii) exponentials (powers) and powers (logarithms) in (1.399b, c) the particular integrals (1.96a, b) [(1.296a, b)].

The transformations (1.399a–c) apply to: (i) the general integral of the unforced equation in the case of simple (1.54; 1.56a, b) [(1.294a–d)] and multiple (1.98a, b; 1.99) [(1.299a–c)] roots; (ii) forcing by exponentials (powers) without (1.129a, b) [(1.328a–c)] or with (1.134a, b) [(1.329a, b)] resonance; (iii) the inverse characteristic polynomial of ordinary (homogeneous) derivatives (1.197a–c) [(1.380a–c)] applied to the product of a smooth function (1.239a) [≡ (1.400a)] by an exponential (1.240b) [power (1.400b)]:

$$J \in \mathcal{D}^{\infty}(|C): \qquad \left\{\frac{1}{P_N(\delta)}\right\} x^a J(x) = x^a \left\{\frac{1}{P_N(\delta + a)}\right\} J(x). \tag{1.400a, b}$$

The series expansion of homogeneous derivatives (1.391) ≡ (1.204; 1.381) = (1.209a–g; 1.382) in (1.400b): (i) terminates if J is a polynomial of logarithms (1.385a, b); (ii) for other smooth functions the series should converge. Even if a is a root of the characteristic polynomial $P_N(a) = 0$ in general, $P_N(\delta + a) \neq 0$ is not, and no resonance occurs in (1.400b).

The proofs (1.54–1.56) of (i), (1.127–1.132) of (ii), and (1.237–1.240) of (iii) for the linear differential equation with constant coefficients need not be repeated for homogeneous coefficients because the transformations (1.399a–c) apply at all stages. Also (1.400a, b) with $J = 1$ proves (1.328a–c) in the non-resonant case; the resonant case (1.400a, b) does not occur for a power or a polynomial of a logarithm unless zero is a root of multiplicity M the characteristic polynomial, in which case like in (1.256a–c; 1.257a, b) the order of the linear homogeneous differential equation can be depressed by M.

1.8.6 Polynomial of Logarithms Multiplied by a Smooth Function

From (1.400a, b) it follows that a linear homogeneous differential equation forced (standard XXXII) by the product of a smooth function (1.400a) and a power (1.401a) has a particular integral (1.401b):

$$\{P(\delta)\} y(x) = x^b J(x), \qquad y_*(x) = x^b \left\{\frac{1}{P_N(\delta + b)}\right\} J(x). \tag{1.401a, b}$$

For the forcing by a smooth function (1.400a) multiplied (standard XXXIII) by the hyperbolic cosine or sine of a logarithm (1.402a, b) with (standard XXXIV), a power as an additional factor (1.402c, d) a particular integral is given respectively by (1.403a–d):

$$B(x) = B\left\{\cosh, \sinh\left(c \log x\right); x^b \cosh, \sinh\left(c \log x\right)\right\} J(x), \quad \text{(1.402a–d)}$$

$$y_*(x) = \frac{B}{2}\left\{\frac{x^c}{P_N(\delta + c)} \pm \frac{x^{-c}}{P_N(\delta - c)}; \frac{x^{b+c}}{P_N(\delta + b + c)} \pm \frac{x^{b-c}}{P_N(\delta + b - c)}\right\} J(x). \quad \text{(1.403a–d)}$$

For the forcing by (standard XXXV) a smooth function (1.400b) multiplied by the circular cosine or sine of a logarithm (1.404a, b) with (standard XXXVI) a power as an additional factor (1.404c, d) a particular integral is respectively (1.405a–d):

$$B(x) = B\left\{\cos, \sin\left(a \log x\right); \quad x^b \cos, \sin\left(a \log x\right)\right\} J(x), \quad \text{(1.404a–d)}$$

$$y_*(x) = \frac{B}{\{2, 2i\}}\left\{\frac{x^{ia}}{P_N(\delta + ia)} \pm \frac{x^{-ia}}{P_N(\delta - ia)}; \frac{x^{b+ia}}{P_N(\delta + b + ia)} \pm \frac{x^{b-ia}}{P_N(\delta + b - ia)}\right\} J(x), \quad \text{(1.405a–d)}$$

allowing for the parameters (a, b) and coefficients $(A_1, \ldots, A_N)$ of the homogeneous characteristic polynomial to be complex. If they are all real (1.406a), the forcing (standard XXXVII) by the product of a smooth function (1.400a) multiplied by a circular cosine or sine of a logarithm as a second factor (1.406b, c), with a power as a third factor (1.406d, e) and a hyperbolic cosine or sine of a logarithm as a fourth factor (1.406f, g):

$$a, b, c, A_1, \ldots, A_N \in |R:$$

$$B(x) = B\left\{\cos, \sin(ax); \quad x^b \cos, \sin(ax); \quad x^b \cos, \sin(ax) \cosh, \sinh(cx)\right\} J(x)$$

$$= B \operatorname{Re}, \operatorname{Im}\left\{x^{ia}, x^{b+ia}, \frac{x^{b+ia+c} \pm x^{b+ia-c}}{2}\right\} J(x), \quad \text{(1.406a–g)}$$

has particular integrals respectively (1.407a–f):

$$y_*(x) = B \operatorname{Re}, \operatorname{Im}\left\{\frac{x^{ia}}{P_N(\delta + ia)}, \frac{x^{b+ia}}{P_N(\delta + b + ia)}, \frac{1}{2}\left[\frac{x^{b+ia+c}}{P_N(\delta + b + ia + c)} \pm \frac{x^{b+ia-c}}{P_N(\delta + b + ia - c)}\right]\right\} J(x). \quad \text{(1.407a–f)}$$

1.8.7 Product of a Power by the Power of a Logarithm

The forcing (standard XXXII) by the product of a power by the power of a logarithm (1.401a, b) is illustrated by the second-order linear homogeneous differential equation (1.321a) with lower sign (1.322a):

$$x^2y'' - xy' + y = x\log x, \tag{1.408}$$

leading to the particular integral:

$$\begin{aligned} y_*(x) &= \frac{1}{1-\delta+\delta(\delta-1)}x\log x = \frac{1}{1-2\delta+\delta^2}x\log x \\ &= \frac{1}{(\delta-1)^2}x\log x = \frac{1}{\delta^2}\log x = \frac{x}{6}\log^3 x, \end{aligned} \tag{1.409}$$

where was used (1.386c) with $n = 2, q = 1$. The differential equation (1.321a) with lower sign has a characteristic polynomial (1.322a) with the double root unity, leading to the general integral (1.322b). Thus, the forcing by the variable x would lead to a resonant particular integral scaling like $x\log^2 x$, and the factor $\log x$ on the RHS of (1.409) leads to an extra power in its particular integral (1.410):

$$y_*(x) = \alpha x\log^3 x. \tag{1.410}$$

Thus, the differential equation (1.408) has a particular integral of the form (1.410), where the constant α is determined by substitution; this leads to $\alpha = 1/6$ in agreement with (1.409), the method of the inverse characteristic polynomial.

1.8.8 Product of a Power by a Hyperbolic Function of a Logarithm

The forcing (standard XXXIII) by the product of a power of a logarithm by the hyperbolic sine of a logarithm (1.402a, b; 1.403b) is applied to the third-order linear homogeneous differential equation (1.324) ≡ (1.411) with lower sign (1.326a):

$$x^3y''' + 2x^2y'' - xy' + y = 2\log x\sinh(2\log x) = (x^2 - x^{-2})\log x. \tag{1.411}$$

Using (1.403a, b; 1.403b) leads to:

$$\begin{aligned}
y_*(x) &= \frac{1}{(\delta-1)^2(\delta+1)}\left[\left(x^2-x^{-2}\right)\log x\right] \\
&= \left\{x^2\frac{1}{(\delta+1)^2(\delta+3)} - x^{-2}\frac{1}{(\delta-3)^2(\delta-1)}\right\}\log x \\
&= \left\{x^2\frac{1}{3+7\delta+O\left(\delta^2\right)} + x^{-2}\frac{1}{9-15\delta+O\left(\delta^2\right)}\right\}\log x \qquad (1.412) \\
&= \left\{\frac{x^2}{3}\left[1-\frac{7}{3}\delta+O\left(\delta^2\right)\right] + \frac{x^{-2}}{9}\left[1+\frac{5}{3}\delta+O\left(\delta^2\right)\right]\right\}\log x \\
&= \left(\frac{x^2}{3}+\frac{1}{9x^2}\right)\log x + \frac{1}{9}\left(\frac{5}{3x^2}-7x^2\right),
\end{aligned}$$

the particular integral (1.412) of (1.411). The differential equation (1.324) with lower sign has a characteristic polynomial (1.326a) with the single (double) root $-1(+1)$, which are distinct from the exponents ± 2 in the RHS of (1.411). Thus, the particular integral is non-resonant of the form:

$$y_*(x) = \alpha_1 x^2 + \frac{\beta_1}{x^2} + \left(\alpha_2\, x^2 + \frac{\beta_1}{x^2}\right)\log x, \qquad (1.413)$$

where the constants $(\alpha_1, \alpha_2, \beta_1, \beta_2)$ are determined by substitution in (1.411). This leads to the same result (1.412), obtained more simply using the inverse characteristic polynomial.

1.8.9 Product of a Power by a Circular Function of a Logarithm

The forcing (standard XXXV) by a power of a logarithm times the circular cosine of a logarithm (1.404a, b; 1.405a, b) is applied to the second-order linear homogeneous differential equation (1.324) ≡ (1.414) with upper sign (1.327a):

$$x^3 y''' + 2\, x^2 y'' + x y' - y = 2\log x \cos\left(2\log x\right) = 2\log x \operatorname{Re}\left(x^{2i}\right). \qquad (1.414)$$

Using (1.404a, 1.405a) leads to (1.414):

$$
\begin{aligned}
y_*(x) &= 2\,\mathrm{Re}\left\{\frac{1}{(\delta-1)(\delta-i)(\delta+i)}\,x^{2i}\log x\right\} \\
&= 2\,\mathrm{Re}\left\{x^{2i}\frac{1}{(\delta-1+2i)(\delta+i)(\delta+3i)}\log x\right\} \\
&= 2\,\mathrm{Re}\left\{x^{2i}\frac{1}{3(1-2i)-(11+4i)\delta+O\left(\delta^2\right)}\log x\right\} \\
&= \frac{2}{3}\,\mathrm{Re}\left\{\frac{x^{2i}}{1-2i}\left[1+\frac{11+4i}{3-6i}\delta+O\left(\delta^2\right)\right]\log x\right\} \\
&= \frac{2}{15}\mathrm{Re}\left\{x^{2i}(1+2i)\left(\log x+\frac{3+26i}{15}\right)\right\} \\
&= \frac{2}{15}\mathrm{Re}\left\{x^{2i}\left[\left(\log x-\frac{49}{15}\right)+i\left(2\log x+\frac{32}{15}\right)\right]\right\} \\
&= \frac{2}{15}\left[\left(\log x-\frac{49}{15}\right)\cos(2\log x)-\left(2\log x+\frac{32}{15}\right)\sin(2\log x)\right],
\end{aligned}
\tag{1.415}
$$

as the particular integral of (1.414). The differential equation (1.324) with lower sign has a characteristic polynomial (1.326a) with simple roots $1, \pm i$ distinct from the exponent $2i$ on the RHS of (1.414). Thus the non-resonant particular integral is of the form:

$$
y_*(x) = \left[\alpha_1+\beta_1\log x\right]\cos\left(2\log x\right)+\left[\alpha_2+\beta_2\log x\right]\sin\left(2\log x\right), \tag{1.416}
$$

where the constants $\left(\alpha_1,\alpha_2,\beta_1,\beta_2\right)$ are obtained by substitution of (1.416) in (1.414). The same result (1.415) is obtained more simply by the method of the inverse characteristic polynomial.

1.8.10 Powers and Logarithms Multiplied by Hyperbolic Functions

The forcing (standard XXXIV) by the triple product of a power times the power of a logarithm times the hyperbolic cosine of a logarithm (1.402c, d; 1.403c, d) is applied to the second-order linear homogeneous differential equation (1.321a) ≡ (1.417) with lower sign (1.322a):

$$x^2y'' - xy' + y = 2x^3\log^2 x\cosh(2\log x) = (x^5 - x)\log^2 x, \tag{1.417}$$

using (1.402c, 1.403c) to obtain:

$$\begin{aligned}
y_*(x) &= \frac{1}{(\delta-1)^2}(x^5 - x)\log^2 x = \left\{x^5\frac{1}{(\delta+4)^2} - x\frac{1}{\delta^2}\right\}\log^2 x \\
&= \frac{x^5}{16}\frac{1}{1+\delta/2+\delta^2/16}\log^2 x - x\frac{1}{\delta^2}\log^2 x \\
&= \frac{x^5}{16}\left[1 - \frac{\delta}{2} - \frac{\delta^2}{16} + \left(\frac{\delta}{2} + \frac{\delta^2}{16}\right)^2 + O\left(\delta^3\right)\right]\log^2 x - \frac{x}{12}\log^4 x \\
&= \frac{x^5}{16}\left[1 - \frac{\delta}{2} + \frac{3}{16}\delta^2 + O\left(\delta^3\right)\right]\log^2 x - \frac{x}{12}\log^4 x \\
&= \frac{x^5}{16}\left(\log^2 x - \log x + \frac{3}{8}\right) - \frac{x}{12}\log^4 x,
\end{aligned} \tag{1.418}$$

as the particular integral (1.418) of (1.417). The differential equation (1.321a) with lower sign has characteristic polynomial (1.322a) with the double root 1, which appears in the second term on the RHS of (1.417); thus, the particular integral has no resonance in the first term and a double resonance in the second term, implying that it is of the form:

$$y_*(x) = x^5\left(\alpha_1\log^2 x + \alpha_2\log x + \alpha_3\right) + \beta x\log^4 x, \tag{1.419}$$

where the constants $(\alpha_1, \alpha_2, \alpha_3, \beta)$ are determined by substitution in (1.417). The same result is obtained more simply using the inverse characteristic polynomial (1.418).

1.8.11 Powers and Logarithms Multiplied by Circular Functions

The forcing (standard XXXVI) by the triple product of a power times the power of a logarithm times the circular sine of a multiple of a logarithm (1.406d, e;1.407c, d) is applied to the second-order linear homogeneous differential equation (1.321a) ≡ (1.420) with upper sign (1.323a):

$$x^2y'' + xy' + y = x\log x\sin(2\log x) = \mathrm{Im}\left\{x^{1+2i}\log x\right\}. \tag{1.420}$$

Using (1.406e; 1.407d) leads to:

$$y_*(x) = \mathrm{Im}\left\{\frac{1}{(\delta - i)(\delta + i)} x^{1+2i} \log x\right\} = \mathrm{Im}\left\{x^{1+2i} \frac{1}{(\delta + 1 + i)(\delta + 1 + 3i)} \log x\right\}$$

$$= \mathrm{Im}\left\{x^{1+2i} \frac{1}{-2(1-2i) + 2(1+2i)\delta + O\left(\delta^2\right)} \log x\right\}$$

$$= -\frac{x}{2}\mathrm{Im}\left\{\frac{x^{2i}}{1-2i} \frac{1}{1-(1+2i)\delta/(1-2i) + O\left(\delta^2\right)} \log x\right\}$$

$$= -\frac{x}{10}\mathrm{Im}\left\{x^{2i}(1+2i)\left[1 + \frac{(1+2i)^2}{5}\delta + O\left(\delta^2\right)\right]\log x\right\}$$

$$= -\frac{x}{10}\mathrm{Im}\left[x^{2i}(1+2i)\left(\log x + \frac{4i-3}{5}\right)\right]$$

$$= -\frac{x}{10}\mathrm{Im}\left\{x^{2i}\left[\log x - \frac{11}{5} + i\left(2\log x - \frac{2}{5}\right)\right]\right\}$$

$$= -\frac{x}{10}\left[\left(\log x - \frac{11}{5}\right)\sin(2\log x) + \left(2\log x - \frac{2}{5}\right)\cos(2\log x)\right], \tag{1.421}$$

as the particular integral (1.421) of (1.420). The differential equation (1.321a) with the upper sign has a characteristic polynomial (1.323a) with simple roots $\pm i$ leading to the general integral (1.323b) ≡ (1.323c) ≡ (1.323d). The roots do not coincide with the exponent $1+2i$ on the RHS of (1.420) and thus, the non-resonant particular integral is of the form:

$$y_*(x) = x\left[\left(\alpha_1 \log x + \beta_1\right)\cos\left(2\log x\right) + \left(\alpha_2 \log x + \beta_2\right)\sin\left(2\log x\right)\right], \tag{1.422}$$

where the constant $(\alpha_1, \alpha_2, \beta_1, \beta_2)$ are determined by substitution of (1.422) in (1.420). This leads with more computations to the same result (1.421) as the inverse characteristic polynomial.

1.8.12 Product of Power by Hyperbolic and Circular Functions of a Logarithm

The forcing (standard XXXVII) by the quadruple product of a power times a logarithm times the hyperbolic sine and circular cosine of a logarithm (1.406a, f, g; 1.407e, f) is applied to the second-order linear homogeneous differential equation (1.321a) ≡ (1.423) with the upper sign (1.323a):

$$x^2y'' + xy' + y = \frac{2}{x^2}\log x \sinh(2\log x)\cos(\log x) = \mathrm{Re}\left[\left(x^i - x^{i-4}\right)\log x\right], \quad (1.423)$$

using (1.406g; 1.407f) leads to:

$$y_*(x) = \mathrm{Re}\left\{\frac{1}{(\delta - i)(\delta + i)}\left(x^i - x^{i-4}\right)\log x\right\}$$

$$= \mathrm{Re}\left\{\left[x^i\frac{1}{\delta(\delta+2i)} - x^{i-4}\frac{1}{(\delta - 4 + 2i)(\delta - 4)}\right]\log x\right\}$$

$$= \mathrm{Re}\left\{\left[\frac{x^i}{2i\delta}\frac{1}{1+\delta/2i} - x^{i-4}\frac{1}{8(2-i) - 2(4-i)\delta + O\left(\delta^2\right)}\right]\log x\right\}$$

$$= \mathrm{Re}\left\{\frac{x^i}{2i\delta}\left[1 - \frac{\delta}{2i} + O\left(\delta^2\right)\right]\log x - \frac{x^{i-4}}{8(2-i)}\left[1 + \frac{4-i}{4(2-i)}\delta + O\left(\delta^2\right)\right]\log x\right\}$$

$$= \mathrm{Re}\left\{\frac{x^i}{2i}\left[\frac{\log^2 x}{2} - \frac{\log x}{2i}\right] - \frac{x^{i-4}}{8}\frac{2+i}{5}\left[\log x + \frac{(4-i)(2+i)}{20}\right]\right\}$$

$$= \mathrm{Re}\left\{\frac{x^i}{4}\log x[1 - i\log x] - \frac{x^{i-4}}{40}\left[(2+i)\log x + \frac{16+13i}{20}\right]\right\}$$

$$= \frac{\log x}{4}[\cos(\log x) + \log x \sin(\log x)]$$

$$-\frac{1}{40x^4}\left[\left(2\log x + \frac{4}{5}\right)\cos(\log x) - \left(\log x + \frac{13}{10}\right)\sin(\log x)\right], \quad (1.424)$$

the particular integral (1.424) of (1.423). The differential equation (1.423) has the characteristic polynomial (1.323a) with roots $\pm i$ leading to the general integral (1.323b). One of the roots i appears in the exponent of the first term on the RHS of (1.423) and thus, the particular integral is resonant (non-resonant) for the first (second) term, leading to the form:

$$y_*(x) = \log x\left[\left(\alpha_1 + \beta_1 \log x\right)\cos\left(\log x\right) + \left(\alpha_2 + \beta_2 \log x\right)\sin\left(\log x\right)\right]$$
$$+\frac{1}{x^4}\left[\left(\alpha_3 + \beta_3 \log x\right)\cos\left(\log x\right) + \left(\alpha_4 + \beta_4 \log x\right)\sin\left(\log x\right)\right]. \tag{1.425}$$

The constants $\left(\alpha_{1-4}, \beta_{1-4}\right)$ in (1.425) are determined by substitution in (1.423), leading with much more labor to the same result (1.424) as the method of the inverse characteristic polynomial.

1.8.13 Superposition of Unforced/Forced Particular Integrals

The principle of superposition applies to the linear homogeneous differential equation (1.285) leading to superposition in the complete integral of: (i) the general integral of the unforced equation; (ii) the particular integrals for each forcing term. Using the parameters ($a = 1$, $b = 2$, $c = 3$) indicates the complete integrals of the linear homogeneous differential equation of: (i) second-order (1.321a) with upper sign (1.323c) with forcing terms (1.332a, 1.333b; 1.392a, 1.395a; 1.420, 1.421; 1.423, 1.424):

$$x^2y'' + xy' + y = 2x^2 + \log^2 x + 2\log x - 1 + x \ \log x \sin\left(2\log x\right)$$
$$+\frac{2}{x^2}\log x \ \sinh\left(2\log x\right) \ \cos\left(\log x\right), \tag{1.426}$$

$$y_*(x) = C_1\cos(\log x) + C_2\sin(\log x) + \frac{2}{5}x^2 + \log^2 x + 2\log x - 3$$
$$-\frac{x}{10}\left(\log x - \frac{11}{5}\right)\sin(2\log x) + \left(2\log x - \frac{2}{5}\right)\cos(2\log x)$$
$$+\frac{\log x}{4}[\cos(\log x) + \log x \ \sin(\log x)] \tag{1.427}$$
$$-\frac{1}{40x^2}\left[\left(2\log x + \frac{4}{5}\right)\cos(\log x) - \left(\log x + \frac{13}{20}\right)\sin(\log x)\right];$$

(ii) second-order (1.321a) with lower sign (1.322a, b) with forcing terms (1.355, 1.357b; 1.392b, 1.395b; 1.408, 1.409; 1.417, 1.418):

$$x^2y'' - xy' + y = 2x^2\cosh\left(3\log x\right) + \log^2 x + 2\log x - 1$$
$$+ x\log x + 2x^3\log^2 x\cosh\left(2\log x\right), \tag{1.428}$$

$$y_*(x) = x(C_1 + C_2 \log x) + \frac{x^2}{32}\left[10\cosh(3\log x) - 6\sinh(3\log x)\right]$$
$$+ \log^2 x + 6\log x + 9 + \frac{x}{6}\log^3 x + \frac{x^5}{16}\left(\log^2 x - \log x + \frac{3}{8}\right) - \frac{x}{12}\log^4 x; \tag{1.429}$$

(iii) third-order (1.324) with the upper sign (1.327a, b) and forcing terms (1.348, 1.351c; 1.392c, 1.397a; 1.414, 1.415):

$$x^3 y''' + 2x^2 y'' + xy' - y = 2\cos(\log x) + \log^2 x + 2\log x - 1 + 2\log x \cos(2\log x), \tag{1.430}$$

$$y_*(x) = C_1 x + C_2 \cos(\log x) + C_3 \sin(\log x)$$
$$- \frac{\log x}{2}\left[\cos(\log x) + \sin(\log x)\right] - \log^2 x - 4\log x - 1 \tag{1.431}$$
$$+ \frac{2}{15}\left[\left(\log x - \frac{49}{15}\right)\cos(2\log x) - 2\left(\log x + \frac{32}{15}\right)\sin(2\log x)\right];$$

(iv) third-order (1.324) with lower signs (1.326a, b) with forcing terms (1.338, 1.339b; 1.392d, 1.397b; 1.411, 1.412):

$$x^3 y''' + 2x^2 y'' - xy' + y = 2\sinh(3\log x) + \log^2 x + 2\log x - 1 + 2\log x \sinh(2\log x), \tag{1.432}$$

$$y_*(x) = x(C_1 + C_2 \log x) + \frac{C_3}{x} + \frac{3}{32}\cosh(3\log x) + \frac{1}{32}\sinh(3\log x)$$
$$+ \log^2 x + 4\log x + 5 + \left(\frac{x^2}{3} + \frac{1}{9x^2}\right)\log x + \frac{1}{9}\left(\frac{5}{3x^2} - 7x^2\right); \tag{1.433}$$

(v) second-order (1.366, 1.369) with forcing terms (1.366, 1.372b; 1.376, 1.378b; 1.392e, 1.398):

$$x^2 y'' - xy' + 2y = 2x\sin(\log x) + x\cos(\log x)\cosh(3\log x) + \log^2 x + 2\log x - 1, \tag{1.434}$$

$$y_*(x) = x\left[C_1 \cos(\log x) + C_2 \sin(2\log x)\right] - x\log x \cos(\log x)$$
$$+ \frac{x}{13}\cos(\log x)\cosh(3\log x) \tag{1.435}$$
$$+ \frac{2x}{39}\sin(\log x)\sinh(3\log x) + \frac{1}{2}\log^2 x + 2\log x + 1.$$

In (1.427, 1.429, 1.435) [(1.431, 1.433)], the arbitrary constants are C_1, C_2 (and C_3).

1.9 Solution of Finite Difference Equations

A finite difference equation of order N relates N successive elements of a sequence $y_n,...,y_{n+N}$; it corresponds to a differential equation for $y_n \to y$ replacing the derivatives $y^{(k)}$ by $y_{n+k} \to y^{(k)}$. Like the differential equations (sections 1.1–1.2), the finite difference equations include, in particular, the linear case with constant coefficients (subsection 1.9.1).The latter leads to the third case of a characteristic polynomial (subsection 1.9.2), comparable to the linear differential equation with constant (homogeneous) coefficients [sections 1.3–1.5 (1.6–1.8)]. The roots of the characteristic polynomial specify the general solution of the linear finite difference equation with constant coefficients (subsection 1.9.3) and also a particular integral for some cases of forcing (subsection 1.9.4). Since a real characteristic polynomial can have complex conjugate roots (subsection 1.9.5) these can appear, for example, in the solution of second-order (fourth-order) linear finite difference equations with constant coefficients [section(s) 1.9.6 (1.9.7–1.9.9)], both forced and unforced. The particular, general and complete integrals of the three types of equations with characteristic polynomials are compared (subsection 1.9.10) in Tables 1.2–1.4.

1.9.1 Classification of Finite Difference Equations

A **finite difference equation** of order N is a relation among N successive elements of a sequence of numbers:

$$n = 1,...,\infty: \qquad F\left(n, y_n, y_{n+1},..., y_{n+N}\right) = 0. \tag{1.436a, b}$$

TABLE 1.2

Three Cases of Equations with Characteristic Polynomials

	Case	I	II	III
Characteristic polynomial	linear equation	differential	differential	finite difference
	coefficients	constant	homogeneous	constant
Unforced equation		section 1.3	section 1.6	section 1.9
Forced equation	direct characteristic polynomial	section 1.4	section 1.7	section 1.9
	inverse characteristic polynomial	section 1.5	section 1.8	–

Note: The method of characteristic polynomials applies to the linear: (i) differential equations with constant coefficients; (ii) differential equations with homogeneous coefficients, that is, with derivatives of order n multiplied by powers with the same exponent n; (iii) finite difference equations with constant coefficients.

TABLE 1.3

General Integral of the Unforced Equation

Case	I	II	III
Linear equation	differential	differential	finite difference
Coefficients	constant	homogeneous	constant
Operator	ordinary derivative	homogeneous derivative	forward difference
Simple roots	1.3.1–1.3.5	1.6.1–1.6.2	1.9.1–1.9.2
Multiple roots	1.3.6–1.3.10	1.6.3–1.6.4	1.9.3–1.9.5
Examples	1.3.11–1.3.14	1.6.5–1.6.10	1.9.6–1.9.10
Section	1.3	1.6	1.9

Note: The characteristic polynomial specifies in all three cases (i) to (iii) in Table 1.2 the linearly independent particular integrals necessary and sufficient to specify the general integral of the unforced equation.

Comparing (1.436b) with (1.1b), an ordinary differential equation of order N, the successive elements are replaced by derivatives of increasing order:

$$y, y', \ldots, y^{(N)} \quad \leftrightarrow \quad y_n, y_{m+1}, \ldots, y_{n+N}. \tag{1.437}$$

Comparison with (1.3) suggests that *the solution of (1.436a, b), a finite difference equation of order N, is a* ***sequence*** *involving N arbitrary constants:*

$$y = y(n; C_1, \ldots, C_N). \tag{1.438}$$

TABLE 1.4

Complete Integral: Direct Characteristic Polynomial

Cases		I	II	III
Forcing function	a	e^{bx}: 1.4.1–1.4.5	x^b: 1.7.1	b^n: 1.9.1
	b	cosh, sinh (cx): 1.4.4	cosh, sinh $(c \log x)$: 1.7.2	cosh, sinh $(n\psi)$: 1.9.10
	c	cos, sin (ax): 1.4.5	cos, sin $(a \log x)$: 1.7.3	cos, sin $(n\varphi)$: 1.9.5
	d	e^{bx} cosh, sinh (cx): 1.4.6	x^b cosh, sinh$(c \log x)$: 1.7.4	b^n cosh, sinh $(n\psi)$: 1.9.10
	e	e^{bx} cos, sin (ax): 1.4.7	x^b cos, sin $(c \log x)$:1.7.5	b^n cos, sin $(n\varphi)$: 1.9.10
	f	e^{bx} cosh, sinh (cx) cos, sin (ax): 1.4.8	x^b cosh, sinh $(c \log x)$ cos, sin $(a \log x)$: 1.7.6	b^n cosh, sinh $(n\psi)$ cos, sin $(n\varphi)$: 1.9.10
Section		1.4	1.7	1.9

Note: The direct method of characteristic polynomial also specifies a particular solution of the equations corresponding to the three cases in Table 1.2, basically for forcing by: (i) an exponential of the variable; (ii) powers of the variable; (iii) powers with fixed base and integral exponent.

The N constants are determined by N compatible and independent initial conditions (1.5a–c) such as the first N values:

$$m = 0, 1, \ldots, N-1: \qquad y_m = C_m. \tag{1.439a, b}$$

An ordinary differential (1.1a, b) [finite difference (1.436a, b)] equation is linear (1.33) [(1.440)] if the function and its derivatives (values of the sequence y_n) appear linearly, that is, there are no power or cross-products:

$$\sum_{k=0}^{N} A_{n,k}\, y_{n+k} = B_n. \tag{1.440}$$

The coefficients may depend on the independent variable (1.33) [on the order k in (1.440)]; if they do not, the linear ordinary differential (1.33) [finite difference (1.440)] equation has constant coefficients (1.52a) [(1.441)]:

$$\sum_{k=0}^{N} A_k\, y_{n+k} = B_n, \tag{1.441}$$

and forcing term that can depend on n.

Introducing the **forward finite difference operator** (1.442a), the linear finite difference equation of order N with constant coefficients (1.441) becomes (1.442b), where (1.442c) is the characteristic polynomial:

$$\Delta y_n \equiv y_{n+1}: \qquad B_n = \sum_{k=0}^{N} A_k\, y_{n+k} = P_N(\Delta) y_n, \quad P_N(\Delta) \equiv \sum_{k=0}^{N} A_k\, \Delta^k. \tag{1.442a–c}$$

The simplest first-order linear finite difference unforced equation is (1.434a), whose solution is the sequence (1.443b):

$$y_{n+1} = \lambda y_n = \Delta y_n, \qquad y_n = \Delta^n y_0 = \lambda^n y_0. \tag{1.443a, b}$$

Thus, the solution of the general unforced linear finite difference equation with constant coefficients (1.444b) is a power (1.444a) whose base is a root of the characteristic polynomial (1.444c):

$$y_n = \lambda^n: \qquad 0 = \sum_{k=0}^{N} A_k\, y_{n+k} = \lambda^n \sum_{k=0}^{N} A_k\, \lambda^k = \lambda^n\, P_N(\lambda), \quad P_N(\lambda) = 0. \tag{1.444a–c}$$

The characteristic polynomial (1.442c) of a linear finite difference equation with constant coefficients (1.441) is the third (section 1.9) and is compared next (subsection 1.9.2) with the first (second) characteristic polynomial (1.52b) [(1.292b, c) ≡ (1.293a, b)] of a linear differential equation with constant (1.52a) [homogeneous (1.285)] coefficients.

1.9.2 Comparison of Three Characteristic Polynomials

The **three characteristic polynomials** relate to: *(i) a linear differential equation with constant coefficients (1.445b), whose unforced particular integrals (1.445c) are exponentials with coefficients that are single roots of the characteristic polynomial (1.445d) of ordinary derivatives (1.445a); (ii) a linear homogeneous differential equation (1.446b), whose unforced partial integrals are powers (1.446c) with exponents that are single roots of the characteristic polynomial (1.446d) of homogeneous derivatives (1.446a); (iii) a linear finite difference equation with constant coefficients (1.447b), whose unforced solutions are powers with integral exponents (1.447c) and whose bases are single roots of a characteristic polynomial (1.447d) of forward finite differences (1.447a):*

$$D \equiv \frac{d}{dx}: \quad 0 = \sum_{n=0}^{N} A_n \frac{d^n y}{dx^n}, \quad y(x) = e^{\lambda x}, \quad P_N(\lambda) = \sum_{n=0}^{N} A_n \lambda^n = 0, \tag{1.445a–d}$$

$$\delta = x\frac{d}{dx}: \quad 0 = \sum_{n=0}^{N} A_n x^n \frac{dy^n}{dx^n}, \quad y(x) = x^{\lambda}, \quad P_N(\lambda) = \sum_{n=0}^{N} A_n \lambda(\lambda-1)\dots(\lambda-n+1) = 0, \tag{1.446a–d}$$

$$\Delta y_n = y_{n+1}: \quad 0 = \sum_{k=0}^{N} A_k y_{n+k}; \quad y_n = \lambda^n, \quad P_N(\lambda) = \sum_{n=0}^{N} A_n \lambda^n = 0. \tag{1.447a–d}$$

All of the preceding particular solutions, either integrals (1.445c; 1.446c) or sequence (1.447c), concern single roots of the characteristic polynomial.

If the characteristic polynomial has (1.448a) a root λ of multiplicity M, then there are M particular integrals or sequences (1.448b), given by (1.448c–e):

$$P_N(\mu) \sim O\left((\mu-\lambda)^M\right); \quad m = 1,\dots,M: \quad y_m(x) = x^{m-1} e^{\lambda x}, \quad y_m(x) = x^{\lambda} \log^{m-1} x,$$
$$y_{n,m} = \lambda^n n^{m-1}, \tag{1.448a–d}$$

namely: (i) the exponentials are multiplied by powers for the linear differential equation with constant coefficients (1.448c); (ii) the powers are multiplied by integral powers of logarithms for the linear homogeneous differential equation (1.448d); (iii) the integral powers are multiplied by powers of n for linear finite difference equation with constant coefficients (1.448e). The solutions (1.448c–e) can be obtained by parametric differentiation (1.449a–c):

$$y_m(x) = \left(\frac{\partial}{\partial\lambda}\right)^{m-1} \exp(\lambda x) = x^{m-1}\exp(\lambda x), \tag{1.449a}$$

$$y_m(x) = \left(\frac{\partial}{\partial\lambda}\right)^{m-1} x^{\lambda} = x^{\lambda}\log^{m-1} x, \tag{1.449b}$$

$$y_{n,m}(x) = \left(\frac{\partial}{\partial\lambda}\right)^{m-1} (\lambda)^n = \lambda^{n-m+1} n(n-1)....(n-m+2), \tag{1.449c}$$

where: (i, ii) coincide (1.449a) ≡ (1.448b) and (1.449b) ≡ (1.448c); (iii) concerning (1.449c) the set of particular integrals (1.438e) is the same, since only the factor n^{m-1} is new for $y_{n,m}$ and all others $1, n, n^2, ..., n^{m-2}$ have appeared before in $(y_n, 1;\ y_{n,2};...;y_{n,m-1})$; also λ^{-m+1} is a constant factor that can be omitted in λ^{n-m+1} leaving only λ^n. This specifies the general (a particular) integral or solution of the unforced (forced) equation [subsection 1.9.3 (1.9.4)].

1.9.3 General Solutions of the Unforced Equations

If the roots of the characteristic polynomial are all distinct (1.450a) the general solution of the unforced equation involves N arbitrary constants $(C_1, ..., C_N)$ *in:*

$$P_N(\lambda) = A_N \prod_{n=1}^{N} (\lambda - \lambda_n): \qquad 0 = \sum_{m=0}^{N} A_N \frac{d^n y}{dx^n}, \quad \sum_{n=0}^{N} A_n x^n \frac{d^n y}{dx^n}, \quad \sum_{n=0}^{N} A_n y_{n+k}, \tag{1.450a–d}$$

$$y(x) = \sum_{m=1}^{N} C_m \exp(\lambda_m x), \qquad y(x) = \sum_{m=1}^{M} C_m x^{\lambda_m}, \quad y_n = \sum_{m=1}^{M} C_m (\lambda_m)^n, \tag{1.451a–c}$$

the linear combination of: (i, ii) exponentials (1.451a) [powers (1.451b)] for the linear differential equation with constant (homogeneous) coefficients (1.450b) [(1.450c)]; (iii) integral powers (1.451e) for (standard XXXVIII) the linear finite difference equation *with constant coefficients (1.450d). If the characteristic polynomial (1.451a, b) has M roots of multiplicities α_m adding to N:*

$$\sum_{m=1}^{M} \alpha_m = N: \qquad P_N(\lambda) = A_N \prod_{m=1}^{M} (\lambda - \lambda_m)^{\alpha_n}, \tag{1.452a, b}$$

the general solution of the unforced equation involves N arbitrary constants $C_{m,k}$ in:

$$y(x) = \sum_{m=1}^{M} \exp(\lambda_m x) \sum_{\beta_m=1}^{\alpha_m} C_{m,\beta_m} x^{\beta_m - 1}, \tag{1.452c}$$

$$y(x) = \sum_{m=1}^{M} x^{\lambda_m} \sum_{\beta_m=1}^{\alpha_m} C_{m,\beta_m} \log^{\beta_m - 1} x, \tag{1.452d}$$

$$y(x) = \sum_{m=1}^{M} (\lambda_m)^n \sum_{\beta_m=1}^{\alpha_m} C_{m,\beta_m} n^{\beta_m - 1}, \tag{1.452e}$$

the linear combination of: (i, ii) products (1.452c) [(1.452d)] of exponentials (powers) by powers (logarithms) for the linear differential equation with constant (homogeneous) coefficients (1.450b) [(1.450c)]; (iii) powers with integral exponents multiplied by powers (1.452e) for (standard XXXIX) the linear finite difference equation with constant coefficients (1.450d).

1.9.4 Particular Solutions of the Forced Equations

The non-resonant forcing not involving a root of the characteristic polynomial (1.453a):

$$P_N(\lambda) \neq 0; \qquad \sum_{n=0}^{N} A_n \frac{dy^n}{dx^n} = e^{\lambda x}: \qquad y(x) = \frac{e^{\lambda x}}{P_N(\lambda)}, \tag{1.453a–c}$$

$$\sum_{m=0}^{N} A_n x^n y^{(n)}(x) = x^{\lambda}: \qquad y(x) = \frac{x^{\lambda}}{P_N(\lambda)}, \tag{1.453d, e}$$

$$\sum_{m=0}^{N} A_m y_{m+n} = \lambda^n, \qquad y_n = \frac{\lambda^n}{P_N(\lambda)}, \tag{1.453f, g}$$

concerns: (i, ii) an exponential (1.453c) [power (1.453e)] for the linear differential equation with constant (homogeneous) coefficients (1.453b) [(1.453d)]; (iii) *a power with integral exponent (1.453g) for (standard XLI) the linear finite difference equation with constant coefficients (1.453f). In the resonant case of a root of multiplicity M of the characteristic polynomial (1.454a) the particular solution is given by (1.454b–d):*

$$P_N(\mu) \sim O\left((\mu-\lambda)^M\right): \quad y_*(x) = \frac{e^{\lambda x} x^M}{P_N^{(M)}(\lambda)}, \quad y_*(x) = \frac{x^\lambda \log^M x}{P_N^{(M)}(\lambda)}, y_{*n} = \frac{\lambda^{n-M} n^M}{P_N^{(M)}(\lambda)}, \tag{1.454a–d}$$

corresponding to: (i, ii) the product (1.454b) [(1.454c)] of an exponential (power) by a power (logarithm) for the linear differential equation with constant (homogeneous) coefficients (1.453b) [(1.453d)]; (iii) the product (1.454d) of a power with integral exponent by a power of n for (standard XLII) the linear finite difference equation with constant coefficients (1.453f). The results (1.454b–d) are obtained respectively from (1.453c, e, g) by applying *L'Hospital* rule of parametric differentiation M times of the numerator and denominator:

$$y_*(x) = \frac{1}{P_N^{(M)}(\lambda)} \frac{\partial^M}{\partial \lambda^M}\left(e^{\lambda x}\right) = \frac{e^{\lambda x} \lambda^M}{P_N^{(M)}(\lambda)}, \tag{1.455a}$$

$$y_*(x) = \frac{1}{P_N^{(M)}(\lambda)} \frac{\partial^M}{\partial \lambda^M}\left(e^{x}\right) = \frac{x^\lambda \log^M x}{P_N^{(M)}(\lambda)}, \tag{1.455b}$$

$$y_{*n} = \frac{1}{P_N^{(M)}(\lambda)} \frac{\partial^M}{\partial \lambda^M}\left(\lambda^n\right) = \frac{\lambda^{n-M}}{P_N^{(M)}(\lambda)} n(n-1)\ldots(n-M+1), \tag{1.455c}$$

where: (i, ii) coincide (1.455a) ≡ (1.454b) and (1.455b) ≡ (1.454c); (iii) concerning (1.445c) only the highest power n^M of n appears in (1.454d), because all lower powers $\left(1, n, n^2, \ldots, n^{M-1}\right)$ are solutions (1.450d) of the unforced equation, and can be included in its general integral (1.451c), adding nothing new to the particular integral of the forced equation.

After the comparison of the general linear differential equation with constant (homogeneous) coefficients with the linear finite difference equation with constant coefficients (subsections 1.9.2–1.9.4), only the latter is considered next for specific examples (subsections 1.9.5–1.9.7).

1.9.5 Pair of Complex Conjugate Roots

If the linear finite difference equation (1.441) has constant real coefficients, the roots of the characteristic polynomial (1.442c) can be: (i) real and distinct

(1.450a); (ii) real and multiple (1.452a, b); (iii) simple or multiple complex conjugate pairs.

A complex conjugate pair of roots (1.456a) with modulus (1.456b) and argument (1.456c):

$$\lambda = a \pm ib = re^{\pm i\phi}: \qquad r = \left|a^2 + b^2\right|^{1/2}, \qquad \phi = arc\tan\left(\frac{b}{a}\right), \tag{1.456a–c}$$

leads (standard XL) to a linear combination of particular sequence of the form:

$$\begin{aligned} y_n &= C_1(a+ib)^n + C_2(a-ib)^n = r^n\left(C_1 e^{in\phi} + C_2 e^{-in\phi}\right) \\ &= r^n\left[D_1\cos(n\phi) + D_2\sin(n\phi)\right] = Er^n\cos(n\phi - \gamma), \end{aligned} \tag{1.456d–g}$$

where the three pairs of arbitrary constant of integration $(C_1, C_2), (D_1, D_2)$, *and* (E, γ) *are related by (1.77a–d; 1.78a–d; 1.81a, b; 1.82a, b).*

Similarly the forcing functions (1.457a, b):

$$\lambda = be^{i\phi}: \quad B_n = b^n\cos,\sin(n\phi) = \frac{b^n}{\{2,2i\}}\left(e^{in\phi} \pm e^{-in\phi}\right) = \frac{1}{\{2,2i\}}\left(\lambda^n \pm \frac{b^{2n}}{\lambda^n}\right), \tag{1.457a, b}$$

in the linear finite difference equation (1.441) lead (standard XLII) to the particular integrals: (i) first (1.457d) for the non-resonant case (1.457e):

$$P_N(\lambda) \neq 0 \neq P_N(b^2/\lambda): \qquad y_n = \frac{1}{\{2,2i\}}\left[\frac{\lambda^n}{P_N(\lambda)} \pm \frac{(b^2/\lambda)^n}{P_N(b^2/\lambda)}\right]; \tag{1.457c, d}$$

second (1.457g) in the resonant case (1.457e, f):

$$O\left((\mu-\lambda)^M\right) \sim P_N(\mu) \sim O\left((\mu - b^2/\lambda)^S\right): \quad y_n = \frac{1}{\{2,2i\}}\frac{\lambda^n n^M}{P_N^{(M)}(\lambda)} \pm \frac{(b^2/\lambda)^n n^S}{P_N^{(S)}(b^2/\lambda)}. \tag{1.457e–g}$$

The preceding theory is applied next to the general quadratic (biquadratic) linear finite difference equations with constant coefficients [subsection 1.9.6 (1.9.7)].

1.9.6 Second-Order Finite Difference Equation

The general linear second-order difference equation with constant coefficients is (1.458a) and has characteristic polynomial (1.458b) with roots (1.458c):

$$0 = y_{n+2} - 2ay_{n+1} + by_n: \qquad \lambda^2 - 2a\lambda + b = 0, \qquad \lambda_\pm - a \pm \sqrt{a^2 - b}, \tag{1.458a–c}$$

leading to three cases: (i) a double root (1.459b) for (1.459a) leading to the solution (1.459c):

$$I: \quad b = a^2: \qquad \lambda_\pm = a, \qquad y_n = a^n \left(C_+ + C_- n\right); \tag{1.459a–c}$$

(ii) for (1.460a) two real roots (1.460b, c) and solution (1.460d):

$$II: \quad b < a^2: \quad \lambda_\pm = a \pm \beta, \quad \beta \equiv \left|a^2 - b\right|^{1/2}; \quad y_n = C_+ \left(a + \beta\right)^n + C_- \left(a - \beta\right)^n; \tag{1.460a–d}$$

(iii) for (1.461a) two complex conjugate roots (1.461b) the solution (1.461c):

$$III: \quad b > a^2: \quad \lambda_\pm = -\alpha \pm i\beta \equiv re^{\pm i\phi}; \quad y_n = r^n \left[C_+ \cos(n\phi) + C_- \sin(n\phi)\right]. \tag{1.461a–c}$$

In all solutions (1.469c, 1.460d, 1.461c) the arbitrary constants $C_\pm$ are determined from initial conditions. An example of a forced equation is (1.462b) whose solution, (i) is (1.462d) in the non-resonant case (1.452a) when c is not a root of the characteristic polynomial (1.462c):

$$c \neq a: \quad y_{n+2} - 2ay_{n+1} + a^2 y_n = c^n, \quad P_2(\lambda) = (\lambda - a)^2, \quad y_n = \frac{c^n}{P_2(c)} = \frac{c^n}{(c - a)^2}; \tag{1.462a–d}$$

$$c = a: \quad y_{n+2} - 2\,ay_{n+1} + a^2 y_n = a^n, \quad y_n = \frac{n^2 a^{n-2}}{P_2''(a)} = \frac{n^2}{2} a^{n-2}, \tag{1.463a–c}$$

(ii) in the resonant case (1.463a, b) of a double root the solution is (1.463c). The particular solution (1.463c) of (1.463b) can be checked as follows:

$$y_{n+2} - 2ay_{n+1} + a^2 y_n = \frac{a^n}{2}\left[(n+2)^2 - 2(n+1)^2 + n^2\right] = a^n. \tag{1.463d}$$

A similar analysis with the substitutions:

$$e^{\lambda x} \quad \leftrightarrow \quad x^{\lambda} \quad \leftrightarrow \quad \lambda^{n}, \tag{1.464}$$

applies to the analogues of (1.465a), which is the general linear second-order differential equation with constant (1.465a) [homogeneous (1.465b)] coefficients:

$$y'' + 2ay' + by = B(x),\ B(x) = \left\{ \left(x\frac{d}{dx} \right)^2 + ax\frac{d}{dx} + b \right\} y(x) = x^2 y'' + (1+a)xy' + by; \tag{1.465a, b}$$

in (1.465b) was used (1.305a).

The complete solution of (1.463b) is the sum of (1.463c) and (1.459c):

$$y_n = a^n \left(C_+ + C_- \, n + \frac{n^2}{2a^2} \right). \tag{1.466}$$

The constants $C_{\pm}$ are determined (1.467c, d) by two compatible and independent initial conditions (1.467a, b):

$$\alpha = y_0 = C_+, \quad \beta = y_1 = a(C_+ + C_-) + \frac{1}{2a}: \quad C_+ = \alpha, \quad C_- = \frac{\beta}{a} - \frac{1}{2a^2} - \alpha; \tag{1.467a–d}$$

substituting (1.467c, d) in (1.466) specifies:

$$y_n = a^n \alpha (1-n) + a^{n-1} \beta n + a^{n-2} \frac{n}{2}(n-1), \tag{1.468}$$

as the complete solution (1.468) of the linear finite difference equation with constant coefficients (1.463b) with initial conditions (1.467a, b).

1.9.7 Unforced Biquadratic Finite Difference Equation

The general linear fourth-order biquadratic finite difference equation with constant coefficients (1.469a) has a characteristic polynomial (1.469b) with squared roots (1.469c):

$$y_{n+4} - 2ay_{n+2} + by_n = 0: \quad P(\lambda) = \lambda^4 - 2\,\lambda^2\, a + b, \quad (\lambda_{\pm})^2 = a \pm \sqrt{a^2 - b}, \tag{1.469a–c}$$

which leads to five cases: (i) the values in (1.469c) are real and positive if (1.469a, b) are met, leading to four real distinct roots (1.470c) and the solution (1.470d):

$$I: \; b<a^2, \; a>0: \qquad \pm\lambda_\pm = \left|a \pm \left|a^2-b\right|^{1/2}\right|^{1/2}, \tag{1.470a–d}$$

$$\begin{aligned} y_n &= C_1(\lambda_+)^n + C_2(-\lambda_+)^n + C_3(\lambda_-)^n + C_4(-\lambda_-)^n \\ &= (\lambda_+)^n\left[C_1+(-)^n C_2\right] + (\lambda_-)^n\left[C_3+(-)^n C_4\right]; \end{aligned} \tag{1.470a–d}$$

(ii) the values in (1.469c) are real and negative if (1.471a, b) are met, leading to pairs of complex conjugate imaginary roots appearing in the solution (1.471c):

$$\begin{aligned} II: \; b<a^2, \; a<0: \; y_n &= C_1(i\lambda_+)^n + C_2(-i\lambda_+)^n + C_3(i\lambda_-)^n + C_4(-i\lambda_-)^n \\ &= i^n\left\{(\lambda_+)^n\left[C_1+(-)^n C_2\right] + (\lambda_-)^n\left[C_3+(-)^n C_4\right]\right\}; \end{aligned} \tag{1.471a–c}$$

(iii, iv) the coincidence in (1.469c) leads to double real (imaginary) roots (1.472c) [(1.473c)] in the case (1.472a, b) [(1.473a, b)], which leads to the solutions (1.472d) [(1.473d)]:

$$\begin{aligned} III: \; b=a^2, a>0: \; \pm\lambda_\pm = |a|^{1/2}, \; y_n &= |a|^{n/2}(C_1+C_2 n) + \left(-|a|^{1/2}\right)^n (C_3+C_4 n) \\ &= |a|^{n/2}\left[C_1+C_2 n+(-)^n(C_3+C_4 n)\right]; \end{aligned} \tag{1.472a–d}$$

$$\begin{aligned} IV: \; b=a^2, a<0: \; \pm\lambda_\pm = i|a|^{1/2}, \; y_n &= \left(i|a|^{1/2}\right)^n (C_1+C_2 n) + \left(-i|a|^{1/2}\right)^n (C_3+C_4 n) \\ &= i^n |a|^{n/2}\left[C_1+C_2 n+(-)^n(C_3+C_4 n)\right]; \end{aligned} \tag{1.473a–d}$$

(v) the remaining case (1.474a) leads for real (a, b) to two pairs of complex conjugate roots (1.474b, c) and to the solution (1.474d):

$$\begin{aligned} &b>a^2: \; a \pm i\left|b-a^2\right|^{1/2} = r^2 \exp^{(i2\phi_\pm)} = (\lambda_\pm)^2, \quad \lambda_{\pm\pm} = r\exp(i\phi_\pm), \\ &y_n = r^n\left[C_1\cos(n\phi_+) + C_2\sin(n\phi_+) + C_3\cos(n\phi_-) + C_4\sin(n\phi_-)\right]. \end{aligned} \tag{1.474a–d}$$

In all the five solutions (1.470d, 1.471c, 1.472d, 1.473d, 1.474d) of (1.469a), the four constants are determined from four independent and compatible initial conditions.

1.9.8 Forced Biquadratic Finite Difference Equation

An example of a forced equation is (1.475b), which has a particular solution (1.475d) in the non-resonant case (1.475a) when c is not a root of the characteristic polynomial (1.475c):

$$c \neq \pm a: \qquad y_{n+4} - 2a^2 y_{n+2} + a^4 y_n = c^n, \tag{1.475a, b}$$

$$P_4(\lambda) = \left(\lambda^2 - a^2\right)^2: \qquad y_n = \frac{c^n}{P_4(c)} = \frac{c^n}{\left(c^2 - a^2\right)^2}. \tag{1.475c, d}$$

There are two resonant cases (1.476a, b) with a particular solution (1.476c):

$$c = \pm a: \quad y_{n+4} - 2a^2 y_{n+2} + a^4 y_n = (\pm a)^n, \quad y_n = \frac{n^2 (\pm a)^{n-2}}{P_4''(\pm a)} = \frac{n^2}{8}(\pm a)^{n-4}, \tag{1.476a–c}$$

since (1.475a) is a double root (1.476g) of the characteristic polynomial (1.475c) ≡ (1.476d) with first-order (1.476e) and second-order (1.476f) derivatives:

$$P_4(\lambda) = \lambda^4 - 2\lambda^2 a^2 + a^4, \qquad P_4'(\lambda) = 4\lambda^3 - 4\lambda a^2,$$
$$P_4''(\lambda) = 12\lambda^2 - 4a^2, \qquad P_4(\pm a) = P_4'(\pm a) = 0 \neq 8a^2 = P_4''(\pm a); \tag{1.476d–g}$$

it can be checked:

$$y_{n+4} - 2a^2 y_{n+2} + a^4 y_n = \frac{(\pm a)^n}{8}\left[(n+4)^2 - 2(n+2)^2 + n^2\right] = (\pm a)^n, \tag{1.476h}$$

that (1.476c) is a particular solution of (1.476b). *A similar analysis with the substitutions (1.464) applies to the analogues of (1.469a), which is the linear biquadratic differential equation with constant (1.477a) [homogeneous (1.477b)] coefficients:*

$$y'''' - 2ay'' + by = B(x), \tag{1.477a}$$

$$x^4 y'''' + 6x^3 y''' + x^2 (7 - 2a) y'' + (1 - 2a) y' + by = B(x). \tag{1.477b}$$

The latter (1.477b) corresponds to:

$$B(x) = \delta^4 - 2a\delta^2 + b = \left\{(xD)^4 - 2a(xD)^2 + b\right\} y(x), \tag{1.478}$$

where (1.305a) and (1.479b) are used, which are inverses of (1.304):

$$\delta^3 = xD(xD)^2 = xD\left(x^2D^2 + xD\right) = x^3D^3 + 3x^2D^2 + xD, \tag{1.479a}$$

$$\delta^4 = xD(xD)^3 = xD\left(x^3D^3 + 3x^2D^2 + xD\right) = x^4D^4 + 6x^3D^3 + 7x^2D^2 + xD. \tag{1.479b}$$

The complete solution of the linear fourth-order finite difference equation with constant coefficients (1.476b) with + sign is the sum of (1.476c) and replacing a by a^2 in (1.472d):

$$y_n = a^n\left[C_1 + C_2\, n + (-)^n (C_3 + C_4 n) + \frac{n^2}{8a^4}\right]. \tag{1.480}$$

1.9.9 Four Initial Conditions for a Finite Difference Equation

Considering the general solution (1.472d) ≡ (1.481d) of the unforced biquadratic linear finite difference equation (1.469a) in the particular case (1.481a–c) ≡ (1.472a–c):

$$b = a^2; a > 0: \quad y_{n+4} - 2\, a y_{n+2} + a^2 y_n = 0, \quad y_n = |a|^{n/2}\left[C_1 + C_2 n + (-)^n (C_3 + C_4 n)\right], \tag{1.481a–d}$$

the four compatible and independent initial conditions (1.482a–d):

$$y_0 = 1, \quad y_1 = y_2 = y_3 = 0: \qquad C_1 = C_3 = \frac{1}{2}, \qquad C_2 = C_4 = -\frac{1}{4}, \tag{1.482a–h}$$

specify the four constants (1.482e–h) as follows: (i) substitution of (1.482a–d) in (1.481d) leads to the system of equations:

$$\begin{gathered} 1 = C_1 + C_3, \quad 0 = C_1 + C_2 - C_3 - C_4, \\ 0 = C_1 + 2C_2 + C_3 + 2C_4, \quad 0 = C_1 + 3C_2 - C_3 - 3C_4; \end{gathered} \tag{1.483a–d}$$

(ii) substituting (1.483a) in (1.483c) gives (1.484a) and subtracting (1.483b) from (1.483d) gives (1.484b), implying (1.484c, d) ≡ (1.482g, h):

$$C_2 + C_4 = -\frac{1}{2}, \qquad C_2 = C_4 : \qquad C_2 = C_4 = -\frac{1}{4}; \tag{1.484a–c}$$

(iii) substituting (1.484b) in (1.483b) gives (1.485a), which together with (1.483a) ≡ (1.485b) implies (1.485c, d) ≡ (1.482e, f):

$$C_1 = C_3, \qquad C_1 + C_3 = 1 : \qquad C_1 = C_3 = \frac{1}{2}. \tag{1.485a–d}$$

It can be checked that (1.484c, d; 1.485c, d) satisfy (1.483a–d). Substituting (1.482e–h) in (1.481c) specifies:

$$y_n = \frac{|a|^{n/2}}{2}\left(1 - \frac{n}{2}\right)\left[1 + (-)^n\right], \tag{1.486a}$$

which is equivalent to:

$$y_{2n+1} = 0, \qquad y_{2n} = |a|^n (1 - n), \tag{1.486b, c}$$

as *the general solution of the unforced linear finite difference equation with constant coefficients (1.481b, c) with the initial conditions (1.482a–d).*

1.9.10 Solutions of the Three Equations with Characteristic Polynomials

The solutions—which are particular, general, and complete integrals or sequences associated with the three equations with characteristic polynomials—are summarized (subsection 1.9.8) in the Tables 1.2–1.5 in three columns comparing similar cases for the: (i) linear differential equations with constant coefficients (sections 1.3–1.5); (ii) homogeneous linear differential equation with power coefficients (sections 1.6-1.8); (iii) linear finite difference equations with constant coefficients (section 1.9).

The general integral of the unforced equations was discussed fully in the text and is listed in Table 1.3. The particular integral of the forced equations was treated fully in the text in the cases (i) and (ii), and is listed in Tables 1.4 and 1.5. Similar methods apply in the case (iii), as outlined next. The baseline case is the linear finite difference equation of order N with power-law forcing (1.453f) for which the solution is (1.453g) [(1.454d)] in the non-resonant (resonant) case when the base λ is not a root (1.453a) [is a root (1.454a) of multiplicity M] of the characteristic polynomial (1.447d). From these follow the forcings by the product of a power by: (i) a circular cosine or sine of a multiple of n in (1.457a, b) leading to (1.457c, d) [(1.457e-g)] in the non-resonant (resonant) case; and (ii) the (standard XLIII) hyperbolic cosine or sine (1.487b) a multiple (1.487a) of n:

$$\lambda \equiv be^{\psi}: \quad B_n = Bb^n \cosh, \sinh(n\psi) = \frac{B}{2} b^n \left(e^{n\psi} \pm e^{-n\psi}\right) = \frac{B}{2}\left[\lambda^n + \left(b^2/\lambda\right)^n\right]; \tag{1.487a, b}$$

(iii) the (standard XLIV) product of hyperbolic and circular cosines and sines (1.488b) of a multiple (1.488a) of n:

$$\lambda_{\pm\pm} = e^{\pm\psi\pm i\phi}: \quad B_n = Bb^n \cosh, \sinh(n\psi)\cos, \sin(n\phi)$$
$$= B\frac{b^n}{\{4, 4i\}}\left(e^{n\psi} \pm e^{-n\psi}\right)\left(e^{in\phi} \pm e^{-in\phi}\right), \tag{1.488a, b}$$

which in the case of all coefficients real (1.489a), simplifies to (1.489b):

$$b, \phi, \psi, A_1, \ldots, A_N \in| R: \qquad B_n = \frac{B}{2} b^n \operatorname{Re}, \operatorname{Im}\left[e^{n(i\phi+\psi)} \pm e^{n(i\phi-\psi)}\right]; \tag{1.489a, b}$$

(iv) the product of hyperbolic and circular cosines and sines (1.489c) of multiples (1.489a) of n:

$$b, \phi, \psi, A_1, \ldots, A_N \in| R; \quad \lambda_{\pm} = e^{i\phi\pm\psi}: \qquad Bb^n \cosh, \sinh(n\psi)\cos, \sin(n\phi)$$
$$= \frac{B}{2} b^n \operatorname{Re}, \operatorname{Im}\left[e^{n(i\phi+\psi)} \pm e^{n(i\phi-\psi)}\right] = \frac{B}{2} b^n \operatorname{Re}, \operatorname{Im}\left[\left(\lambda_+\right)^n \pm \left(\lambda_-\right)^n\right], \tag{1.489a–c}$$

assuming all coefficients are real (1.489a). The solutions corresponding to the power law forcing (1.453f) are given by [(1.453g) (1.454d)] in the non-resonant (resonant) case. A differential equation (1.1b) can be discretized as a finite difference equation (1.436b) and their solutions compared (notes 5.4–5.8). There are five methods to obtain a particular integral of the linear differential equation with constant coefficients forced by an arbitrary function (notes 1.1–1.28).

NOTE 1.1: Five Methods of Solution of Forced Differential Equations

Considerable analogies were demonstrated among (Table 1.2) the three classes of equations with characteristic polynomials: [I(II)] the linear

TABLE 1.5

Complete Integral: Inverse Characteristic Polynomial

Cases		I	II
General		1.5.1–1.5.7	1.8.1–1.8.4
	a	e^{bx}: 1.5.8–1.5.13	x^b: 1.8.5–1.8.7
	b	cosh, sinh (cx): 1.5.14	cosh, sinh $(c \log x)$: 1.8.8
forcing function: smooth $J \in D^\infty$ multiplied by: $J(x)x$....	c	cos, sin (ax): 1.5.15	cos, sin $(a \log x)$: 1.8.9
	d	e^{bx} cosh, sinh (cx): 1.5.16	x^b cosh, sinh $(a \log x)$: 1.8.10
	e	e^{bx} cos, sin (ax): 1.5.17	x^b cos, sin $(a \log x)$: 1.8.11
	f	e^{bx} cosh, sinh (cx) cos, sin (ax): 1.5.18	x^b cosh, sinh $(a \log x)$ cos, sin $(a \log x)$: 1.8.12
Example		1.5.19	1.8.13
Section		1.5	1.8

Note: The inverse method of characteristic polynomials also supplies a particular integral of a linear differential equation with (i) constant [(ii) homogeneous] coefficients forced by the product of an exponential (power) by a smooth function, which is infinitely differentiable.

ordinary differential equations with constant (homogeneous) coefficients [l.o.d.e.c.c (l.o.d.e.h.c.)] in the sections 1.3–1.5 (1.6–1.8); (III) the linear finite difference equations with constant coefficients (l.f.d.e.c.c.) in section 1.9. In each case: (a) the general integral of the unforced equation is specified by the simple or multiple roots of the characteristic polynomial (Table 1.3); (b) the characteristic polynomial also specifies cases of resonant and resonant forcing by elementary functions and their products using the direct (inverse) characteristic polynomial [Table 1.4 (1.5)]. The method of the inverse characteristic polynomial (Table 1.5) applies in the cases I(II) of linear differential equations with constant (homogeneous) coefficients to forcing by an arbitrary smooth function (A). This is one of the six cases (Table 1.6) of the solution of a linear differential equation with an arbitrary forcing function. For linear ordinary differential equations with variable coefficients (l.o.d.e.v.c.) two methods apply, namely, (B) variation of parameters [(C) Green or influence function] for forcing by an arbitrary integrable (continuous) function [notes 1.2–1.4 (1.5–1.8)]. In the case of linear differential equations with constant coefficients, three more methods apply for arbitrary forcing by: (D) a function of bounded fluctuation in a finite interval using Fourier series (notes 1.9–1.10); (E) a function of bounded fluctuation and absolutely integrable on the real line using the Fourier integral (notes 1.11–1.14); (F) a function absolutely integrable on the finite positive real line and of fast decay at infinity using the Laplace transform (notes 1.15–1.22). These restrictions for ordinary forcing

TABLE 1.6

Solution of Differential Equations with Arbitrary Forcing

	A	B	C	D	E	F
Method	Inverse characteristic polynomial	Variation of parameters	Green or influence function	Fourier series	Fourier integral	Laplace transform
forcing function	$\mathcal{D}^\infty$ smooth	$\mathcal{E}$ integrable	$\mathcal{C}$ continuous	$\mathcal{F}$ bounded fluctuation	$\mathcal{F}\cap\mathcal{L}^1$ bounded fluctuation and absolutely integrable	$\mathcal{L}^1(0,L)\cap\underline{\mathcal{V}}(L,\infty)$ absolutely integrable and of slow growth
domain	any	any	any	finite interval $(-L,+L)$	real line $(-\infty,+\infty)$	positive real line $(0,+\infty)$
linear differential equation with	section 1.5 (1.8) constant (homogeneous) coefficients	notes 1.2–1.4 variable coefficients	notes 1.5–1.8	notes 1.9–1.10	notes 1.11–1.14 constant coefficients	notes 1.15–1.28

Note: Besides the method of the (A) inverse characteristic polynomial there are five other methods to obtain solutions of forced differential equations, namely (B) variation of parameters, (C) Green function, Fourier (D) series or (E) integral and (F) Laplace transform. These methods may differ in the domain of application: (i) to differential equations with variable, homogeneous, or constant coefficients; (ii) to forcing functions that may be integrable, continuous, smooth, or of bounded oscillation; (iii) to domains that may be arbitrary intervals, a finite interval, the whole real line, or the positive real line.

functions can be removed by considering the forcing by generalized functions (volume III), such as the unit jump and impulse, and their derivatives (notes 1.23–1.28).

NOTE 1.2: Method of Variation of Parameters

Consider a linear ordinary differential equation of order N with variable coefficients (1.33) consisting of: (i) a linear operator (1.34b) of the independent variable x; (ii) applied to the dependent variable y; (iii) equated to a forcing function of the independent variable. The general integral (1.490e) of the unforced equation (1.490d) is a linear combination (1.490a) of N linearly independent (1.490c) particular integrals (1.490b):

$$n=1,\dots,N: \qquad \left\{L\left(\frac{d}{dx}\right)\right\}y_n(x)=0, \qquad W(y_1,y_2,\dots y_N)\neq 0:$$

$$\left\{L\left(\frac{d}{dx}\right)\right\}y(x)=0 \quad\Rightarrow\quad y(x)=\sum_{n=1}^{N}C_n y_n(x), \tag{1.490a–e}$$

where $(C_1,...,C_N)$ are arbitrary constants and (1.490c) is the Wronskian (1.40a–c) of the particular integrals. The **method of variation of parameters** (standard XLV) seeks a particular integral of the forced equation (1.491a) of the same form (1.490e) replacing the constants by functions (1.491b):

$$\left\{L\left(\frac{d}{dx}\right)\right\}y_n(x)=B(x): \qquad y(x)=\sum_{n=1}^{N}C_n(x)y_n(x). \tag{1.491a, b}$$

In order to determine the coefficient functions $(C_1(x),....,C_2(x))$ in (1.491b) must be imposed N independent and compatible condition namely: (i) satisfying the forced differential equation (1.491a); (ii) an additional $(N-1)$ conditions can be chosen at will.

In the case of a forced linear differential equation of the first (second) order, $N=1(N=2)$ no $N-1=0$ (one $N-1=1$) additional condition (ii) is needed [section 3.3 (note 2.1)]. The method of solution is outlined next for the forced linear differential equation of order N, in which case are chosen (ii) the $N-1$ conditions (1.492a, b):

$$k=0,...,N-2: \qquad \sum_{n=1}^{N}C_n'(x)\frac{d^k}{dx^k}\left[y_n(x)\right]=0. \tag{1.492a, b}$$

The conditions (1.492a, b) imply that when differentiating (1.491b) m times all derivatives go to the particular integrals (1.493a, b):

$$m=1,...,N-1: \qquad \frac{d^m}{dx^m}\left[y(x)\right]=\sum_{n=1}^{N}C_n(x)\frac{d^m}{dx^m}\left[y_n(x)\right]; \tag{1.493a, b}$$

$$\frac{d^N}{dx^N}\left[y(x)\right]=\sum_{n=1}^{N}C_n(x)\frac{d^N}{dx^N}\left[y_n(x)\right]+C_n'(x)\frac{d^{N-1}}{dx^{N-1}}\left[y_N(x)\right], \tag{1.494}$$

this is no longer the case for the derivative of order N in (1.494).

NOTE 1.3: Forced/Unforced Linear Differential Equations

Substituting (1.493a, b; 1.494) in the forced differential equation (1.491a) gives:

$$\begin{aligned} B(x)&=\left\{L\left(\frac{d}{dx}\right)\right\}\sum_{n=1}^{N}C_n(x)y_n(x) \\ &=\sum_{n=1}^{N}C_n(x)\left\{L\left(\frac{d}{dx}\right)\right\}y_n(x)+\sum_{n=1}^{N}C_n'(x)\frac{d^{N-1}}{dx^{N-1}}\left[y_n(x)\right], \end{aligned} \tag{1.495a}$$

where the first term on the RHS of (1.495a) vanishes by (1.490b), leaving only the last term:

$$B(x) = \sum_{n=1}^{N} C_n'(x) \frac{d^{N-1}}{dx^{N-1}} \left[y_n(x) \right]. \tag{1.495b}$$

The system of N linear equations (1.493a, b; 1.495b) for the N unknowns $(C_1', \ldots, C_N')$:

$$\begin{bmatrix} y_1(x) & y_2(x) & \cdots & y_{N-1}(x) & y_N(x) \\ y_1'(x) & y_2'(x) & \cdots & y_{N-1}'(x) & y_N'(x) \\ \vdots & \vdots & & \ddots & \vdots \\ y_1^{(N-2)}(x) & y_2^{(N-2)}(x) & \cdots & y_{N-1}^{(N-2)}(x) & y_N^{(N-2)}(x) \\ y_1^{(N-1)}(x) & y_2^{(N-1)}(x) & \cdots & y_{N-1}^{(N-1)}(x) & y_N^{(N-1)}(x) \end{bmatrix} \begin{bmatrix} C_1'(x) \\ C_1'(x) \\ \vdots \\ C_{N-2}'(x) \\ C_{N-1}'(x) \end{bmatrix} = \begin{bmatrix} 0 \\ 0 \\ \vdots \\ 0 \\ B(x) \end{bmatrix}, \tag{1.496}$$

has the for determinant of the matrix of coefficients (1.497c) the Wronskian (1.497d) $\equiv$ (1.40c) that is not zero because the particular integrals $\left[y_1(x), \ldots, y_N(x) \right]$ are linearly independent:

$$n = 1, \ldots, N; \; m, \, l = 0, \ldots, N-1: \; Y_n^m \equiv y_n^{(m)}(x), \; \operatorname{Det}\left[y_n^{(m)}(x) \right] = \operatorname{Det}\left(Y_n^m \right) = W \neq 0. \tag{1.497a–d}$$

In the unforced case (1.498a): (i) the linear system (1.496) is homogeneous with non-zero determinant (1.497d), hence the only solution is trivial (1.498b, c); (ii) thus, all functions reduce to arbitrary constants (1.498d) and (1.491b) becomes the general integral (1.490e) of the unforced differential equation:

$$B(x) = 0: \qquad n = 1, \ldots . N: \qquad C_n'(x) = 0, \qquad C_n(x) = const. \tag{1.498a–d}$$

In the forced case (1.499a), since the determinant is non-zero (1.497d), there exists an inverse matrix (1.499b) specifying the solution (1.499c) of (1.496):

$$B(x) \neq 0: \qquad Y_\ell^m(x) Z_n^\ell(x) = \delta_n^m, \qquad C_n'(x) = Z_n^N(x) B(x) \equiv f_n(x). \tag{1.499a–c}$$

In (1.499b) appears the identity matrix δ_n^m and the integration of (1.499c) gives:

$$B \in \mathcal{E}(|C): \qquad C_n(x) = C_n + f_n(x), \qquad f_n(x) \equiv \int^x Z_n^N(\xi) B(\xi) d\xi. \tag{1.500a–c}$$

Substituting (1.500b) in (1.491b): (i) the constant part first on the RHS of (1.500b) leads to the general integral (1.490e) of the unforced equation (1.490d); (ii) the non-constant part second on the RHS of (1.500b) specifies a particular integral (1.501b) of the forced equation (1.501a):

$$\left\{L\left(\frac{d}{dx}\right)\right\}y_*(x)=B(x): \qquad y_*(x)=\sum_{n=1}^{N} y_n(x)\int^x f_n(\xi)d\xi. \qquad (1.501\text{a, b})$$

It has been shown that *if N linearly independent (1.490a, c) particular integrals (1.490b) of the unforced linear differential equation (1.490d) with variable coefficients (1.34a, b) are known then (standard XLV): (i) the general integral of the unforced equation (1.490d) is a linear combination with constant coefficients (1.490e); (ii) a particular integral (1.501a) of the equation forced by an arbitrary integrable function (1.500a) is a similar linear combination (1.501b) replacing the constants by (1.500b, c) the primitives of the functions (1.499c) that are solutions (1.499b) of the linear system of N equations (1.496) ≡ (1.497a–d).* The method simplifies for the linear differential equation of first (second) order with variable (constant) coefficients [section 3.3 (2.9)]. Next is considered, as an example, a linear second-order differential equation with variable coefficients (note 1.4).

NOTE 1.4: Forced Solution of an Equation with Variable Coefficients

As an example is considered the forcing by an arbitrary integrable function (1.502a) of the differential equation (1.502b) ≡ (1.42a):

$$B\in\mathcal{E}(|C): \qquad (x-1)y''-xy'+y=B(x), \qquad (1.502\text{a, b})$$

which is linear of second-order with variable coefficients, but not of the homogeneous type (1.285). Two linearly independent (1.43a) particular integrals of the unforced equation (1.42a) are (1.42b, c) leading to the general integral (1.43b), where (C_1,C_2) are arbitrary constants. A particular integral of the same equation (1.42a) ≡ (1.502b) with forcing by an arbitrary integrable function (1.502a) is sought in the same form (1.43b), replacing the constants (C_1,C_2) by functions $\left[C_1(x),C_2(x)\right]$ in (1.503a), subject to the condition (1.492a, b) ≡ (1.1503b):

$$y(x)=xC_1(x)+e^xC_2(x), \qquad 0=xC_1'(x)+e^xC_2'(x). \qquad (1.503\text{a, b})$$

The functions $\left[C_1(x),C_2(x)\right]$ in (1.503a) must satisfy the differential equation (1.502b) and the condition (1.503b). The latter condition implies (1.504a, b):

$$y'(x)=C_1(x)+e^xC_2(x), \qquad y''(x)=C_1'(x)+e^x\left[C_2(x)+C_2'(x)\right], \qquad (1.504\text{a, b})$$

where only first-order derivatives appear in (1.504b).

Substituting (1.503a; 1.504a, b) in the differential equation (1.502b) gives:

$$B(x)=(x-1)\left[C_1'+e^x\left(C_2+C_2'\right)\right]-x\left(C_1+e^xC_2\right)+C_1x+C_2e^x=(x-1)\left[C_1'+e^xC_2'\right]. \tag{1.505}$$

The linear inhomogeneous system of two equations (1.503b; 1.505) may be solved for (C_1', C_2') leading to:

$$-(x-1)^2 C_1'(x)=B(x), B(x)=(x-1)\left(1-\frac{1}{x}\right)e^xC_2'(x)=\frac{(x-1)^2}{x}e^xC_2'(x). \tag{1.506a, b}$$

The integration of (1.506a, b) specifies:

$$C_1(x)=C_1-\int^x\frac{B(\xi)}{(\xi-1)^2}d\xi, \qquad C_2(x)=C_2+\int^x\frac{\xi e^{-\xi}}{(\xi-1)^2}B(\xi)d\xi, \tag{1.507a, b}$$

the coefficient functions (1.507a, b) appearing in the complete integral (1.503a) of the linear second-order differential equation with variable coefficients (1.502b) forced by an arbitrary integrable function (1.502a). For example, the forced differential equation (1.508a) has complete integral (1.508b):

$$(x-1)y''-xy'+y=(x-1)^2e^x: \qquad y(x)=C_1x+C_2e^x+e^xx\left(\frac{x}{2}-1\right), \tag{1.508a, b}$$

where (C_1, C_2) are arbitrary constants, determined by boundary conditions. For example, the two-point boundary conditions (1.509a, b) lead to the values (1.509a, c) for the arbitrary constants appearing in the complete integral (1.508b), implying (1.509d):

$$\alpha=y(0)=C_2, \qquad \beta=y(1)=C_1+e\left(C_2-\frac{1}{2}\right)=C_1+e\left(\alpha-\frac{1}{2}\right):$$
$$y(x)=e^x\left(\frac{x^2}{2}-x+\alpha\right)+x\left(\beta-e\alpha+\frac{e}{2}\right). \tag{1.509a–d}$$

The passage from the complete integral (1.503a; 1.507a, b) of the differential equation (1.502b) to the particular case (1.508a) uses the forcing function (1.510a), leading to the integrals (1.507a, b) ≡ (1.510b, c):

$$B(x)=(x-1)^2e^x: \; C_1(x)-C_1=-\int^x e^\xi\, d\xi=-e^x, \; C_2(x)-C_2=\int^x\xi\, d\xi=\frac{x^2}{2}; \tag{1.510a–c}$$

substitution of (1.510b, c) in (1.503a) gives (1.508b).

NOTE 1.5: Influence or Green Function as the Fundamental Solution

The **influence or Green function** is the **fundamental solution** of a linear differential equation forced by a unit impulse (III.7.71a) ≡ (1.511):

$$\left\{L\left(\frac{d}{dx}\right)\right\}G(x;\xi) \equiv \sum_{n=1}^{N} A_n(x)\frac{d^n}{dx^n}\left[G(x;\xi)\right] = \delta(x-\xi), \tag{1.511}$$

and depends also on the boundary conditions. *The principle of superposition holds (subsection III.7.6.2 ≡ subsection 1.2.1) for a linear differential operator, and supplies (standard XLVI) the complete integral (1.512a) for arbitrary forcing by a continuous function (1.513a) in terms of the influence function (1.512b):*

$$\left\{L\left(\frac{d}{dx}\right)\right\}y(x) = B(x): \qquad y(x) = \int B(\xi)G(x;\xi)d\xi. \tag{1.512a, b}$$

The proof of (1.511; 1.512a, b) is based on the property (1.513b) ≡ (III.3.15a) of the unit impulse relative to a continuous function (1.513a) ≡ (III.3.12):

$$B \in C(|R): \qquad \int_{-\infty}^{+\infty} B(\xi)\delta(x-\xi)d\xi = B(x). \tag{1.513a, b}$$

The proof assumes that the integral (1.512b) is uniformly convergent with regard to x and thus, (I.13.40) the derivatives with regard to x can be brought out of the integration sign:

$$\begin{aligned} B(x) &= \int_{-\infty}^{+\infty} B(\xi)\left\{L\left(\frac{d}{dx}\right)\right\}G(x;\xi)d\xi \\ &= \left\{L\left(\frac{d}{dx}\right)\right\}\int_{-\infty}^{+\infty} B(\xi)G(x;\xi)d\xi = \left\{L\left(\frac{d}{dx}\right)\right\}y(x); \end{aligned} \tag{1.514a, b}$$

thus, substituting (1.511) in (1.513b) yields (1.514a), which proves (1.514b) ≡ (1.512b). The influence function may also be defined for a non-linear differential equation:

$$F\left(G(x;\xi)\frac{d}{dx}\left[G(x;\xi)\right],\ldots,\frac{d^N}{dx^N}\left[G(x;\xi)\right]\right) = \delta(x-\xi), \tag{1.515}$$

but in this case, the principle of superposition (1.512b) does not generally hold. The linear (non-linear) influence functions have been obtained for a concentrated transverse force applied to: (i) an elastic string supported at both ends and causing its deflection with small (large) slope (chapter III.2); (ii) an elastic bar with clamped, pinned, sliding, free, or other means of support at the ends and subject to weak (strong) bending (chapter III.4). The influence function has also been obtained for the Laplace operator in two, three, or higher dimensions (chapter III.9). All these are applications of the generalized function unit impulse in one (chapters III.1 and III.3) and several (chapter III.5) dimensions to the Green function (chapter III.7) of differential equations. The influence or Green function for the linear differential equation (1.511) of order N with variable coefficients can be determined from the solution of the unforced equation, assuming that the latter is known (note 1.6).

NOTE 1.6: Continuity and Jump Conditions for the Green Function

Assume that the solution of the unforced linear differential equation with variable coefficients (1.516a) is known (1.516b):

$$\left\{L\left(\frac{d}{dx}\right)\right\}y(x)=0: \qquad y(x)=f(x;C_1,\ldots,C_N), \tag{1.516a, b}$$

involving N arbitrary constants of integration $(C_1,\ldots,C_N)$. Since the unit impulse is zero for non-zero argument (1.517a, b) ≡ (III.1.34a, b):

$$\delta(x-\xi)=\begin{cases} 0 & \text{if} \quad x\neq\xi, & (1.517a)\\ \infty & \text{if} \quad x=\xi, & (1.517b)\end{cases}$$

the solution (1.516b) applies to the Green function (1.511) both before $x<\xi$ (after $x>\xi$) the point $x=\xi$ with generally distinct sets of N constants of integration $(D_1,\ldots,D_N)\left[(E_1,\ldots,E_N)\right]$ in (1.518a) [(1.518b):

$$\delta(x-\xi)=\begin{cases} f(x;D_1,\ldots,D_N) & \text{if} \quad x<\xi, & (1.518a)\\ f(x;E_1,\ldots,E_N) & \text{if} \quad x>\xi. & (1.518b)\end{cases}$$

In (1.518a, b) there are a total of $2N$ constants of integration, whereas the general integral of a differential equation of order N can have only N arbitrary constants determined from boundary conditions. Thus, these must be another N independent and compatible conditions holding across $x=\xi$, where (1.516a, b) or (1.518a, b) do not hold.

The primitive of the Dirac unit impulse (1.517a, b) is the Heaviside unit jump (1.519a–c) ≡ (III.1.28a–c):

$$H(x-\xi) \equiv \delta^{(-1)}(x-\xi) = \int_0^x \delta(\eta-\xi)\,d\eta = \begin{cases} 0 & \text{if} \quad x<\xi, & (1.519a) \\ 1/2 & \text{if} \quad x=\xi, & (1.519b) \\ 1 & \text{if} \quad x>\xi, & (1.519c) \end{cases}$$

which has a unit jump at $x=\xi$. The n-th order primitive of the Heaviside unit jump (1.519a–c) is the **n-th power ramp function** (1.519d, e) ≡ (III.3.70a, b):

$$H^{(-n)}(x-\xi) = \delta^{(-1-n)}(x-\xi) = \begin{cases} 0 & \text{if} \quad x \le \xi, & (1.519d) \\ \dfrac{(x-\xi)^n}{n!} & \text{if} \quad x \ge \xi, & (1.519e) \end{cases}$$

which is continuous at $x=\xi$. It follows *that the Green or influence function of an n-th order differential* equation (1.511)*: (i) has a unit jump at $x=\xi$ for the derivative of order $N-1$ in (1.520a):*

$$G^{(N-1)}(\xi+0;\xi) - G^{(N-1)}(\xi+0;\xi) = 1;\ M=0,\ldots,N-2: G^{(M)}(\xi+0;\xi) = G^{(M)}(\xi-0;\xi). \tag{1.520a–c}$$

(ii) the Green function and all the derivatives (1.520b) up to order $N-2$ are continuous (1.520c). Thus, the fundamental solution or influence, or Green function of a differential equation (1.511) forced by a unit impulse applied at $x=\xi$, consists of the unforced (1.516a) solutions (1.516b) before (1.518a) and after (1.518b) involving two sets of N constants of integration $(D_1,\ldots,D_N)$ and $(E_1,\ldots,E_N)$: (i) the second set is related to the first by N matching conditions across $x=\xi$ stating the continuity of the Green function and its first $N-2$ derivatives (1.520b, c) and the unit jump (1.520a) of the derivative of order $N-1$; (ii) the first set is determined from N independent and compatible boundary conditions.

NOTE 1.7: Matching and Boundary Conditions for the Green Function

Consider as example the linear second-order differential equation (1.521), where the coefficient of the higher-order derivative is unity:

$$y'' + \frac{1}{x}y' - \frac{1}{x^2}y = B(x). \tag{1.521}$$

The corresponding unforced (1.522a) differential equation (1.522b) has homogeneous coefficients:

$$B(x)=0: \qquad x^2y''+xy'-y=0, \tag{1.522a, b}$$

leading to the characteristic polynomial (1.523a) and hence, (subsection 1.6.2) general integral (1.523b):

$$0=P_2(\delta)=\delta(\delta-1)+\delta-1=\delta^2-1=(\delta-1)(\delta+1): \quad y(x)=C_1x+\frac{C_2}{x}. \tag{1.523a, b}$$

The Green function (1.524b) of the linear second-order homogeneous differential equation (1.521) corresponds to forcing (1.524a) by a unit impulse with the same factor unity as the higher-order derivative:

$$B(x)=\delta(x-\xi): \qquad \left\{\frac{d^2}{dx^2}+\frac{1}{x}\frac{d}{dx}-\frac{1}{x^2}\right\}G(x;\xi)=\delta(x-\xi). \tag{1.524a, b}$$

For $x>\xi\,(x<\xi)$ the RHS of (1.524b) is zero and thus the general integral is (1.523b) with distinct constants of integration $(D_1,D_2)[(E_1,E_2)]$ in (1.525a) [(1.525b)]:

$$G(x;\xi)=\begin{cases} D_1\,x+\dfrac{D_2}{x} & \text{if} \quad 0\le x<\xi, \qquad (1.525a)\\[2ex] E_1\,x+\dfrac{E_2}{x} & \text{if} \quad \xi<x\le L. \qquad (1.525b)\end{cases}$$

The four constants (D_1,D_2,E_1,E_2) may be determined by: (i) two boundary conditions at the ends of the interval $(0, L)$; (ii) two matching conditions at $x=\xi$.

Choosing zero boundary condition (1.526a) [(1.526c)] at the ends of the interval $(0, L)$:

$$0=G(0;\xi) \;\Rightarrow\; D_2=0, \quad 0=G(L;\xi)=E_1L+\frac{E_2}{L} \;\Rightarrow\; E_2=-E_1L^2, \tag{1.526a–d}$$

determines one constant (1.526b) [relates two constants (1.526d)] in the Green function (1.525a) [(1.525b)] leading to (1.527a) [(1.527b)]:

$$G(x;\xi)=\begin{cases} D_1\,x & \text{if} \quad 0\le x\le\xi, \qquad (1.527a)\\[2ex] E_1\left(x-\dfrac{L^2}{x}\right) & \text{if} \quad \xi\le x\le L. \qquad (1.527b)\end{cases}$$

The matching conditions at $x=\xi$ are the continuity of the Green function (1.528a) and the unit jump of its first-order derivative (1.528b):

$$0=G(\xi+0;\xi)-G(\xi-0;\xi)=E_1\left(\xi-\frac{L^2}{\xi}\right)-D_1\,\xi, \tag{1.528a}$$

$$1=G'(\xi+0;\xi)-G'(\xi-0;\xi)=E_1\left(1+\frac{L^2}{\xi^2}\right)-D_1. \tag{1.528b}$$

Solving (1.528a, b) for (D_1, E_1):

$$E_1=\frac{\xi^2}{2\,L^2},\qquad D_1=\frac{1}{2}\left(\frac{\xi^2}{L^2}-1\right), \tag{1.529a, b}$$

specifies the remaining constants of integration in the (1.527a, b) Green function (1.530a, b):

$$G(x;\xi)=\begin{cases}\dfrac{x}{2}\left(\dfrac{\xi^2}{L^2}-1\right) & \text{if}\quad 0\le x\le\xi, \quad (1.530a)\\[2ex] \dfrac{\xi^2}{2L^2}\left(x-\dfrac{L^2}{x}\right) & \text{if}\quad \xi\le x\le L. \quad (1.530b)\end{cases}$$

The derivative (1.531a, b) of the Green function (1.530a, b):

$$G'(x;\xi)\equiv\frac{d}{dx}\left[G(x;\xi)\right]=\begin{cases}\dfrac{1}{2}\left(\dfrac{\xi^2}{L^2}-1\right) & \text{if}\quad 0\le x<\xi, \quad (1.531a)\\[2ex] \dfrac{\xi^2}{2L^2}\left(1+\dfrac{L^2}{x^2}\right) & \text{if}\quad \xi<x\le L, \quad (1.531b)\end{cases}$$

confirms that the slopes after (1.532a) and before (1.532b) $x=\xi$ differ by unity (1.528b):

$$G'(\xi+0;\xi)=\frac{\xi^2}{2L^2}+\frac{1}{2},\quad G'(\xi-0;\xi)=\frac{\xi^2}{2L^2}-\frac{1}{2};\quad G(\xi;\xi)=\frac{\xi}{2}\left(\frac{\xi^2}{L^2}-1\right), \tag{1.532a–c}$$

the continuity (1.528a) of the Green function (1.530a, b) at $x=\xi$ is satisfied with the value (1.532c). The boundary condition (1.526a) [(1.526c)] is satisfied by (1.530a) [(1.530b)] completing the check that (1.530a, b) has all the properties of a Green function.

NOTE 1.8: General and Particular Forcing Functions

It has been shown that *the linear second-order differential equation (1.521) ≡ (1.533d) forced by a function (1.533a) continuous in the interval (0, L) and with boundary conditions (1.533b, c):*

$$B \in C(0,L); \qquad y(0)=0=y(L): \qquad y'' - \frac{1}{x}y' + \frac{1}{x^2}y'' = B(x), \tag{1.533a–d}$$

has solution:

$$y(x) = \left(x - \frac{L^2}{x}\right)\int_0^x \frac{\xi^2}{2L^2} B(\xi)\, d\xi + \frac{x}{2}\int_x^L \left(\frac{\xi^2}{L^2} - 1\right) B(\xi)\, d\xi, \tag{1.534}$$

obtained substituting the Green or influence function (1.530a) [(1.530b)] in the superposition principle, and noting that it applies for $x<\xi$ $(x>\xi)$ that is in the interval (x, L) [(0, x)]. The particular forcing function (1.535a) leads to the solution (1.535c) of the differential equation (1.535b) with boundary conditions (1.533b, c):

$$B(x)=1: \qquad x^2y'' - xy' + y = x^2, \qquad y(x) = \frac{x}{3}(x-L). \tag{1.535a–c}$$

The result (1.535c) is obtained by substituting (1.535a) in (1.534):

$$\begin{aligned} y(x) &= \left(x - \frac{L^2}{x}\right)\int_0^x \frac{\xi^2}{2L^2}\, d\xi + \frac{x}{2}\int_x^L \left(\frac{\xi^2}{L^2} - 1\right) d\xi \\ &= \frac{x^3}{6L^2}\left(x - \frac{L^2}{x}\right) + \frac{x}{2}\left[\frac{\xi^3}{3L^2} - \xi\right]_x^L = \frac{x}{3}(x-L). \end{aligned} \tag{1.536}$$

The method of the Green function provides the solution of the differential equation (1.533d) forced by an arbitrary continuous function (1.533a); the particular case (1.535b) can be solved by an alternative method as a check on the solution (1.153c). The linear second-order differential equation (1.535c) has homogeneous coefficients and a characteristic polynomial (1.523a), and hence the particular integral of the forced equation is (1.537a):

$$y_*(x) = \frac{x^2}{P_2(2)} = \frac{x^2}{3}; \qquad y(x) = C_1 x + \frac{C_2}{x} + \frac{x^2}{3}, \tag{1.537a, b}$$

adding to (1.537a) the general integral (1.523b) of the unforced equation (1.522b) specifies the complete integral (1.537b) of the forced equation. The boundary conditions (1.526a, c) ≡ (1.538a, c) specify the constants (1.538b, d):

$$0 = y(0) \Rightarrow C_2 = 0; \qquad 0 = y(L) \Rightarrow C_1 = -\frac{L}{3}; \qquad y(x) = \frac{x}{3}(x - L), \quad (1.538\text{a–e})$$

substitution of (1.538b, d) in (1.537b) yields (1.538e) ≡ (1.535c), confirming the result obtained via the Green function.

NOTE 1.9: **Fourier Series for Forcing in a Finite Interval**

A finite interval can be mapped by translation to have the origin as the middle point (1.539a) and a **partition** of the interval is an increasing sequence of points (1.539b):

$$-L \le x \le L: \qquad -L \equiv x_0 < x_1 < x_2 < .... < x_N \equiv +L. \qquad (1.539\text{a, b})$$

The **oscillation** of a function in the interval (1.539a) for the partition (1.539b) is the sum of the moduli of successive differences:

$$F\left(f(x); x_0, ..., x_N\right) = \sum_{n=1}^{N} \left| f(x_n - 0) - f(x_{n-1} + 0) \right|, \qquad (1.539\text{c})$$

where the function need not be continuous. The **functions of bounded oscillation** in the interval have a finite oscillation for any partition:

$$\mathcal{F}(-L_1 + L) \equiv \left\{ f(x): \;\; F\left(f(x); -L \equiv x_0, x_1, ..., x_{N-1}, x_N \equiv +L\right) \le C < \infty \right\}. \qquad (1.539\text{d})$$

A function with **bounded oscillation** in a symmetric interval (1.540a) has (II.5.168a–c) a **Fourier series** (1.540b) with coefficients (1.540c):

$$B \in \mathcal{F}) - L, +L): \;\; B(x) = \sum_{n=-\infty}^{+\infty} B_n \exp\left(\frac{in\pi x}{L}\right), \;\; B_n = \frac{1}{2L} \int_{-L}^{+L} B(x) \exp\left(-\frac{in\pi x}{L}\right) dx. \qquad (1.540\text{a–c})$$

Thus, *the forcing of a linear differential equation with constant coefficients (1.52a) by a function of bounded oscillation (1.540a) ≡ (1.539a–d) in a finite interval, and specified by its Fourier series (1.540b, c), leads (standard XLVII) to the particular integral (1.541b) assuming there are no resonant terms (1.541a):*

$$P_N\left(\frac{in\pi}{L}\right) \ne 0: \qquad y_*(x) = \sum_{n=-\infty}^{+\infty} \frac{B_n}{P_N(in\pi / L)} \exp\left(\frac{inx}{L}\right); \qquad (1.541\text{a, b})$$

if any term has a resonance (1.541a) of order M for one value m of n:

$$P_N(D) \sim O\left(\left(D - \frac{im\pi}{L}\right)^M\right): \qquad y_*(x) = \sum_{\substack{n=-\infty \\ n \neq m}}^{+\infty} \frac{B_n e^{in\pi x/L}}{P_N(in\pi/L)} + \frac{B_m x^M e^{im\pi/L}}{P_N^{(M)}(im\pi/L)}, \tag{1.542a, b}$$

then: (i) all terms in (1.541b) with $m \neq n$ are retained in (1.542a) in the form (1.129a, b); (ii) only the resonant n-th term is replaced in the form (1.134a, b).

NOTE 1.10: Non-Resonant and Resonant Terms in a Discrete Spectrum

As an example of the preceding theory (note 1.9), consider a linear biquadratic differential equation with constant coefficients (1.543b) forced by an arbitrary function with finite oscillation in a finite interval (1.543a) ≡ (1.539a–d):

$$B \in \mathcal{F})-L,+L): \qquad y'''' + \left(a^2 + b^2\right)y'' + a^2b^2y = B(x). \tag{1.543a, b}$$

The characteristic polynomial:

$$P_4(D) = D^4 + \left(a^2 + b^2\right)D^2 + a^2b^2 = \left(D^2 + a^2\right)\left(D^2 + b^2\right), \tag{1.544}$$

leads to the following particular integrals corresponding to **discrete spectra**: (i) in the absence of resonance (1.545b) when (1.545a) applies for all integers n:

$$\pm a \neq \frac{n\pi}{L} \neq \pm b: \qquad y_*(x) = \sum_{n=-\infty}^{+\infty} \frac{B_n e^{in\pi x/L}}{\left(a^2 - n^2\pi^2/L^2\right)\left(b^2 - n^2\pi^2/L^2\right)}; \tag{1.545a, b}$$

(ii) if there is (1.546a), one resonant term $n = m$ for a (or b) with $b \neq a$, the corresponding n-th term in (1.545b) is replaced by (1.546b):

$$\frac{m\pi}{L} = a \neq b: \qquad \frac{B_m}{b^2 - m^2\pi^2/L^2} \lim_{a \to m\pi/L} \frac{(\partial/\partial a)\, e^{iax}}{(\partial/\partial a)\left(a^2 - m^2\pi^2/L^2\right)}$$

$$= \frac{B_m}{b^2 - m^2\pi^2/L^2} \lim_{a \to m\pi/L} \frac{ix}{2a} e^{iax} = i\frac{B_m L}{2m\pi} \frac{x e^{im\pi x/L}}{b^2 - m^2\pi^2/L^2}; \tag{1.546a, b}$$

(iii) if $a = b$ and one value m of n satisfies (1.547a) then the n-th term in (1.545b) is replaced by (1.547b):

$$\frac{m\pi}{L} = a = b: \qquad B_m \lim_{a \to m\pi/L} \frac{\left(\partial^2/\partial a^2\right) e^{iax}}{\left(\partial^2/\partial a^2\right)\left[\left(a^2 - m^2\pi^2/L^2\right)^2\right]}$$

$$= \frac{B_m}{4} \lim_{a \to m\pi/L} \frac{(ix)^2 e^{iax}}{3a^2 - m^2\pi^2/L^2} = -\frac{B_m L^2}{8m^2\pi^2} x^2 e^{im\pi x/L}, \tag{1.547a, b}$$

corresponding to a double resonance.

NOTE 1.11: **Fournier Integral for Forcing on the Real Line**

A function is **absolutely integrable** if its modulus is integrable:

$$\mathcal{L}^1(|R) \equiv \left\{ f(x): \int_{-\infty}^{+\infty} |f(x)|\, dx \le C < \infty \right\}. \tag{1.548}$$

A function of bounded oscillation (1.539a–d) ≡ (1.549a) and absolutely integrable (1.548) on the real line (1.549b) has **direct (inverse) Fourier transform** (1.549c) [(1.549d)]:

$$B \in \mathcal{F} \cap \mathcal{L}^1(|R): \qquad B(x) = \int_{-\infty}^{+\infty} \tilde{B}(k)\, e^{ikx} dk, \quad \tilde{B}(k) = \frac{1}{2\pi} \int_{-\infty}^{+\infty} B(x)\, e^{-ikx} dx. \tag{1.549a–d}$$

The forcing of a linear differential equation with constant coefficients (1.33) ≡ (1.34a, b) is considered, assuming that the particular integral also has a Fourier transform (1.550a) with derivatives (1.550c) up to order (1.550b):

$$y(x) = \int_{-\infty}^{+\infty} \tilde{y}(k)\, e^{ikx} dk; \qquad n = 1, \ldots, N: \quad y^{(n)}(x) = \int_{-\infty}^{+\infty} \tilde{y}(k)\, e^{ikx} (ik)^n\, dk. \tag{1.550a–c}$$

Substituting (1.549c; 1.550a, c) in the linear forced differential equation with constant coefficients (1.52a) leads to (1.551a):

$$0 = \int_{-\infty}^{+\infty} \left[\tilde{B}(k) - \tilde{y}(k) \sum_{n=0}^{N} A_n (ik)^n \right] e^{ikx} dk = \int_{-\infty}^{+\infty} \left[\tilde{B}(k) - \tilde{y}(k)\, P_N(ik) \right] e^{ikx}\, dk, \tag{1.551a, b}$$

which involves (1.551b) the characteristic polynomial (1.52b) of variable *ik*. The integral (1.551b) vanishes for arbitrary x if the term in square brackets vanishes, leading to the algebraic identity (1.552a):

$$\tilde{y}(k) = \frac{\tilde{B}(k)}{P_N(ik)}: \qquad y(x) = \int_{-\infty}^{+\infty} \frac{\tilde{B}(k)}{P_N(ik)} e^{-ikx} dk, \tag{1.552a, b}$$

substituting (1.552a) in (1.550a) leads to the (standard XLVIII) *particular integral (1.552b) of the linear differential equation with constant coefficients (1.52a) forced by a function of bounded oscillation (1.539a–d) ≡ (1.540a) and absolutely integrable (1.548) on the real line (1.549a). The Fourier integral (1.552b) can be evaluated by residues (section I.17.5)*, for example, to calculate the influence function (notes III.3.11–III.3.12) in the case of a linear differential equation of: i(ii) first (second) order in general form [note(s) III.3.13 (III.3.14-III.3.17)]; (iii) fourth-order in a particular form (example E. III.10.9); (iii) in the case of a forced biquadratic linear differential equation (note 1.12).

NOTE 1.12: Discrete (Continuous) Spectrum in a Finite (Infinite) Interval

A biquadratic linear differential equation (1.553b), similar to (1.543b) with a change of sign, is considered in a finite (1.543a) [infinite (1.553a)] interval leading to a **discrete (continuous) spectrum**:

$$B \in \mathcal{F} \cap \mathcal{L}^1(|R): \qquad y'''' - \left(a^2 + b^2\right) y'' + a^2 b^2 y = B(x), \tag{1.553a, b}$$

where the forcing function has bounded oscillation (1.539a–c) [and is absolutely integrable (1.548)]. Substituting the characteristic polynomial:

$$P_4(ik) = (ik)^4 - \left(a^2 + b^2\right)(ik)^2 + a^2 b^2 = \left(k^2 + a^2\right)\left(k^2 + b^2\right), \tag{1.554}$$

in (1.552b) specifies the particular solution of the forced equation (1.553b) as a Fourier integral:

$$y_*(x) = \int_{-\infty}^{+\infty} \frac{e^{ikx}\,\tilde{B}(k)}{\left(k^2 + a^2\right)\left(k^2 + b^2\right)} dk. \tag{1.555}$$

It is assumed that the integrand satisfies the condition (I.17.29) ≡ (1.556), allowing the path of integration along the real line to be closed by a half-circle of infinite radius:

$$\lim_{|k| \to \infty} \left| \frac{\tilde{B}(k)}{\left(k^2 + a^2\right)\left(k^2 + b^2\right)} \right| = \lim_{|k| \to \infty} \frac{\left|\tilde{B}(k)\right|}{O\left(k^4\right)} = 0; \tag{1.556}$$

furthermore:

$$|\exp(ikx)| = |\exp[ix\mathrm{Re}(k) - x\mathrm{Im}(k)]| = \exp[-x\mathrm{Im}(k)], \tag{1.557}$$

implies that the path of integration should be closed in the upper (lower) complex-k half-plane:

$$0 = \lim_{|K|\to\infty} |\exp(ikx)| \text{ for } \begin{cases} \mathrm{Im}(k) > 0 \text{ if } x > 0, & (1.558a) \\ \mathrm{Im}(k) < 0 \text{ if } x < 0, & (1.558b) \end{cases}$$

for x positive (1.558a) [negative (1.558b)].

NOTE 1.13: Evaluation of the Fournier Integral by Residues

For positive values (1.559b) of x, and $a \neq b$ in (1.559c) there are two simple poles $(+ia, +ib)$ in the upper-half complex k-plane (Figure 1.9), whose sum of residues multiplied by $2\pi i$ evaluates (1.559a) the integral (1.555) ≡ (I.17.32):

$$g(k) \equiv \frac{e^{ikx}\tilde{B}(k)}{(k^2 + a^2)(k^2 + b^2)}; \quad x >< 0; \quad a \neq b: \quad y_*(x) = \pm 2\pi i \left[g_{(1)}(\pm ia) + g_{(1)}(\pm ib) \right], \tag{1.559a–d}$$

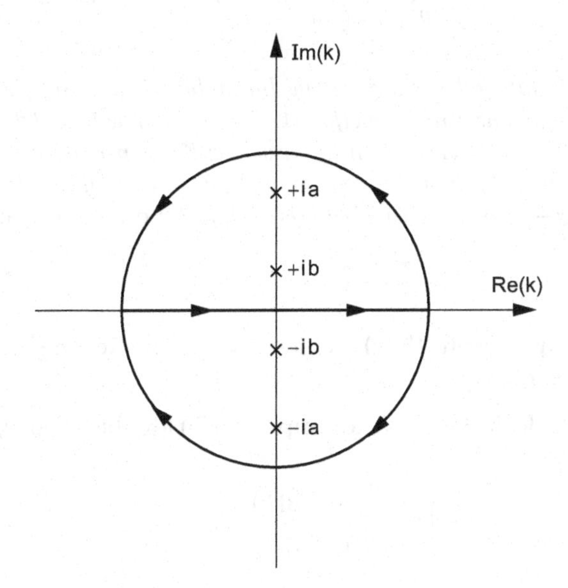

FIGURE 1.9
The particular integral of a linear differential equation with constant coefficients forced by an arbitrary function absolutely integrable and of bounded fluctuation on the real line can be obtained using the Fourier transform; this leads to an integral along the real axis that may be closed by a large half-circle in the upper or lower complex half-plane and evaluated by the residues in the interior, in the present case four simple poles that can coalesce to two double poles.

with integrand (1.559a); a similar expression (1.559d) holds for $x<0$ changing $\left(\pm 2\pi i, \pm ia, \pm ib\right)$. The residues at the simple poles $\pm ia$ are given (I.15.24b) ≡ (1.205) by (1.560):

$$g_{(1)}(\pm ia) = \lim_{k\to\pm ia}(k\mp ia)\,g(k) = \lim_{k\to\pm ia}\frac{e^{ikx}\,\tilde{B}(k)}{(k\pm ia)(k+ib)(k-ib)}$$
$$= \frac{e^{\mp ax}\;\tilde{B}(\pm ia)}{\pm 2ia\,(\pm ia-ib)(\pm ia+ib)} = \pm\frac{ie^{\mp ax}\;\tilde{B}(\pm ia)}{2a\left(a^2-b^2\right)}. \quad (1.560)$$

The residues at the simple poles at $\pm ib$ are evaluated (1.561b) interchanging (a, b) in (1.560) ≡ (1.561a):

$$g_{(1)}(\pm ia) = \pm\frac{ie^{\mp ax}\tilde{B}(\pm ia)}{2a\left(a^2-b^2\right)}, \qquad g_{(1)}(\pm ib) = \pm\frac{ie^{\mp bx}\tilde{B}(\pm ib)}{2b\left(b^2-a^2\right)}. \quad (1.561\text{a, b})$$

Substituting (1.561a, b) in (1.559d) leads to:

$$a\neq b;\quad x><0:\qquad y_*(x) = \frac{\pi}{b^2-a^2}\left[\frac{e^{\mp ax}}{a}\,\tilde{B}(\pm ia) - \frac{e^{\mp bx}}{b}\,\tilde{B}(\pm ib)\right], \quad (1.562\text{a–c})$$

as the particular integral (1.562c) of the linear biquadratic differential equation (1.553b), forced by an arbitrary function (1.553a) of bounded oscillation (1.539a–d) and absolutely integrable (1.548) on the real line; the upper (lower) sign holds for positive (negative) x, and in both cases the solution vanishes at infinity $|x|\to\infty$*, that is, for* $x\to+\infty\,(x\to-\infty)$*. The case* $a=b$ *is excluded,* because it leads to double poles (note 1.14).

NOTE 1.14: Simple (Multiple) Poles for Non-Resonant (Resonant) Responses

The case (1.562a) [(1.563a)] leads to simple (1.555) [double (1.563b)] poles:

$$a=b:\qquad y_*(x) = \int_{-\infty}^{+\infty}\frac{e^{ikx}\;\tilde{B}(k)}{\left(k^2+a^2\right)^2}\,dk, \quad (1.563\text{a, b})$$

and implies non-resonant (resonant) responses [note 1.13 (1.14)]. The same arguments (1.556; 1.557; 1.558a, b) allow the evaluation of (1.563b):

$$x><0:\qquad y_*(x) = \pm 2\pi i g_{(2)}(\pm ia), \quad (1.564\text{a, b})$$

using the residue at the double pole (II.15.33b) ≡ (1.210) at $\pm ia$:

$$g_{(2)}(\pm ia) = \lim_{k \to \pm ia} \frac{d}{dk}\left[(k \mp ia)^2 g(k)\right] = \lim_{k \to \pm ia} \frac{d}{dk}\left[\frac{e^{ikx}\tilde{B}(k)}{(k \pm ia)^2}\right]; \qquad (1.565a)$$

the residue consists of three terms:

$$\begin{aligned} g_{(2)}(\pm ia) &= \lim_{k \to \pm ia} e^{ikx}\left[-\frac{2\tilde{B}(k)}{(k \pm ia)^3} + \frac{ix\tilde{B}(k) + \tilde{B}'(k)}{(k \pm ia)^2}\right] \\ &= e^{\mp ax}\left\{\mp i\frac{\tilde{B}(\pm ia)}{4a^3} - \frac{1}{4a^2}\left[ix\tilde{B}(\pm ia) + \tilde{B}'(\pm ia)\right]\right\}. \end{aligned} \qquad (1.565b)$$

Substituting (1.565b) in (1.563b) specifies:

$$x >< 0: \qquad y_*(x) = e^{\mp ax}\frac{\pi}{2a^2}\left[\left(\frac{1}{a} \pm x\right)\tilde{B}(\pm ia) \mp i\tilde{B}'(\pm ia)\right], \qquad (1.566)$$

as the *particular integral of the biquadratic (1.553a, b) linear differential equation with constant coefficients with (1.567b) double roots (1.567a) of the characteristic polynomial (1.554) ≡ (1.567c):*

$$a = b: \qquad y'''' - 2a^2 y'' + a^4 y = B(x), \qquad P_4(ik) = \left(k^2 + a^2\right)^2, \qquad (1.567a–c)$$

leading to double poles and the resonant response (1.566) involving a growing amplitude factor x dominated as $|x| \to \infty$ *by the exponential* $\exp(-a|x|) \to 0$. *The forcing function is of bounded oscillation and absolutely integrable on the real line (1.553a); the resonance implies also the appearance of the derivative* $\tilde{B}'(k)$ *of the spectrum* $\tilde{B}(k)$ *at the double poles* $k = \pm ia$.

NOTE 1.15: Laplace Transform for Forcing on the Positive Real Line

In order to compare with the harmonic oscillator (chapter 2), the independent (dependent) variable is chosen to be time t (position x) in the linear differential equation of order N with constant coefficients:

$$\left\{P_N\left(\frac{d}{dt}\right)\right\}x(t) = B(t), \qquad P_N\left(\frac{d}{dt}\right) = \sum_{n=0}^{N} A_n \frac{d^n}{dt^n}. \qquad (1.568a, b)$$

The solution will be sought using both for the **response** $x(t)$ and the **forcing** $B(t)$ using the representation as a **Laplace transform**:

$$\bar{B}(s) \equiv \mathcal{L}\left[B(t); t \to s\right] \equiv \int_0^\infty B(t)\, e^{-st}\, dt. \tag{1.569}$$

Bearing in mind that:

$$\left|e^{-st}\right| = \left|\exp\left[-t\,\mathrm{Re}(s) - it\mathrm{Im}(s)\right]\right| = \left|\exp\left[-t\,\mathrm{Re}(s)\right]\right| \left|\exp\left[-it\mathrm{Im}(s)\right]\right| = \exp\left[-t\,\mathrm{Re}(s)\right], \tag{1.570}$$

it follows that for a function absolutely integrable (1.548) on the positive real line (1.571a):

$$f \in \mathcal{L}^1(0,+\infty); \quad \mathrm{Re}(s) > 0: \quad \left|\bar{B}(s)\right| \le \int_0^\infty \left|B(t)\, e^{-st}\right| dt$$

$$\le \int_0^\infty \left|B(t)\right|\, e^{-t\,\mathrm{Re}(s)}\, dt \le \int_0^\infty \left|B(t)\right| dt < C, \tag{1.571a–c}$$

the Laplace transform is bounded (1.571c) in the RHS complex-s half-plane (1.571b):

$$f \in \mathcal{L}^1(0,+\infty) \quad \Rightarrow \quad \bar{B} \in \mathcal{B}\left(\mathrm{Re}(s) > 0\right). \tag{1.572a, b}$$

A function is **bounded** in a set A if its modulus does not exceed a finite value at any point:

$$B(A) \equiv \left\{ f(x): \qquad \exists_{M \in |R} \forall_{x \in A} \quad \Rightarrow \quad \left|f(x)\right| < M \right\}. \tag{1.573}$$

A function absolutely integrable (1.548) on the positive real line must vanish at infinity. The condition of absolute integrability is too strict, since there are functions not absolutely integrable in the positive real axis that have a Laplace transform. The simplest example is the constant function unity (1.574a), which has Laplace transform (1.574c) on the RHS complex-s half-plane (1.574b):

$$f(x) = 1: \qquad \mathrm{Re}(s) > 0: \qquad \bar{f}(s) = \int_0^\infty e^{-st} dt = -\frac{1}{s}\left[e^{-st}\right]_0^\infty = \frac{1}{s}. \tag{1.574a–c}$$

A more general set of sufficient conditions for the existence of the Laplace transform is given next.

For the existence of the Laplace transform (1.569) of a function it is sufficient that it satisfies the following three conditions: (i) the scaling at the origin (1.575b) is at most like a power with real part of the exponent (1.575a) greater than minus unity; (ii) it is absolutely integrable in a finite interval (1.575c); (iii) the asymptotic scaling does not exceed that of an exponential (1.575e), in which case the Laplace transform exists (Figure 1.10) *for (1.575d):*

$$\operatorname{Re}(a) > -1: \quad f(t) \sim O\left(t^a\right); \quad \int_A^B |f(t)|\, dt < M < \infty; \tag{1.575a–c}$$

$$\operatorname{Re}(s) \geq \mu > 0, \quad \exists_{\mu \in |R} \forall_{t \geq B}: \quad f(t) \leq C e^{\mu t}. \tag{1.575d–e}$$

The proof is made dividing the Laplace integral (1.569) in three intervals (1.576a, b):

$$|\bar{f}(s)| \leq \left|\int_0^A f(t) e^{-st} dt\right| + \left|\int_A^B f(t) e^{-st} dt\right| + \left|\int_B^\infty f(t) e^{-st} dt\right| \equiv I_1 + I_2 + I_3, \tag{1.576a, b}$$

where: (i) the first integral has upper bound (1.576d) for (1.575a) ≡ (1.576a):

$$\operatorname{Re}(a) > -1: \quad I_1 \leq \int_0^A t^a \left|e^{-st}\right| dt \leq \int_0^A t^a\, dt = \left[\frac{t^{a+1}}{a+1}\right]_0^A = \frac{A^{a+1}}{a+1}; \tag{1.576c, d}$$

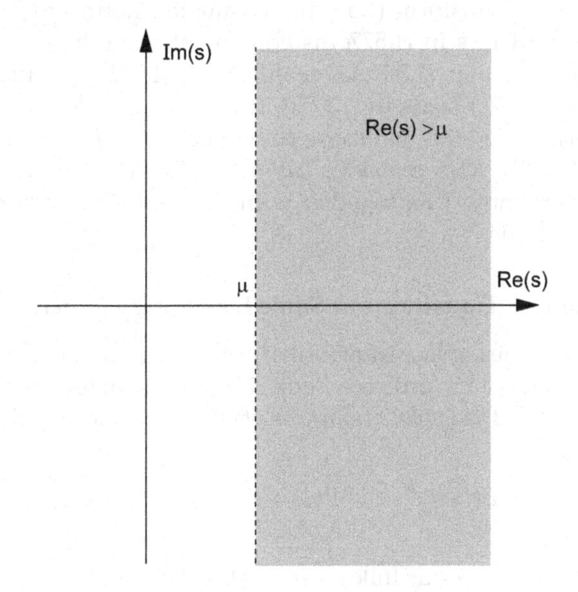

FIGURE 1.10
The complete integral of a linear differential equation forced by an arbitrary function absolutely integrable on the finite positive real line and of slow growth at infinity may be obtained using the Laplace transform, which is usually valid in a complex-s half-plane to the right of a fixed value $\operatorname{Re}(s) > \mu$ for example, $\mu = 0$.

(ii) the last integral has upper bound (1.576f) for (1.575d) ≡ (1.576e):

$$\operatorname{Re}(s) > \mu > 0: \quad I_3 \le \int_0^\infty |f(t)|\,|e^{-st}|\,dt \le C\int_B^\infty \exp\{[\mu - \operatorname{Re}(s)]t\}\,dt = \frac{C}{\mu - \operatorname{Re}(s)}. \tag{1.576e, f}$$

(iii) the middle integral has upper bound (1.576h) for (1.575d) ≡ (1.576g):

$$\operatorname{Re}(s) > 0: \quad I_2 \le \int_A^B |f(t)|\,|e^{-st}|\,dt \le \int_A^B |f(t)|\,e^{-t\operatorname{Re}(s)}\,dt \le \int_A^B |f(t)|\,dt < M. \tag{1.576g, h}$$

The sum (1.576b) of three bounded terms (1.576d, f, h) is bounded. QED. For example, the power (1.577a) with non-negative integer exponent (1.577a) grows slower than any exponential at infinity (1.575e) and thus, the Laplace transform exists (1.575d) for (1.577c):

$$n \in |N_0, \qquad f(t) = t^n, \qquad \operatorname{Re}(s) > 0: \tag{1.577a–c}$$

$$\bar{f}(t) = \int_0^\infty t^n e^{-st}\,dt = \left(-\frac{d}{ds}\right)\int_0^\infty e^{-st}\,dt = \left(-\frac{d}{ds}\right)^n \frac{1}{s} = \frac{n!}{s^{n+1}}, \tag{1.577d–f}$$

where the Laplace transform (1.577d) is evaluated noting that: (i) differentiation with regard to s in (1.577e) is equivalent to multiplication by $-t$ in (1.577d); (ii) the integral in (1.577e) is evaluated by (1.574c); (iii) the differentiation n times in (1.577e) leads to (1.577f). It follows that *the Laplace transform (1.569) of a power (1.577b) is an inverse power (1.577f) with a factorial coefficient and is bounded on the RHS complex-s half-plane (1.577c).* This result (1.577a–f) is confirmed next (note 1.16) together with the Laplace transforms of other elementary functions.

NOTE 1.16: Laplace Transforms of Some Elementary Functions

Rather than invert the Laplace transform (1.569) a small Table 1.7 (1.8) of Laplace transforms of elementary ordinary (note 1.16) [generalized (note 1.24)] functions is established. *The Laplace transform of an exponential (1.578b) is (1.578c):*

$$\operatorname{Re}(s) > \operatorname{Re}(b): \qquad B(t) = e^{bt}, \qquad \bar{B}(s) = \frac{1}{s-b}, \tag{1.578a–c}$$

valid for (1.578a) ≡ (1.579a), as follows from (1.579b):

$$\operatorname{Re}(s) > \operatorname{Re}(b): \qquad \int_0^\infty e^{-(s-b)t}\,dt = \left[-\frac{e^{-(s-b)t}}{s-b}\right]_0^\infty = \frac{1}{s-b}; \tag{1.579a, b}$$

TABLE 1.7

Laplace Transforms of Some Elementary Ordinary Functions

Ordinary Function	**Laplace Transform**	**Domain of Validity**
$f(x)$	$\bar{f}(s)$	$s \in D$
1	$\frac{1}{s}$	$\text{Re}(s) > 0$
x^n	s^{-1-n}	$\text{Re}(s) > 0$
e^{bx}	$\frac{1}{s-b}$	$\text{Re}(s) > \text{Re}(a)$
$x^n e^{bx}$	$(s-b)^{-1-n}$	$\text{Re}(s) > \text{Re}(b)$
$\cosh(cx)$	$\frac{s}{s^2-c^2}$	$\text{Re}(s) > \lvert\text{Re}(c)\rvert$
$\sinh(cx)$	$\frac{c}{s^2-c^2}$	$\text{Re}(s) > \lvert\text{Re}(c)\rvert$
$\cos(ax)$	$\frac{s}{s^2+a^2}$	$\text{Re}(s) > \lvert\text{Im}(a)\rvert$
$\sin(ax)$	$\frac{a}{s^2+a^2}$	$\text{Re}(s) > \lvert\text{Im}(a)\rvert$
$x\cosh(cx)$	$\frac{s^2+c^2}{\left(s^2-c^2\right)^2}$	$\text{Re}(s) > \lvert\text{Re}(c)\rvert$
$x\sinh(cx)$	$\frac{2cs}{\left(s^2-c^2\right)^2}$	$\text{Re}(s) > \lvert\text{Re}(c)\rvert$
$x\cos(ax)$	$\frac{s^2-a^2}{\left(s^2+a^2\right)^2}$	$\text{Re}(s) > \lvert\text{Im}(a)\rvert$
$x\sin(ax)$	$\frac{2as}{\left(s^2+a^2\right)^2}$	$\text{Re}(s) > \lvert\text{Im}(a)\rvert$
$e^{bx}\cosh(cx)$	$\frac{s-b}{(s-b)^2-c^2}$	$\text{Re}(s) > \text{Re}(b \pm c)$
$e^{bx}\sinh(cx)$	$\frac{c}{(s-b)^2-c^2}$	$\text{Re}(s) > \text{Re}(b \pm c)$
$e^{bx}\cos(ax)$	$\frac{s-b}{(s-b)^2+a^2}$	$\text{Re}(s) > \text{Re}(b \pm ia)$
$e^{bx}\sin(ax)$	$\frac{a}{(s-b)^2+a^2}$	$\text{Re}(s) > \text{Re}(b \pm ia)$
$\cosh(cx)\cos, \sin(ax)$	$\text{Re}, \text{Im}\left[\frac{s-ia}{(s-ia)^2-c^2}\right]$	$\text{Re}(s) > \lvert c\rvert$*

(Conitnued)

TABLE 1.7 (Conitnued)

Ordinary Function	Laplace Transform	Domain of Validity
sinh (cx) cos, sin (ax)	$\text{Re, Im}\left[\frac{c}{(s-ia)^2-c^2}\right]$	Re $(s) > \|c\|$*
e^{bx} cosh (cx) cos, sin(ax)	$\text{Re, Im}\left[\frac{s-b-ia}{(s-b-ia)^2-c^2}\right]$	Re $(s) > b \pm c$*
e^{bx} sinh (cx) cos, sin(ax)	$\text{Re, Im}\left[\frac{c}{(s-b-ia)^2-c^2}\right]$	Re $(s) > b \pm c$*

* *for real $a, b, c \in |R$*

Note: Laplace transforms of some elementary functions and their products indicating their domain of validity in the complex plane in all cases, allowing for complex parameters (a, b, c); the cases restricted to (a, b, c) real are marked with an asterisk.

the condition (1.579a) is necessary for the primitive in (1.579b) to vanish at infinity. This integral (1.579b) is uniformly convergent with regard to b, and thus, (I.13.40) differentiating n times with regard to b leads to *the Laplace transforms (1.580a, c) of a power times an exponential (1.580b):*

$$\operatorname{Re}(s) > \operatorname{Re}(b): \quad B(t) = t^n e^{bt} = \frac{\partial^n}{\partial b^n}\left(e^{bt}\right), \quad \bar{B}(s) = \frac{\partial^n}{\partial b^n}\frac{1}{s-b} = \frac{n!}{(s-b)^{n+1}}. \tag{1.580a–c}$$

The particular case $b = 0$ of (1.580a–c) confirms the Laplace transform of the power (1.577a–f). *From the Laplace transform of the exponential (1.578a–c), power (1.577a–f), and their product (1.580a–c) follow those of: (i)(ii) the hyperbolic (circular) cosine and sine (1.581a–c) [(1.582a–c)]:*

$$\operatorname{Re}(s) > |\operatorname{Re}(c)|: \qquad B(t) = \cosh, \sinh(ct) \equiv \frac{e^{ct} \pm e^{-ct}}{2},$$
$$\bar{B}(s) = \frac{1}{2}\left(\frac{1}{s-c} \pm \frac{1}{s+c}\right) = \frac{\{s, c\}}{s^2 - c^2}, \tag{1.581a–c}$$

$$\operatorname{Re}(s) > |\operatorname{Im}(a)|: \qquad B(t) = \cos, \sin(at) \equiv \frac{e^{iat} \pm e^{-iat}}{\{2, 2i\}},$$
$$\bar{B}(s) = \frac{1}{\{2, 2i\}}\left(\frac{1}{s-ia} \pm \frac{1}{s+ia}\right) = \frac{\{s, a\}}{s^2 + a^2}. \tag{1.582a–c}$$

(iii)(iv) the product of (i)(ii) by an exponential (1.583a–c) [(1.584a–c)]:

$$\mathrm{Re}(s) > \mathrm{Re}(b \pm c): \qquad B(t) = e^{bt}\cosh,\sinh(ct) = \frac{e^{(b+c)t} \pm e^{(b-c)t}}{2}$$

$$\bar{B}(s) = \frac{1}{2}\left(\frac{1}{s-b-c} \pm \frac{1}{s-b+c}\right) = \frac{\{s-b, c\}}{(s-b)^2 - c^2}, \tag{1.583a–c}$$

$$\mathrm{Re}(s) > \mathrm{Re}(b \pm ia): \qquad B(t) = e^{bt}\cos,\sin(ct) = \frac{e^{(b+ia)t} \pm e^{(b-ia)t}}{2}$$

$$\bar{B}(s) = \frac{1}{\{2, 2i\}}\left(\frac{1}{s-b-ia} \pm \frac{1}{s-b+ia}\right) = \frac{\{s-b, a\}}{(s-b)^2 + a^2}; \tag{1.584a–c}$$

(v) the product of an exponential by a hyperbolic and a circular cosine or sine (1.585a–d):

$$a, b, c \in |R; \quad \mathrm{Re}(s) > \mathrm{Re}(b \pm c \pm ia):$$

$$B(t) = e^{bt}\cosh,\sinh(ct)\cos,\sin(at) = \mathrm{Re},\mathrm{Im}\left[\frac{e^{(b+ia+c)t} \pm e^{(b+ia-c)t}}{2}\right];$$

$$\bar{B}(s) = \mathrm{Re},\mathrm{Im}\left\{\frac{1}{2}\left(\frac{1}{s-b-ia-c} \pm \frac{1}{s-b-ia+c}\right)\right\} = \mathrm{Re},\mathrm{Im}\left[\frac{\{s-b-ia, c\}}{(s-b-ia)^2 - c^2}\right], \tag{1.585a–d}$$

where $\mathrm{Re}(\mathrm{Im})$ *apply to the circular cosine (sine), and {cosh, sinh} correspond to the upper(lower) sign.* Differentiation of (1.581b, c) [(1.582b, c)] with regard to the parameter *c(a)* leads to *the Laplace transform of the product of a variable by the hyperbolic (1.586a–c) [circular (1.587a–c)] cosine and sine:*

$$\mathrm{Re}(s) > |\mathrm{Re}(\pm a)|: \qquad B(t) = t\cosh,\sinh(ct) = \frac{\partial}{\partial c}[\sinh,\cosh(ct)]$$

$$\bar{B}(s) = \frac{\partial}{\partial c}\left[\frac{\{c, s\}}{s^2 - c^2}\right] = \frac{\{s^2 + c^2, 2sc\}}{\left(s^2 - c^2\right)^2}, \tag{1.586a–c}$$

$$\mathrm{Re}(s) > |\mathrm{Im}(a)|: \qquad B(t) = t\cos,\sin(at) = \pm\frac{\partial}{\partial a}[\sin,\cos(at)]$$

$$\bar{B}(s) = \pm\frac{\partial}{\partial a}\left[\frac{\{a, s\}}{s^2 + a^2}\right] = \frac{\{s^2 - a^2, 2sa\}}{\left(s^2 + a^2\right)^2}. \tag{1.587a–c}$$

The parameters (a, b, c) may be complex in (1.579a, b; 1.580a–c; 1.581a–c; 1.582a–c; 1.583a–c; 1.584a–c; 1.586a–c; 1.587a–c) and are real (1.585a) in (1.585b–d). The conditions (1.581a) ≡ (1.588b) [(1.582a) ≡ (1.588d)]:

$$\operatorname{Re}(s) > \operatorname{Re}(\pm a) \quad \Rightarrow \quad \operatorname{Re}(s) > |\operatorname{Re}(a)|, \quad \operatorname{Re}(s) > \operatorname{Re}(\pm ia) \Rightarrow \operatorname{Re}(s) > |\operatorname{Im}(a)|, \tag{1.588a–d}$$

follow from (1.588a) [(1.588c)].

NOTE 1.17: Laplace Transform of Derivatives

In order to apply Laplace transforms to a differential equation the Laplace transforms of derivatives are needed for all orders. Starting with the first-order, an integration by parts:

$$\begin{aligned} L\{x'(t); t \to s\} &\equiv \int_0^\infty x'(t)\, e^{-st}\, dt = \int_0^\infty \left\{ \left[x(t)\, e^{-st}\right]' + s\,\bar{x}(t) e^{-st} \right\} dt \\ &= \left[x(t)\, e^{-st}\right]_0^\infty + s \int_0^\infty x(t)\, e^{-st}\, dt = -x(0) + s\,\bar{x}(s). \end{aligned} \tag{1.589a}$$

introduces one initial value:

$$y(t) = x'(t): \qquad \bar{y}(s) = s\bar{x}(s) - x(0). \tag{1.589b, c}$$

A second application of (1.589b, c) leads to (1.589d, e):

$$\begin{aligned} z(t) = y'(t) = x''(t): \qquad \bar{z}(s) &= s\bar{y}(s) - y(0) = s\left[s\bar{x}(s) - x(0)\right] - x'(0) \\ &= s^2\bar{x}(s) - sx(0) - x'(0). \end{aligned} \tag{1.589d, e}$$

The same result applied recursively n times leads to:

$$\begin{aligned} u(t) = \frac{d^n x}{dt^n}: \quad \bar{u}(s) &= s^n\bar{x}(s) - s^{n-1}x(0) - s^{n-2}x'(0) - \dots - x^{(n-1)}(0) \\ &= s^n\bar{x}(s) - \sum_{k=0}^{n-1} s^{n-k-1} x^{(k)}(0), \end{aligned} \tag{1.590a, b}$$

which can be proved by induction: (i) it holds (1.590a, b) for $n = 1$ in (1.589a–c); (ii) if it holds (1.590a, b) for n, it also holds for $n + 1$:

$$v(t) = u'(t) = \frac{d^{n+1}x}{dt^{n+1}}: \qquad \bar{v}(s) = s\,\bar{u}(s) - u(0)$$
$$= s^{n+1}\bar{x}(s) - \sum_{k=0}^{n-1} s^{n-k}x^{(k)}(0) - x^{(n)}(0) \qquad (1.590\text{c, d})$$
$$= s^{n+1}\bar{x}(s) - \sum_{k=0}^{n} s^{n-k}x^{(k)}(0),$$

since (1.590d) coincides with (1.590b), replacing n by $n + 1$. Thus, the *Laplace transform (1.590b) of the n-th order derivative of a function (1.590a) consists of: (i) the Laplace transform of the function multiplied by* s^n*; (ii) minus all derivatives of lower order k of the function at the origin multiplied by* s^{n-k-1}.

NOTE 1.18: Differential Equation and Initial Conditions

Using (1.569) and (1.590a, b), the Laplace transform of the linear differential equation with constant coefficients (1.568a, b) is (1.591):

$$\bar{B}(s) = \sum_{n=0}^{N} A_n \left[s^n\bar{x}(s) - \sum_{k=0}^{n-1} s^{n-k-1}x^{(k)}(0) \right]; \qquad (1.591)$$

this is an algebraic relation:

$$\bar{B}(s) = P_N(s)\bar{x}(s) - \sum_{m=1}^{N} D_m s^{m-1}, \qquad D_m \equiv \sum_{\ell=m}^{N} A_\ell\, x^{(\ell-m)}(0), \quad (1.592\text{a, b})$$

consisting (1.592a) of: (i) the Laplace transform of the integral times the characteristic polynomial (1.52b) ≡ (1.568b); (ii) minus a polynomial of degree $N - 1$ with coefficients (1.592b). The proof of (ii) follows from:

$$\sum_{n=0}^{N} A_n \sum_{k=0}^{n-1} s^{n-k-1}x^{(k)}(0) = A_1x(0) + A_2\left[x'(0) + s\,x(0)\right] + ... +$$
$$A_N\left[x^{(N-1)}(0) + s\,x^{(N-2)}(0) + ... + s^{N-1}x(0)\right]$$
$$= A_1x(0) + A_2x'(0) + ... + A_N x^{(N-1)}(0) \qquad (1.592\text{c})$$
$$+ s\left[A_2x(0) + A_3x'(0) + ... + A_N x^{(N-2)}(0)\right]$$
$$+ .... + x^{N-1}A_N x(0)$$
$$= D_1 + D_2\,s + D_3\,s^2 + ... + D_N\,s^{N-1} = \sum_{m=1}^{N} D_m\,s^{m-1}.$$

Thus, *the Laplace transform of the complete integral of the forced linear differential equation of order N with constant coefficients (1.568a, b) is (standard XLIX):*

$$\bar{x}(s) = \frac{\bar{B}(s)}{P_N(s)} + \frac{Q_{N-1}(s)}{P_N(s)}, \qquad Q_{N-1}(s) = \sum_{m=1}^{N} D_m s^{m-1}, \qquad (1.593a, b)$$

the sum (1.593a) of: (i) the ratio by the characteristic polynomial (1.52b) of the Laplace transform of the forcing function (1.569), corresponding to the particular integral of the forced equation; (ii) plus a rational function whose denominator is the characteristic polynomial of degree N and numerator is a polynomial of lower degree N − 1 with (1.593b) with coefficients (1.592b) involving the initial conditions, corresponding to the general integral of the unforced equation.

Concerning (ii) the general integral of the unforced linear differential equation with constant coefficients there are two cases: (ii-1) if all roots of the characteristic polynomial are simple (1.594a) ≡ (1.54) the rational function in the second term on the RHS of (1.593b) has partial fraction decomposition (1.203a–d) ≡ (1.204) ≡ (1.594b) with simple poles:

$$P_N(s) = A_N \prod_{n=1}^{N} (s - a_n): \qquad \bar{x}(s) - \bar{x}_*(s) = \frac{Q_{N-1}(s)}{P_N(s)} = \sum_{k=1}^{N} \frac{C_n}{s - a_n},$$

$$x(t) - x_*(t) = \sum_{k=1}^{N} C_n \exp(a_n t), \qquad (1.594a–c)$$

and the general integral of the unforced equation is a linear combination (1.594c), of exponentials (1.578a–c) in agreement with (1.56b); (ii-2) if the characteristic polynomial has M roots (1.595b) of multiplicities α_m adding to N in (1.595a):

$$\sum_{m=1}^{M} \alpha_m = N; \qquad P_N(s) = A_N \prod_{n=1}^{M} (s - a_N)^{\alpha_m}: \qquad (1.595a, b)$$

$$\bar{x}(s) - \bar{x}_*(s) = \frac{Q_{N-1}(s)}{P_N(s)} = \sum_{M=1}^{M} \sum_{\beta_m=1}^{\alpha_m} \frac{(k-1)!C_{m,\beta_m}}{(s - a_m)^{\beta_m}}, \qquad (1.595c)$$

$$x(t) - x_*(t) = \sum_{m=1}^{M} \exp(a_m t) \sum_{\beta_m=1}^{\alpha_m} C_{m,\beta_m} t^{\beta_m - 1} \qquad (1.595d)$$

the rational function second on the RHS of (1.593b) has (1.209a–d) ≡ (1.595c), the partial fraction decomposition corresponding to the general integral of the unforced equation (1.596d) involving products of powers and exponentials

(1.580a–c) in agreement with (1.99). The use of the characteristic polynomial (1.54; 1.56a, b) and (1.98a, b; 1.99) [the Laplace transform (1.595a–d)] give the same general integral of the unforced linear differential equation with constant coefficients (1.568a, b) with $B(t) = 0$, involving arbitrary constants [which are expressed in terms (1.592b) of N single-point boundary conditions (1.5a, b)]. The Laplace transform specifies both the general (a particular) integral of the unforced (forced) linear differential equation with constants coefficients, as shown next for the second-order equation, corresponding to an oscillator with constant parameters [notes 1.19–1.22 (1.23–1.28)].

NOTE 1.19: Harmonic Oscillation with Constant Amplitude

As a first example of a second-order linear differential equation with constant coefficients is considered the harmonic oscillator (section 2.2), with constant natural frequency ω_0 in (1.597a), for which the characteristic polynomial (1.597b) has simple conjugate imaginary roots (1.597c):

$$\frac{d^2x}{dt^2} + \omega_0^2 x = 0, \qquad P_2(s) = s^2 + \omega_0^2 = (s - i\omega_0)(s + i\omega_0). \quad (1.597a–c)$$

Using (1.590a, b) with $n = 2$ leads to (1.589d, e) ≡ (1.598a, b):

$$y(t) = \frac{d^2x}{dt^2}: \qquad \bar{y}(s) = s^2\bar{x}(s) - sx(0) - x'(0), \quad (1.598a, b)$$

the Laplace transform of the differential equation (1.597a) is (1.599a):

$$0 = \left(s^2 + \omega_0^2\right)\bar{x}(s) - sx(0) - x'(0), \qquad \bar{x}(s) = \frac{sx(0) + x'(0)}{s^2 + \omega_0^2}, \quad (1.599a, b)$$

or equivalently (1.599b). The latter involves the Laplace transforms (1.582a–c):

$$x(t) = x(0)\cos(\omega_0 t) + \frac{x'(0)}{\omega_0}\sin(\omega_0 t). \quad (1.600a)$$

$$x'(t) = \frac{dx}{dt} = -\omega_0 x(0)\sin(\omega_0 t) + x'(0)\cos(\omega_0 t). \quad (1.600b)$$

Thus, *the second-order linear differential equation with constant coefficients (1.597a) corresponds to an oscillator with* ***natural frequency*** ω_0, *with initial displacement*

$x(0)$ [velocity $x'(0)$] at time $t = 0$, and displacement (1.600a) [velocity (1.600b)] at arbitrary time t.

NOTE 1.20: Condition of Critical Attenuation or Amplication

Adding an extra term to (1.597a), it becomes the general linear second-order differential equation with constant coefficients (1.465a) ≡ (1.601a), corresponding (section 2.3) to the harmonic oscillator with damping:

$$\frac{d^2x}{dt^2} + 2\lambda\frac{dx}{dt} + \omega_0^2 x = 0: \qquad P_2(s) = s^2 + 2\lambda s + \omega_0^2 = (s - s_-)(s - s_+). \tag{1.601a, b}$$

The characteristic polynomial (1.601b) appears in the Laplace transform (1.602a) of the differential equation (1.601a) leading to (1.602b):

$$0 = P_2(s)\bar{x}(s) - sx(0) - x'(0) - 2\lambda x(0), \tag{1.602a}$$

$$\bar{x}(s) = \frac{sx(0) + x'(0) + 2\lambda x(0)}{P_2(s)} = \frac{x'(0) + (s + 2\lambda)x(0)}{(s - s_-)(s - s_+)}. \tag{1.602b}$$

The characteristic polynomial (1.601b) has roots (1.603a):

$$s_\pm = -\lambda \pm \sqrt{\lambda^2 - \omega_0^2}, \qquad \bar{\omega} \equiv \left|\omega_0^2 - \lambda^2\right|^{1/2}, \quad \bar{\omega}^2 + \lambda^2 = \omega_0^2, \tag{1.603a–c}$$

with the **oscillation frequency** (1.603b) as discriminant satisfying (1.603c). This leads to three cases: (I) double root (note 1.20); (II) two real roots (note 1.21); (III) pair of complex conjugate roots (note 1.22). The case (II) of a double root (1.604a, b) leads (1.602b) to (1.604c):

$$\lambda = \omega_0; \quad s_\pm = -\lambda: \quad \bar{x}(s) = \frac{sx(0) + 2\lambda x(0) + x'(0)}{(s+\lambda)^2} = \frac{x(0)}{s+\lambda} + \frac{x'(0) + \lambda x(0)}{(s+\lambda)^2}; \tag{1.604a–c}$$

the Laplace transform (1.604c) is inverted using (1.579a, b; 1.580a–c):

$$x(t) = e^{-\lambda t}\left\{x(0) + \left[x'(0) + \lambda\, x(0)\right]t\right\}, \tag{1.605a}$$

$$v(t) = \frac{dx}{dt} = e^{-\lambda t}\left\{x'(0) - \lambda\left[x'(0) + \lambda x(0)\right]t\right\}. \tag{1.605b}$$

Thus, *the general second-order linear differential equation with constant coefficients (1.465a) ≡ (1.601a) in the* ***critical case*** *II of (1.604a) of a double root (1.604b) of the characteristic polynomial (1.601b) represents an* ***amplification*** $\lambda < 0$ ***(attenuation*** $\lambda > 0$*), since the exponential dominates the displacement (1.605a) and velocity (1.605b) for large time.*

NOTE 1.21: Case of Supercritical Decay or Growth

For the differential equation (1.601a) the case of two real roots (1.606a, b) of the characteristic polynomial (1.601b) leads (1.602b) to (1.606c):

$$\lambda > \omega_0; \quad s_\pm = -\lambda \pm \bar{\omega} < 0: \quad \bar{x}(s) = \frac{s x(0) + x'(0) + 2\lambda x(0)}{(s+\lambda+\bar{\omega})(s+\lambda-\bar{\omega})} = \frac{(s+\lambda)x(0) + x'(0) + \lambda x(0)}{(s+\lambda)^2 - \bar{\omega}^2}. \tag{1.606a–c}$$

The Laplace transform (1.606c) is inverted using (1.583a–c) leading to:

$$x(t) = e^{-\lambda t}\left[x(0)\cosh(\bar{\omega}t) + \frac{x'(0)+\lambda x(0)}{\bar{\omega}}\sinh(\bar{\omega}t)\right], \tag{1.607a}$$

$$x'(t) \equiv \frac{dx}{dt} = e^{-\lambda t}\left[x'(0)\cosh(\bar{\omega}t) - \frac{\lambda x'(0) + \omega_0^2 x(0)}{\bar{\omega}}\sinh(\bar{\omega}t)\right]. \tag{1.607b}$$

Thus, *the general linear second-order differential equation (1.465a) ≡ (1.601a) in the case I of (1.606a) real distinct roots (1.606b) represents a* ***growth*** $\lambda < 0$ *(* ***decay*** *$(\lambda > 0)$ in time since the displacement (1.607a) and velocity (1.607b) scale for large time respectively, like* $\exp\left[\left(|\lambda| + \omega\right)t\right]$ and $\exp\left[\left(-|\lambda| + \omega\right)t\right]$ with $|\lambda| > \omega$.

NOTE 1.22: Damped or Overstable Oscillation

For the differential equation (1.601a), the case (1.608a) of a pair of complex conjugate roots (1.608b) of the characteristic polynomial (1.601b) leads (1.602b) to (1.608c):

$$\lambda < \omega_0; \quad s_\pm = -\lambda \pm i\bar{\omega}: \quad \bar{x}(s) = \frac{s x(0) + 2\lambda x(0) + x'(0)}{(s+\lambda-i\bar{\omega})(s+\lambda+i\bar{\omega})} = \frac{(s+\lambda)x(0) + x'(0) + \lambda x(0)}{(s+\lambda)^2 + \bar{\omega}^2}. \tag{1.608a–c}$$

The Laplace transform (1.608c) is inverted using (1.584a–c):

$$x(t) = e^{-\lambda t}\left[x(0)\cos(\bar{\omega}t) + \frac{x'(0)+\lambda x(0)}{\bar{\omega}}\sin(\bar{\omega}t)\right], \tag{1.609a}$$

$$x'(t) \equiv \frac{dx}{dt} = e^{-\lambda t}\left[x'(0)\cos(\bar{\omega}t) - \frac{\lambda x'(0)+\omega_0^2 x(0)}{\bar{\omega}}\sin(\bar{\omega}t)\right]. \tag{1.609b}$$

In the first-order derivative (1.607b) [(1.609b)] in the case I(III) appears (1.603a, b) the growth factor (1.609c) [oscillation frequency (1.609e)] leading to the common factor (1.609d) [(1.609f)]:

$$I: \qquad \bar{\omega} = \sqrt{\lambda^2 - \omega_0^2}: \quad \lambda^2 - \bar{\omega}^2 = \omega_0^2;$$
$$III: \qquad \bar{\omega} = \sqrt{\omega_0^2 - \lambda^2}: \quad \lambda^2 + \bar{\omega}^2 = \omega_0^2. \tag{1.609c–f}$$

Thus, *the general second-order linear differential equation with constant coefficients (1.465a) ≡ (1.601a), in the case III in (1.608a) of a pair of complex conjugate roots (1.608b) of the characteristic polynomial represents for* $\lambda > 0 (\lambda < 0)$ *a* ***damped (overstable) oscillator*** *with frequency (1.603b) and exponentially decaying (growing) amplitude. The oscillation frequency (1.603b) varies from zero* $\bar{\omega} = 0$ *for critical damping (1.604a) to the natural frequency (1.610c) for* ***weak*** *(1.610a)* ***damping (overstability)*** *when (1.609a, b) simplify to (1.610b, d):*

$$\lambda^2 << \omega_0^2: \qquad x(t) = e^{-\lambda t}\left[x(0)\cos(\omega_0 t) + \frac{x'(0)+\lambda x(0)}{\omega_0}\sin(\omega_0 t)\right], \tag{1.610a–d}$$

$$\omega = \omega_0, \qquad x'(t) = e^{-\lambda t}\left\{x'(0)\cos(\omega_0 t) - \omega_0\left[x(0) + \frac{\lambda}{\omega_0}x'(0)\right]\sin(\omega_0 t)\right\}. \tag{1.610c, d}$$

In the absence $\lambda = 0$ *of damping or amplification (1.610c, d), simplify to (1.600a, b) with constant amplitude.* The Laplace transform applies both to ordinary (generalized) functions [notes 1.15–1.22 (1.23–1.27)].

NOTE 1.23: Unit Jump, Impulse, and Derivatives

The convergence of the Fourier series (notes 1.9–1.10) and integrals (notes 1.11–1.14) and of the Laplace transforms (notes 1.15–1.22) involves restrictions when applied to ordinary functions. These restrictions can be lifted by considering generalized functions, as shown next for the Laplace transform (notes 1.23–1.28). The generalized functions, like the Dirac delta

(1.517a, b), do not have a Riemann integral (section I.13.2) and thus, their Laplace transform (1.569) does not exist, and its direct calculation is merely indicative (note 1.23). A rigorous definition of a generalized function (chapters III.1 and III.2) is needed (notes 1.24–1.26) to obtain in an equally rigorous manner their Laplace transforms, as is the case [notes III.3.3–III.3.6 (III.3.7–III.3.9)] for Fourier series (integrals)]. The Laplace transform of a power (1.577b) is an inverse power (1.577a, c). In order to obtain Laplace transforms that are powers, hence divergent as $s \to \infty$, it is necessary to consider generalized functions.

The simplest is *the unit jump (1.519a–c) whose Laplace transform (1.569) coincides with the Laplace transform of unity:*

$$\bar{H}(s) = \int_0^\infty e^{-st}\, dt = \left[-\frac{e^{-st}}{s}\right]_0^\infty = \frac{1}{s}, \tag{1.612}$$

which is the same as the power (1.577a–f) with zero exponent $n = 0$.

The unit impulse (III.1.34a, b) ≡ (1.517a, b) ≡ (1.613a) is the derivative of the unit jump and has Laplace transform equal to unity (1.613b):

$$\delta(t) = \frac{d}{dt}\left[H(t)\right] = \begin{cases} 0 & \text{if} \quad x \neq 0 \\ \infty & \text{if} \quad x = 0 \end{cases}, \qquad \bar{\delta}(s) = 1, \tag{1.613a, b}$$

as follows from (1.589c), using (1.612, 1.614a):

$$H(-0) = 0: \qquad \bar{\delta}(s) = s\bar{H}(s) - H(-0) = 1. \tag{1.614a, b}$$

Using the fundamental property of the unit impulse (III.3.11c) ≡ (1.512b) ≡ (1.615b) relative to a continuous test function (1.615a) ≡ (III.3.11a):

$$\Phi \in C(|R): \qquad \left[\delta(t), \Phi(t)\right] \equiv \int_{-\infty}^{+\infty} \delta(t)\Phi(t)\, dt = \Phi(0), \tag{1.615a, b}$$

$$\bar{\delta}(s) = \int_{-0}^{\infty} \delta(t) e^{-st}\, dt = \lim_{t \to 0} e^{-st} = 1, \tag{1.615c}$$

leads to the same result (1.615c) ≡ (1.614b) ≡ (1.613b). In (1.614b) [(1.615c)] the unit jump (lower limit of the integrals) was taken at –0.

The ***n*-th derivative unit impulse** (1.616a) has Laplace transform, a power with exponent n in (1.616b):

$$f(t) \equiv \delta^{(n)}(t): \qquad \bar{f}(s) = s^n, \tag{1.616a, b}$$

as follows from (1.590b):

$$\bar{f}(s) = s^n \bar{\delta}(s) - \sum_{k=0}^{n-1} s^{n-k-1} \delta^{(k)}(-0) = s^n. \tag{1.617}$$

The fundamental property of the n-th derivative unit impulse (III.3.21b) ≡ (1.618b) relative to a test function with continuous n-th derivative (1.618a):

$$\Phi \in C^n(|R): \qquad \left[\Phi(t), \delta^{(n)}(t)\right] \equiv \int_{-\infty}^{+\infty} \delta^{(n)}(t)\Phi(t)dt = (-)^n \Phi^{(n)}(0), \tag{1.618a, b}$$

leads to:

$$L\left[\delta^{(n)}(t), t \to s\right] \equiv \int_{-\infty}^{+\infty} \delta^{(n)}(t) e^{-st} dt = (-)^n \lim_{t \to 0} \frac{d^n}{dt^n}\left(e^{-st}\right) = s^n \lim_{t \to 0} e^{-st} = s^n, \tag{1.619a, b}$$

in agreement with (1.619b) ≡ (1.616b). The preceding derivations (note 1.23) provide simple and straightforward predictions of correct result, although they are questionable as proofs, for example, as the Dirac unit impulse (1.517a, b) and its derivatives are not bounded and the integrals (1.615c;1.618b) do not exist as Riemann integrals (I.13.9). A rigorous proof (note 1.26) requires a rigorous definition of generalized function (note 1.24) and of its derivatives of all orders (note 1.25). The definition of generalized function as a linear functional (chapters III.3 and III.5) is preferred to the non-uniform limit of a family of functions (chapter III.1). The same results obtained in a heuristic (rigorous) [note(s) 1.23 (1.24–1.26)] are applied to the forcing of a harmonic oscillator (note 1.27).

NOTE 1.24: Linear Functional Over Test Functions

*The **support** of a function is the set of points where it does not vanish:*

$$S\left[f(x)\right] \equiv \left\{x: \quad f(x) \neq 0\right\}. \tag{1.620}$$

For example, the support of the Heaviside (Dirac) unit jump (1.518a–c) [impulse (1.617a, b)] is the positive real line (1.621a) [one point, namely the origin (1.621b)]:

$$S\left[H(x)\right] = |R^+ = (0,+\infty); \qquad S\left[\delta(x)\right] = \{0\}. \tag{1.621a, b}$$

A function with **compact support** vanishes outside a finite interval (III.3.26) ≡ (1.622):

$$J^0 \equiv \left\{ f(x):\ \exists_{a(b\in|R}:\ x<a \text{ or } x>b \ \Rightarrow\ f(x)=0 \right\}. \tag{1.622}$$

The **test functions** are (III.3.32) ≡ (1.623) smooth, that means are infinitely differentiable (1.327a):

$$\mathcal{V}_\infty^\infty(|C) = \left\{ f(x):\ \forall_{x\in|C,n\in|N} \exists f^{(n)}(x) \wedge \exists_{a<b}:\ x<a \text{ or } x>b:\ f^{(n)}(x)=0 \right\}, \tag{1.623}$$

and all derivatives have compact support (1.622).

A **generalized function** (III.3.44a) ≡ (1.624a) is a linear (III.3.45a–d) and continuous (III.3.46a–c) functional, which assigns to each test function (1.623) ≡ (III.3.44b) ≡ (1.624b) of number (III.3.44c) ≡ (1.624c):

$$f \in \mathcal{J}: \qquad \Phi \in \mathcal{V}_\infty^\infty(|R) \ \rightarrow\ \left[F(x),\Phi(x)\right] \equiv \int_{-\infty}^{+\infty} F(x)\Phi(x)dx \in |R. \tag{1.624a–c}$$

For example, the Dirac unit impulse (1.613a) assigns to each continuous test function (1.513a) ≡ (1.625a) its value at the origin (1.513b) ≡ (1.625b):

$$\Phi \in C(|R): \qquad \left[\delta(x),\Phi(x)\right] \equiv \int_{-\infty}^{+\infty} \delta(x)\Phi(x)dx = \Phi(0); \tag{1.625a, b}$$

in this case the set of test functions (1.623) can be extended to the continuous functions (1.625a). The Heaviside unit jump (1.519a–c) assigns to each integrable function (1.626a) its integral along the positive real line (1.626b):

$$\Phi \in \mathcal{E}(|R): \qquad \left[H(x),\Phi(x)\right] \equiv \int_{-\infty}^{+\infty} H(x)\Phi(x)dx = \int_{0}^{+\infty} \Phi(x)dx; \tag{1.626a, b}$$

in this case the set of test functions (1.623) can be extended to the integrable functions (1.626a). The n-th derivative of the unit impulse (1.618b) assigns to each function with continuous n-th order derivative (1.618a) ≡ (1.627a) its n-th derivative at the origin (1.627b) with +(−) sign for n even (odd):

$$\Phi \in C^n(|R): \qquad \left[\delta^{(n)}(x), \Phi(x)\right] \equiv \int_{-\infty}^{+\infty} \delta^{(n)}(x)\Phi(x)\,dx = (-)^n \Phi^{(n)}(0); \tag{1.627a, b}$$

in this case the set of test functions (1.623) can be extended to the functions with continuous n-th order derivatives (1.627a). The advantage of a more restrictive set of test functions (1.623) is that it allows differentiation of a generalized function to any order (note 1.25).

NOTE 1.25: Derivatives of all Orders of a Generalized Function

Two ordinary differentiable functions (1.628a) satisfy the **rule of integration by parts** (1.628b):

$$F, \Phi \in \mathcal{D}(|R): \qquad \int_{-\infty}^{+\infty} F'(x)\Phi(x)\,dx = \left[F(x)\Phi(x)\right]_{-\infty}^{+\infty} - \int_{-\infty}^{+\infty} F(x)\Phi'(x)\,dx; \tag{1.628a, b}$$

this can be extended to a generalized function (1.629a) and a test function (1.629b), with the first term on the RHS of (1.628b) equal to zero in (1.629c) because the test function (1.623) has compact support:

$$F \in \mathcal{J}(|R), \Phi \in \mathcal{V}_\infty^\infty(|R): \qquad \left[F'(x),\ \Phi(x)\right] \equiv \int_{-\infty}^{+\infty} F'(x)\,\Phi(x)\,dx$$

$$= -\int_{-\infty}^{+\infty} F(x)\ \Phi'(x)\,dx = -\left[F(x),\ \Phi'(x)\right]. \tag{1.629a–c}$$

The property (1.629a–c) ≡ (1.630a, b, d) can be extended to derivatives of all orders (1.630c) because the test function (1.623) is infinitely differentiable and all the derivatives have compact support:

$$F, \in \mathcal{J}(|R), \Phi \in \mathcal{V}_\infty^\infty(|R), \forall_{n \in |N}: \qquad \left[F^{(n)}(x), \Phi(x)\right] \equiv (-)^n \left[F(x), \Phi^{(n)}(x)\right], \tag{1.630a–d}$$

Thus, *the derivative of any order (1.630c) of a generalized function (1.630a) is defined (1.630d) by transferring in the inner product (1.624a–c) the derivative to the test function (1.630b), which is smooth with compact support (1.623). For example, the derivative of the Heaviside unit jump (1.626a, b) is given by:*

$$\begin{aligned}\left[H'(x),\Phi(x)\right] &\equiv -\left[H(x),\Phi'(x)\right] \equiv -\int_{-\infty}^{+\infty} H(x)\Phi'(x)dx \\ &= -\int_{0}^{+\infty}\Phi'(x)dx = -\left[\Phi'(x)\right]_0^{\infty} = \Phi(0) = \left[\delta(x),\Phi(x)\right],\end{aligned} \tag{1.631}$$

which proves (1.613a) that it equals the unit impulse $H'(x)=\delta(x)$. The n-th derivative of the unit impulse is given by:

$$\left[\delta^{(n)}(x),\Phi(x)\right] = (-)^n\left[\delta(x),\Phi^{(n)}(x)\right] = (-)^n\int_{-\infty}^{+\infty}\delta(x)\Phi^{(n)}(x)dx = (-)^n\,\Phi^{(n)}(0), \tag{1.632}$$

which proves rigorously (1.627a, b). The same method provides a rigorous definition and calculation of Laplace transforms of generalized functions (note 1.26).

NOTE 1.26: Laplace Transform of a Generalized Function

The test functions (1.623) which are smooth with compact support are also bounded (1.573) and of slow growth (1.575d, e), so their Laplace transform exists. They can be extended to the latter when defining the **Laplace transform of a generalized function** *(1.633a) by transferring the Laplace transform (1.569) ≡ (1.633d) to the test function (1.633a, b) assumed to be bounded (1.573) and of slow growth (1.574) on the positive real line where the inner product is taken over the positive real line (1.633e):*

$$\begin{aligned}F\in\mathcal{J}(|R),\quad \Phi\in\mathcal{B}\cap\mathcal{V}^n(|R):\quad &\left[\bar{F}(s)\,,\Phi(s)\right]\equiv\left[F(s)\,,\bar{\Phi}(s)\right] \\ &\equiv\int_0^{\infty}F(s)\Phi(s)ds.\end{aligned} \tag{1.633a–e}$$

For example, the Laplace transform of the Heaviside unit jump with a translation (1.634a) is (1.634b):

$$B(t)=H(t-T):\qquad \bar{B}(s)=\frac{e^{-sT}}{s}, \tag{1.634a, b}$$

as follows from:

$$\begin{aligned}\left[\bar{B}(s),\Phi(s)\right]&\equiv\left[B(s),\bar{\Phi}(s)\right]\\&=\int_0^\infty H(s-T)\,\bar{\Phi}(s)\,ds=\int_T^\infty\bar{\Phi}(s)\,ds=\int_T^\infty ds\int_0^\infty dt\;\Phi(t)\;e^{-st}\\&=\int_0^\infty dt\;\Phi(t)\left[-\frac{e^{-st}}{t}\right]_T^\infty=\int_0^\infty\Phi(t)\;\frac{e^{-tT}}{t}\;dt\\&=\int_0^\infty\frac{e^{-sT}}{s}\;\Phi(s)\;ds=\left[\frac{e^{-sT}}{s},\;\Phi(s)\right];\end{aligned} \tag{1.635}$$

thus, (1.635) proves rigorously (1.634a, b), which includes (1.612) as the particular case without translation T = 0. *The Laplace transform of the Dirac delta function with a translation (1.636a) is (1.636b):*

$$B(t)=\delta(t-T):\qquad B(s)=e^{-sT}, \tag{1.636a, b}$$

as follows from:

$$\begin{aligned}\left[\bar{B}(s),\Phi(s)\right]&\equiv\left[B(s),\bar{\Phi}(s)\right]\\&=\int_0^\infty\delta(s-T)\;\bar{\Phi}(s)\,ds\\&=\int_0^\infty ds\;\delta(s-T)\int_0^\infty dt\;\Phi(t)\;e^{-st}=\int_0^\infty dt\;\Phi(t)\int_0^\infty ds\;\delta(s-T)\;e^{-st}\\&=\int_0^\infty dt\;\Phi(t)\lim_{s\to T}e^{-st}=\int_0^\infty dt\;\Phi(t)e^{-tT}\\&=\int_0^\infty\Phi(s)\;e^{-sT}\,ds=\left[\;e^{-sT},\Phi(s)\right];\end{aligned} \tag{1.637}$$

thus, (1.637) proves rigorously (1.636a, b) and includes the particular case (1.613a, b) ≡ (1.614a, b) without translation $T=0$.

NOTE 1.27: Translation Property for Ordinary and Generalized Functions

The Laplace transform of the n-th derivative of a unit impulse with a translation (1.638a) is (1.638b):

$$B(t)=\delta^{(n)}(t-T):\qquad \bar{B}(s)=s^n e^{-sT}, \tag{1.638a, b}$$

as follows from:

$$\begin{aligned}\left[\bar{B}(s),\Phi(s)\right] &\equiv \left[B(s),\bar{\Phi}(s)\right] = \int_0^\infty \delta^{(n)}(s)\,\bar{\Phi}(s-T)\,ds \\ &= \int_0^\infty ds\,\delta^{(n)}(s-T)\int_0^\infty dt\,\Phi(t)\,e^{-st} = \int_0^\infty dt\,\Phi(t)\int_0^\infty ds\,e^{-st}\,\delta^{(n)}(s-T) \\ &= \int_0^\infty dt\,\Phi(t)\,(-)^n \lim_{s\to T}\frac{d^n}{ds^n}\left(e^{-st}\right) = \int_0^\infty dt\,\Phi(t)\,t^n\,e^{-tT} \\ &= \int_0^\infty e^{-sT}\,s^n\,\Phi(s)\,ds = \left[s^n\,e^{-sT},\Phi(s)\right];\end{aligned} \tag{1.639}$$

thus, (1.639) proves rigorously (1.638a, b), which includes (1.616a, b) ≡ (1.617) ≡ (1.619a, b) as the particular case without translation $T = 0$.

Table 1.8 summarizes a few Laplace transforms of the simplest generalized functions. The comparison of the Laplace transform with (without) translation for the Heaviside unit jump (1.634a, b; 1.635) [(1.612)], Dirac unit jump (1.636a, b; 1.637) [(1.613a, b) ≡ (1.614a, b) ≡ (1.615a–c)] and its derivatives (1.638a, b; 1.639) [(1.616a, b) ≡ (1.617) ≡ (1.619a, b)] suggests the **translation rule** *(1.640b) for the Laplace transform (1.640a) of ordinary or generalized functions:*

$$f(t) = B(t-T): \qquad \bar{f}(s) = e^{-sT}\,\bar{B}(s), \tag{1.640a, b}$$

TABLE 1.8

Laplace Transforms of Some Generalized Functions

Name	Generalized Function	Laplace Transform
Heaviside unit jump	$H(x)$	$\frac{1}{s}$
Dirac unit impulse	$\delta(x)$	1
n-th derivative of unit impulse	$\delta^{(n)}(x)$	s^n
unit jump with translation	$H(x-\xi)$	$\frac{e^{-s\xi}}{s}$
unit impulse with translation	$\delta(x-\xi)$	$e^{-s\xi}$
n-th derivative unit impulse with translation	$\delta^{(n)}(x-\xi)$	$s^n e^{-s\xi}$

Note: Laplace transforms of a few of the most important generalized functions.

which is proved differently: (i) for (1.641d) an ordinary function absolutely integrable on the finite real line (1.641a) and of fast decay at infinity (1.641b) and zero (1.641d) on the negative real line (1.641c) the change of variable (1.641e) leads to (1.641f–i):

$$B \in \mathcal{L}^1(0,L) \cap \underline{\mathcal{V}}(L,+\infty(; x<0 \Rightarrow \quad B(x)=0; \quad u=t-T: \tag{1.641a–e}$$

$$\bar{f}(s)=\int_0^\infty B(t-T)e^{-st}\,dt=\int_T^\infty B(t-T)e^{-st}\,dt = e^{-sT}\int_0^\infty B(u)e^{-su}\,du=e^{-sT}\bar{B}(s); \tag{1.641f–i}$$

(ii) for a generalized function (1.642a) whose support (1.620) is the positive real line (1.641b, c) ≡ (1.642b;1.620) a similar (1.641s) change of variable (1.642c) leads to (1.642d–j):

$$\begin{aligned} B\in\mathcal{J}; S(B(t))=(0,+\infty(; \; u=s-T:\left[\bar{f}(s),\Phi(s)\right]&\equiv\left[f(s),\bar{\Phi}(s)\right] \\ &=\int_0^\infty B(s-T)\,\Phi(s)\,ds \\ &=\int_T^\infty ds\,B(s-T)\int_0^\infty dt\,\Phi(t)\,e^{-st} \\ &=\int_0^\infty dt\,\Phi(t)\,e^{-tT}\int_0^\infty du\,e^{-ut}\,B(u) \\ &=\int_0^\infty dt\,\Phi(t)\,e^{-tT}\,\bar{B}(t)=\int_0^\infty \Phi(s)\,e^{-sT}\,\bar{B}(s)\,ds \\ &=\left[e^{-sT}\,\bar{B}(s),\,\Phi(s)\right]. \end{aligned} \tag{1.642a–j}$$

The forcing of a differential equation may correspond to either an ordinary or a generalized (note 1.28) function.

NOTE 1.28: Oscillator Forced by a Derivative of the Unit Impulse

As an example, consider the forcing of an undamped harmonic oscillator (1.597a) by the n-th derivative of the unit impulse (1.643a):

$$\frac{d^2x}{dt^2}+\omega_0^2 x=\delta^{(n)}(t): \qquad \left(s^2+\omega_0^2\right)\bar{x}(s)-sx(0)-x'(0)=s^n, \tag{1.643a, b}$$

using (1.589d, e) and (1.616a, b) ≡ (1.617) ≡ (1.638a, b) leads to (1.643b). The case $n=0$ of forcing by a unit impulse corresponds to the Green or influence function (1.644a):

$$\frac{d^2G}{dt^2}+\omega_0^2 G=\delta(t): \qquad \bar{x}(s)=\frac{sx(0)-x'(0)}{s^2+\omega_0^2}, \tag{1.644a, b}$$

and leads to a Laplace transform (1.644b), which coincides with (1.599b), and hence has the same inverse (1.600a, b). It follows that *a unit impulse forcing an undamped harmonic oscillator excites (1.643b) ≡ (1.645a) the forced oscillations (1.645c) in addition to the free oscillations (1.645b) due to initial conditions:*

$$\bar{x}(s)=\bar{x}_f(s)+\bar{x}_*(s): \qquad \bar{x}_f(s)=\frac{sx(0)+x'(0)}{s^2+\omega_0^2}, \qquad \bar{x}_*(s)=\frac{s^n}{s^2+\omega_0^2}. \tag{1.645a–c}$$

The free oscillations (1.645b) ≡ (1.599a) correspond to (1.600a, b), that is to a circular cosine (sine) for the amplitude in the case of initial displacement (1.646a–d) [velocity (1.647a–d)].

$$x(0)\neq 0=x'(0): \qquad \{x_f(t), v_f(t)\}=x(0)\{\cos(\omega_0 t), -\omega_0\sin(\omega_0 t)\}, \tag{1.646a–d}$$

$$x(0)=0\neq x'(0): \qquad \{x_f(t),\ v_f(t)\}=x'(0)\left\{\frac{\sin(\omega_0 t)}{\omega_0},\ \cos(\omega_0 t)\right\}. \tag{1.647a–d}$$

In the case (1.648a) of forcing by the Dirac unit impulse (1.648b), the response is the Green function (1.648c) for the harmonic oscillator:

$$n=0: \qquad \frac{d^2G}{dt^2}+\omega_0^2\,G=\delta(t), \qquad G(t)=\frac{\sin(\omega_0 t)}{\omega_0}. \tag{1.648a–c}$$

In the case of forcing by the n-th derivative of the unit impulse (1.643a), the response (1.645c) is (1.589a, b) the n-th derivative of the Green function (1.649):

$$x(t)=\frac{d^n}{dt^n}\left[\frac{\sin(\omega_0 t)}{\omega_0}\right]=\frac{d^nG}{dt^n}, \tag{1.649}$$

as follows comparing (1.648a–c) with (1.643a). The differentiations in (1.649) lead to cosines (1.650c) [sines (1.651c)] for even (1.650a, b) [odd (1.651a, b) order:

$$n=2m: \qquad \frac{d^2G}{dt^2}+\omega_0^2\,x=\delta^{(2m)}(t), \qquad x(t)=(-)^m\,\omega_0^{2m-1}\sin(\omega_0 t), \tag{1.650a–c}$$

$$n=2m+1: \qquad \frac{d^2x}{dt^2}+\omega_0^2\,x=\delta^{(2m+1)}(t), \qquad x(t)=(-)^{m+1}\,\omega_0^{2m}\cos(\omega_0 t). \tag{1.651a–c}$$

The Green's function can be extended from the undamped (notes 1.19 and 1.28) to the damped or amplified oscillator (notes 1.20–1.22) using: (i) the Laplace transform (notes 1.15–1.28); (ii) the method of variation of parameters (section 2.9); (iii) the Fourier transform (notes 2.2–2.12). The mathematical approach to the free or forced motion of the linear or damped oscillator using Laplace transform (notes 1.15–1.28) serves as an introduction to the more detailed study of physical oscillators (chapter 2) based on the characteristic polynomial (sections 1.3–1.5).

Conclusion 1

The general integral of a differential equation of order N involves N arbitrary constants of integration; choosing values for these constant gives particular integrals. For example, a first-order differential equation specifies the slope(s) at each point of the plane (Figure 1.1): (i) the general integral is a family of integral curves with a parameter C; (ii) each value of C corresponds to a particular curve of the family that is a particular integral of the differential equation; (iii) through each regular point passes one curve of the family, corresponding to a unique particular integral for a given boundary condition. There may exist singular points of the first (second) kind through no (several) singular curve(s) pass, for example, the y-axis (all points of the plane) in the Figure 1.2(1.3). A differential equation of order N may have a special integral involving less than N arbitrary constants of integration and not included in the general integral. An example of a first-order differential equation is the envelope (Figure 1.4) of a family of curves: (i) it satisfies the differential equation since it has the same tangent or slope at the points of contact with each integral curve; (ii) it does not coincide with any integral curve, and thus, it is not a particular integral that is included in the general integral; (iii) it is a single curve that does not involve any constant of integration. An example of an envelope is a pair of horizontal lines tangent to the circles with constant radius and centers on the real axis (Figure 1.5): the circles (horizontal lines) are the integral curves (envelopes), that is, the particular (special) integrals, that are contained (not contained) in the general integral.

A differential equation may involve parameters; it has a bifurcation relative to a parameter if the number or nature of the solutions changes as the parameter crosses the bifurcation value. For example, a monotonic potential (Figure 1.6a) leads to closed orbits (Figure 1.6b) for $C > 0$, a point $C = 0$ and no orbit for $C < 0$, so that $C = 0$ is a bifurcation value of the parameter (Figure 1.6c); another example is a non-monotonic potential (Figure 1.7a) leading to closed orbits with or without a double point (Figure 1.7b), or points or non-existent orbits (Figure 1.7c) so that there are two bifurcation values $C = 0$ and $C = C_0$ of the parameter C. The first (second) example [Figure 1.6b (Figure 1.7b, c)] includes a bifurcation of a quadratic (cubic) potential [Figure 1.6a (1.7a)] across which [Figure 1.6c (1.8)] the raths disappear (change in topology). The special integrals and bifurcations do not occur for linear differential equations with constant coefficients, which may be solved with forcing by an absolutely integrable function (also of bounded oscillation) on the real positive (real) line using the Laplace (Fourier) transform; the Fourier (Laplace) transform leads to contour integrals (is valid in a right-hand half) in the complex plane [Figure 1.9 (1.10)].

The linear differential equation with (i) constant [(ii) homogeneous] coefficients has in common with (iii) the linear finite difference equation, the existence of a characteristic polynomial (Table 1.2) in all three cases that (i) to (iii) specify: (a) the general integral of the unforced equation (Table 1.3); (b) a particular integral of the equation with special forcing functions (Table 1.4). The use of the inverse characteristic polynomial of ordinary (homogeneous) derivatives supplies a particular integral of linear differential equation with constant (homogeneous) coefficients involving forcing by an arbitrary smooth function (Table 1.5). Five other methods, namely variation of parameters, Green function, Fourier series, and integral and Laplace transform (Table 1.6) apply to: (α) linear differential equations with variable, homogeneous, or constant coefficients; (β) forcing by different classes of functions in distinct domains. Some examples of the Laplace transforms of elementary (generalized) functions used to solve linear differential equations with constant coefficients are given in Table(s) 1.7 (1.8). The general integral of a differential equation of order N of any type (linear or non-linear, constant or variable coefficients, forced or unforced) involves N arbitrary constants of integration, determined by N compatible or independent boundary conditions; the case of second-order differential equations $N = 2$ allows the consideration of single-point two-point, and mixed boundary conditions (Table 1.1).

2

The Damped/Amplified and Forced Oscillator

The motion of a mechanical oscillator is specified (section 2.1) by balancing the inertia force, equal to the product of mass by acceleration, against three forces: the restoring force, which depends on position; the friction force, which depends on velocity; and the external applied force, which depends on time. The inertia and restoring forces are associated, respectively, with the kinetic and potential energies, whose sum is the total energy; the friction force is associated with dissipation, which reduces the energy, whereas the activity or work per unit time, of the external applied force, may increase the energy. An analogous problem is the quasi-stationary electrical circuit, for which the inertia, friction, restoring, and applied forces are replaced, respectively, by the inductive, resistive, capacitive, and external electromotive force. The kinetic and potential energies are replaced, respectively, by the magnetic and electric energies. The balance of forces (electromotive forces) for the mechanical (electrical) circuit relates the particle displacement (electric charge) to its first two derivatives.

In the case of small oscillations, the differential equation is linear, and the solution consists of: (i) the general integral of the homogeneous equation, that is, the free oscillations (sections 2.2–2.6), in the absence of an external applied force, following a perturbation in initial conditions, leading to a motion which may be monotonic or oscillatory and whose amplitude may be constant, decaying, or amplified; (ii) the particular integral of the forced equation, for example, for sinusoidal forcing, represents the oscillations driven (sections 2.7–2.9) by an external harmonic force, which may have constant, sinusoidal, or growing amplitude, namely the latter two cases correspond, respectively, to the phenomena of beats and resonance.

2.1 Linear Electromechanical Circuits

A mechanical circuit consists of a mass, a spring, and a damper, associated, respectively, (subsections 2.1.1–2.1.3) with inertia, restoring, and friction forces. The energies corresponding to the inertia (restoring) force are the kinetic (potential) energy, whose sum is the total energy (subsection 2.1.4); the latter is dissipated by friction whereas applied forces may have no effect or increase or decrease the total energy. The total energy is conserved (subsections 2.1.5) if the work of the applied forces is positive and balances dissipate, or if there is no dissipation and the applied forces do no work. An electrical circuit (subsections 2.1.6) consists of a self, a resistor, and a capacitor, and is associated with (subsections 2.1.7) electrical and magnetic energies and Joule dissipation. The analogy between electrical and mechanical circuits applies both (subsections 2.1.8) to the free motion (forced response) under no (under) applied external or electromotive force. The equation of the mechanical circuit follows from Newton's law of motion (subsection 2.1.1) and can be linearized for small displacements and velocities (subsections 2.1.2–2.1.5). The equation of the linear electric circuit is analogous (subsections 2.1.6–2.1.8) and can be obtained (subsection 2.1.13) from the Maxwell equations of the electromagnetic field (subsection 2.1.9) in the quasi-stationary approximation (subsection 2.1.12), which is intermediate between steady (unsteady) fields [subsection 2.1.10 (2.1.11)].

2.1.1 Mass, Motion, and Inertia Force (Newton, 1686)

Consider a particle of **mass** m, that can move one-dimensionally along a coordinate $x(t)$, that specifies the **displacement** x as a function of time t; the first (second) derivatives specify the **velocity** (2.1a) [**acceleration** (2.1b)]:

$$\mathrm{v} = \dot{x} \equiv \frac{dx}{dt}, \qquad a \equiv \ddot{x} = \frac{d^2x}{dt^2} = \frac{d\mathrm{v}}{dt} = \dot{\mathrm{v}}. \tag{2.1a, b}$$

For a ***mechanical system*** (Figure 2.1), *the* ***Newton law (1686)*** *states that the* ***inertia force****, equal to mass times acceleration:*

$$m\ddot{x} = j(x) + h(\dot{x}) + F_m(t), \tag{2.2}$$

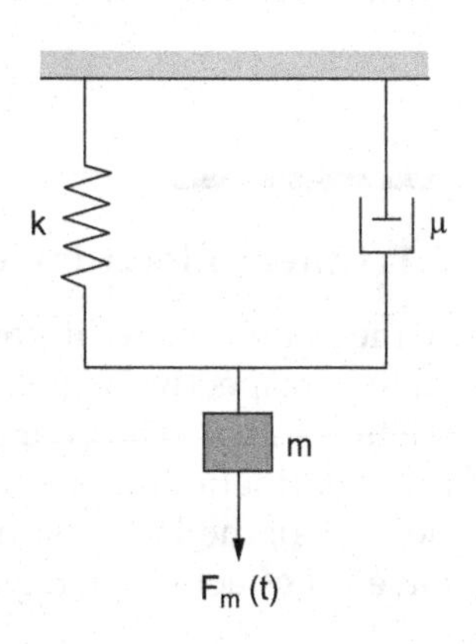

FIGURE 2.1
The linear second-order system with constant coefficients consists in mechanics of a constant mass, a linear damper, and a linear spring specifying respectively, the inertia/friction/restoring force when multiplied by the acceleration/velocity/displacement, and balanced by an external forcing by a mechanical force that is an ordinary or generalized function of time.

is balanced by: (i) the ***restoring force*** *$j(x)$, due to* ***a spring****, that depends on position; (ii) the* ***friction force*** *$h(\dot{x})$, due to a* ***damper****, that depends on velocity; (iii) the* ***applied force*** *$F_m(t)$, due to external forcing, that depends on time.*

2.1.2 Spring, Restoring Force, and Potential Energy

Assuming that the origin $x = 0$ is a position of equilibrium, the restoring force is a regular function of position in its neighborhood, and can expand in a MacLaurin (I.23.34b) ≡ (2.3) power series:

$$j(x) = -\sum_{n=0}^{\infty} k_n x^n = k_0 - k_1 x - k_2 x^2 - k_3 x^3 + O\left(x^4\right); \tag{2.3}$$

the restoring force is **attractive (repulsive)** if negative (positive). A force that depends only on position is conservative, and is associated with a **mechanical potential energy**:

$$\begin{aligned} \Phi_m(x) &= -\int_0^x j(\xi)\,d\xi = \sum_{n=0}^{\infty} k_n \frac{x^{n+1}}{n+1} \\ &= k_0 x + k_1 \frac{x^2}{2} + k_2 \frac{x^3}{2} + k_3 \frac{x^4}{4} + O\left(x^5\right). \end{aligned} \tag{2.4}$$

The five leading terms in the power series for the restoring force (2.3) and potential energy (2.4), may be interpreted as follows: (i) if $x = 0$ is an equilibrium position, the restoring force must vanish there $0 = j(0) = -k_0$ and the potential energy (2.4) has no linear term; (ii) if $x = 0$ is a position of **stable** equilibrium, the restoring force $-k_1 x$ must oppose small displacements $k_1 > 0$, in which case the potential energy is quadratic, and has a minimum (Figure 2.2a) at the equilibrium position, for a linear spring of **resilience** $k \equiv k_1 > 0$, corresponding to an **attractor** at the origin; (iii) for a quadratic potential with negative coefficient $k_1 < 0$, the potential is maximum at the origin, which is a position of **bilateral unstable** equilibrium (Figure 2.2b) since any displacement positive or negative leads to further displacement away from the **repeller** at the origin; (iv) if $k_2 \neq 0$, then the restoring force $-k_2 x^2$ is repulsive (attractive) for both directions, it increases (decreases) the displacement for $k_2 < 0 (k_2 > 0)$, the potential energy is a cubic $-k_3 x^3/3$ and has an inflexion at $x = 0$, showing (Figure 2.2c) that the equilibrium is **unilateral unstable** in one direction; (iv) if $k_2 = 0 \neq k_3$, the cubic restoring force $-k_3 x^3$ and quartic potential term in the energy $k_3 x^4/4$, are consistent

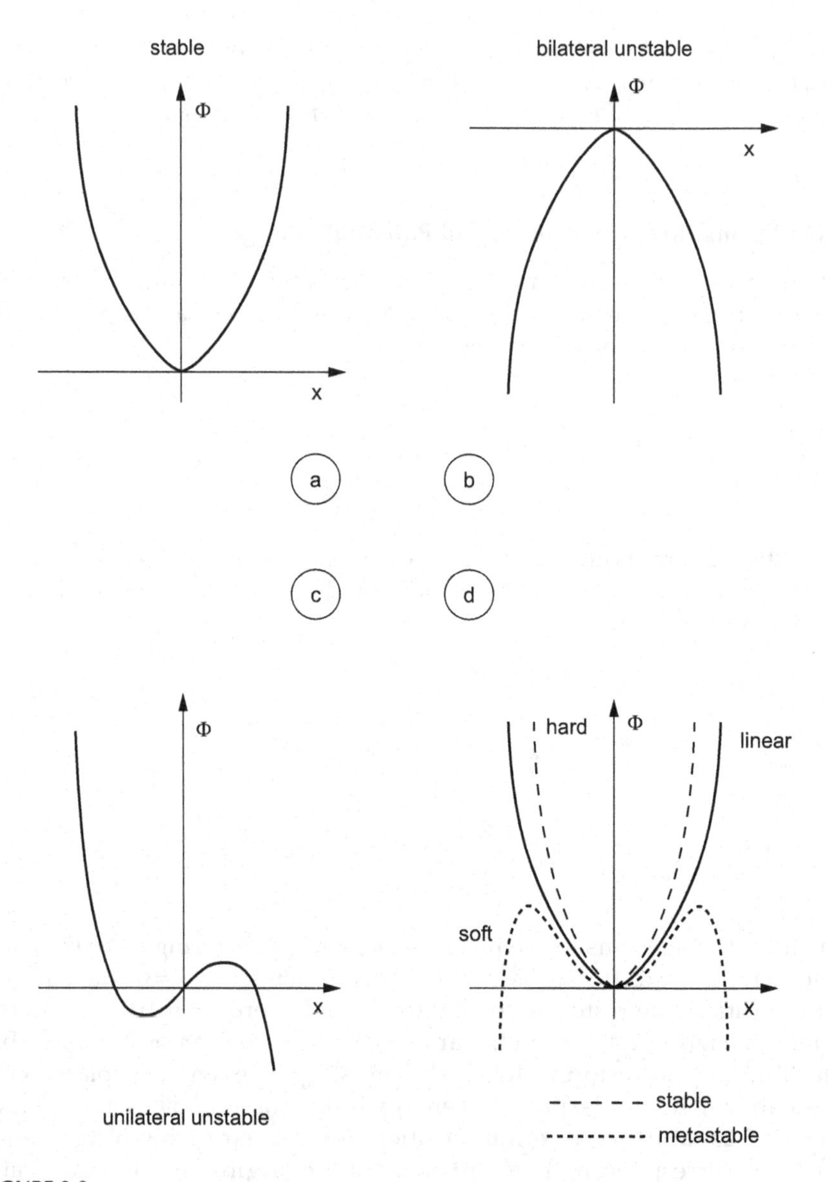

FIGURE 2.2
The potential of the restoring force: (i)(ii) if it is a quadratic function of position with a positive (negative) coefficient, and has a minimum (maximum) at the origin that is a position of stable (unstable) equilibrium corresponding [Figure 2.2a(b)] to an attractor (repeller); (iii) if it is cubic and has an inflexion at the origin that is a position (Figure 2.2c) of unstable equilibrium in one direction; (iv) if it biquadratic with both coefficients positive and it corresponds to hard spring that reinforces stability for all displacements small or large (Figure 2.2d); (v) if it is biquadratic with positive quadratic and negative biquadratic coefficient, and it corresponds to a soft spring that is stable (unstable) for small displacements below (beyond) a threshold, and hence is metastable (Figure 2.2d).

with stable equilibrium for small displacements, but for large displacements lead to a **non-linear spring**, that is **hard (soft)** relative to the linear case (Figure 2.2d) if $k_3 > 0 (k_3 < 0)$ implying that it remains stable for arbitrary large displacements (it becomes unstable for large displacements beyond a threshold, and therefore is **metastable**). Thus:

$$k_1 \equiv k > 0: \qquad \Phi_m(x) = \frac{1}{2} kx^2 + O(x^4), \qquad j(x) = -\frac{d\Phi_m}{dx} = -kx + O(x^3), \tag{2.5a–c}$$

specify *the potential energy (2.5b) and restoring force (2.5c), for a translational spring of resilience (2.5a), about a position x = 0 of stable equilibrium*. The linear (non-linear) oscillator is considered in the chapter 2.4.

2.1.3 Damper, Friction Force, and Dissipation Function

The **friction force** is a regular function for small velocities $\dot{x}$, and hence it has the power series:

$$h(\dot{x}) = -\sum_{n=0}^{\infty} \mu_n \dot{x}^n = -\mu_0 - \mu_1 \dot{x} - \mu_2 \dot{x}^2 - \mu_3 \dot{x}^3 + O(\dot{x}^4); \tag{2.6}$$

minus the **activity** or **power** of work per unit time of the friction force:

$$\begin{aligned} \Psi_m(\dot{x}) &= -h(\dot{x}) \frac{dx}{dt} = -h(\dot{x})\dot{x} = \sum_{n=0}^{\infty} \mu_n \dot{x}^{n+1} \\ &= \mu_0 \dot{x} + \mu_1 \dot{x}^2 + \mu_2 \dot{x}^3 + \mu_3 \dot{x}^4 + O(\dot{x}^5), \end{aligned} \tag{2.7}$$

specifies the **dissipation function** $\Psi(\dot{x})$. The leading terms in the power series for the friction force (2.6) [dissipation function (2.7)] may be interpreted as follows: (i) $\mu_0 = -h(0)$ is the **static friction force**, that is the friction force in the absence of motion $\dot{x} = 0$; (ii) the leading term for the **kinetic friction force** is $-\mu_1 \dot{x}$, and since it must oppose the motion $\mu_1 > 0$, that is for a linear damper with **damping** $\mu \equiv \mu_1 > 0$, the dissipation function $\mu \dot{x}^2$ is quadratic and positive; (iii) if $\mu_2 \neq 0$, the force $-\mu_2 \dot{x}^2$ would oppose velocities in both directions and the dissipation $\mu_2 \dot{x}^3$ for $\dot{x} > 0$ could be positive for $\mu_2 > 0$ or negative for $\mu_2 < 0$, that is positive dissipation for a damper that extracts energy, and negative dissipation for an **active element** that supplies energy, for example, a muscular cell that can amplify a nervous signal to exert a force; (iv) if $\mu_3 \neq 0$, then $-\mu_3 \dot{x}^3$ corresponds to a **non-linear damper**, that is **compliant (stiff)** relative to the linear case if $\mu_3 < 0 (\mu_3 > 0)$. Thus:

$$\mu \equiv \mu_1 > 0: \qquad \Psi_m(\dot{x}) = \mu \dot{x}^2 + O(\dot{x}^4), \qquad h(\dot{x}) = -\frac{\Psi_m(\dot{x})}{\dot{x}} = -\mu \dot{x} + O(\dot{x}^3), \tag{2.8a–c}$$

specify *the dissipation function (2.8b) and the kinematic friction force (2.8c) for a linear damper with decay (2.8a).*

2.1.4 Kinetic Energy, Dissipation, and Work

Multiplying the general, non-linear equation of motion (2.2), by the velocity $\dot{x}$, leads to:

$$0 = m\ddot{x}\dot{x} - \dot{x}\, j(x) - \dot{x}h(\dot{x}) - \dot{x}F_m(t) = \frac{d}{dt}\left\{\frac{1}{2}m\dot{x}^2 - \int^x j(\xi)\, d\xi\right\} + \Psi_m(\dot{x}) - A, \tag{2.9}$$

where the potential energy (2.4) [dissipation function (2.7)] may be identified in the second (third) term on the righthand side (RHS). The first term involves the **kinetic energy** (2.10b), which is equal to one-half the product of the constant mass (2.10a) by the square of velocity:

$$m = \text{const}: \qquad E_v = \frac{1}{2}mv^2, \qquad E_t = E_v + \Phi_m(x), \tag{2.10a–c}$$

and added to the potential energy $\Phi(x)$, specifies the **total energy** (2.10c). The fourth term is (2.11a) the activity A, or **power** or **work** dW per unit time dt of the external force (2.11b):

$$A = F_m(t)\dot{x}(t) = F_m(t)\frac{dx}{dt} = \frac{dW}{dt}, \qquad dW = F_m(t)\, dx. \tag{2.11a, b}$$

The equation (2.9), with (2.4; 2.7; 2.10a, b; 2.11a) states that:

$$\frac{dE_t}{dt} = -\Psi_m(\dot{x}) + A, \tag{2.12}$$

the *rate of change in time of the total energy (2.10c), with constant mass (2.10a), which is kinetic (2.10b) plus potential (2.4) is determined by: (i) the dissipation function (2.7), that causes energy to decay $dE/dt < 0$; (ii) the activity (2.11a) of* *the external forces, that may not affect $A = 0$, may increase $A > 0$ or decrease $A < 0$ energy, depending on whether they do no work, or do positive or negative work. The* ***energy balance*** *(2.12) applies both in the linear (2.5a–c; 2.8a–c) [non-linear (2.3, 2.4; 2.6, 2.7)] cases of the equation of motion (2.2) with the external force performing the work (2.11b) or activity (2.11a).*

2.1.5 Conservation of the Total Energy

Thus, ***conservation of energy*** *(2.13b) is possible: (i) in the absence of dissipation and external forces, that is, for undamped free motion; (ii) in the presence of damping and external forces, such that the dissipation and activity exactly balance (2.13a):*

$$\Psi_m = A: \qquad const = E_t = \frac{1}{2} m v^2 + \Phi_m(x). \qquad (2.13a, b)$$

The kinetic energy is a quadratic function of velocity (2.10a), but for a general, non-linear spring, the potential is not a purely quadratic function of displacement (2.4); it becomes so for a linear spring (2.5b), when the total energy becomes a sum of squares:

$$E_t = \frac{1}{2} m v^2 + \frac{1}{2} k x^2, \qquad (2.14)$$

and the dissipation function is also quadratic (2.8b) for a linear damper. Thus, the equation of motion (2.2) is (problem 1) linearized (2.5c; 2.8c) for small displacements and velocities:

$$m\ddot{x} + \mu\dot{x} + kx = F_m(t), \qquad (2.15)$$

for a mass m, acted by a damper of decay (2.8a) and a spring of resilience (2.5a) plus an external force F(t).

2.1.6 Electrical Circuit: Self, Resistor, and Capacitor

Whereas the equations of dynamics are non-linear, and have to be linearized for small displacements and velocities, the Maxwell equations are linear in general; thus, a linear differential equation like (2.15) should apply to a quasi-stationary **electrical circuit** (Figure 2.3), consisting of a self, a resistor, a capacitor, and a **battery**, once appropriate analogies or identifications are made. The electrical circuit is specified by non-linear equations in the presence of other elements, such as transistors or valves. *The variable for a mechanical (electrical) circuit is the particle displacement x(t) [electric charge q(t)], and its*

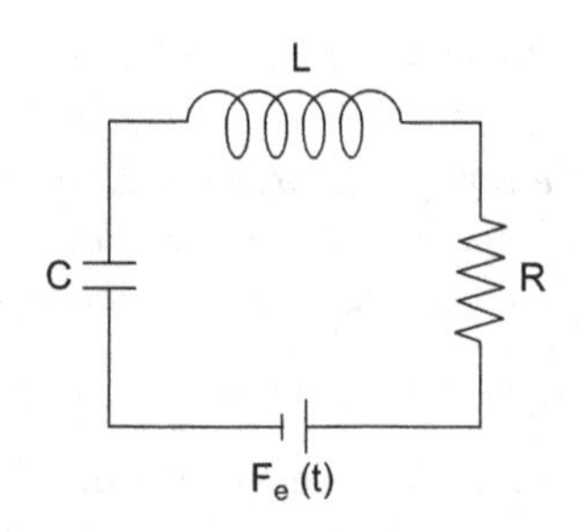

FIGURE 2.3
The linear second-order system with constant coefficients corresponds to an electric circuit consisting of a self, a resistor, and a capacitor through which flow an electric current, that is the time derivative of the electric charge, and is supplied by a battery acting as a forcing term through the electromotive force.

derivative with regard to time is the particle velocity $v = \dot{x}$ *[electric current* $j = \dot{q}$*] and driver is* $F_m\left(F_e\right)$ *the mechanical* ***(electromotive) force*** (2.16c):

$$x, \quad v \equiv \dot{x} \quad \leftrightarrow \quad q, \quad j \equiv \dot{q}, \qquad F_m(t) \leftrightarrow F_e(t); \tag{2.16a–c}$$

further analogies between mechanical (electrical) circuits include the mass m ***(induction*** *L) of a body (self), the decay* μ ***(resistance*** *R) of a damper (resistor), and the resilience k (inverse* ***capacity*** *1/C) of a spring (condenser):*

$$m, \mu, k \leftrightarrow L, R, \frac{1}{C}, \tag{2.17a–c}$$

which were discussed in detail before (chapters I.2, I.4, I.6).

2.1.7 Electric and Magnetic Energies and Dissipation (Joule)

Thus, *the analogue of the kinetic (2.10a) [potential (2.5b)] energy is the* ***magnetic*** *(2.18a) [(****electric*** *(2.18b)]* ***energy*** *associated with a* ***self (capacitor)****:*

$$E_v \leftrightarrow E_m = \frac{1}{2}Lj^2, \qquad \Phi \leftrightarrow E_e = \frac{q^2}{2C}. \tag{2.18a, b}$$

The total energy is ***electromagnetic*** *(2.19a):*

$$E_{em} \equiv E_m + E_e = \frac{1}{2}Lj^2 + \frac{q^2}{2C}, \qquad \Psi_e = Rj^2, \tag{2.19a, b}$$

and energy dissipation is due to the ***Joule effect*** *(2.19b), which is due to electric currents in* ***resistors****. The electromotive force* $F_e(t)$*, due to a battery, may not affect, increase, or decrease the electromagnetic energy, according to:*

$$\frac{dE_{em}}{dt} = -\Psi_e + jF_e(t), \tag{2.20}$$

which is the analogue of the mechanical energy equation (2.12).

2.1.8 Free Motion and Forced Response

The analogue of the equation of motion (2.15) for a mechanical system states that (problem 2) *in an electrical circuit* (Figure 2.3) *the electromotive force due to the battery drives (2.21) an electric charge through the capacitor, an electric current through the resistance, and a time rate of the electric current through the self:*

$$L\ddot{q} + R\dot{q} + \frac{q}{C} = F_e(t). \tag{2.21}$$

Comparing (2.15) and (2.21), it follows that *mechanical system and electrical circuit are described by the same equation:*

$$\ddot{x} + 2\lambda\dot{x} + \omega_0^2 x = f(t), \tag{2.22}$$

in terms of ***decay factor*** λ, ***natural frequency*** ω_0, *and* ***forcing function*** $f(t)$, *defined respectively by:*

$$\omega_0 \equiv \sqrt{\frac{k}{m}}, \frac{1}{\sqrt{LC}}; \qquad \lambda = \frac{\mu}{2m}, \frac{R}{2L}; \qquad f(t) = \frac{F_m(t)}{m}, \frac{F_e(t)}{L}. \tag{2.23a–c}$$

The natural frequency (2.23a) for: (i) the mechanical system increases with increasing resilience of the spring and decreasing mass; (ii) the electrical circuit increases with decreasing induction of the self and capacity of the capacitor. The damping factor (2.23b) for the mechanical system (electrical circuit) increases with increasing damping (resistance) and decreasing mass (induction). The forcing function (2.23c) for the mechanical system (electrical circuit) increases with increasing mechanical applied (electromotive) force and decreasing mass (induction).

The ***total motion*** *corresponding to the particle displacement (analogous to the electric charge) for a mechanical system (electrical circuit) corresponds to the complete integral of the forced differential equation (2.22), and consists of two parts: (i) the general integral of the unforced equation, corresponds to (2.22) in the absence of external forcing* $f(t) = 0$, *that is the* ***free motion,*** *following an initial disturbance, for example, in displacement (2.24a) and velocity (2.24b):*

$$x_0 = x(0), \qquad x_0 = \dot{x}(0) = v_0; \tag{2.24a, b}$$

(ii) the simplest particular integral of the forced equation (2.22) that is independent of initial conditions, is the ***forced motion*** *in response to the forcing function.*

After introducing the **electromechanical** analogy (section 2.1), next are considered the various cases of the free motion (sections 2.7–2.6) and of forced response (sections 2.7–2.9). For definiteness, the terminology of mechanical systems is used in the sequel, with occasional reference to the analogue electrical circuit when needed. The electromechanical analogy also applies in other situations like sound (electromagnetic wave) propagation and dissipation in tubes (waveguides) for wavelength larger than the transverse dimensions (notes 7.1–7.55). The equations of the linear mechanical system (electric circuit) follow from the Newton law of motion (Maxwell equations of the electromagnetic field) using the assumption of linearity (quasi-stationary field) in the subsections 2.1.1–2.1.5 (2.1.9–2.1.13). The equation of the linear electric circuit (2.21): (i) was introduced by analogy (2.16a, b; 2.17a–c) with the linear mechanical circuit (2.15); (ii) is obtained next (subsection 2.1.13) for the Maxwell equations of the electromagnetic field (subsection 2.1.9) in the quasi-stationary case (subsection 2.1.12), which is intermediate between electrostatics and magnetostatics (subsection 2.1.10) and propagation and diffusion of electromagnetic waves (subsection 2.1.11).

2.1.9 Unsteady Electromagnetic Field (Maxwell, 1863)

The **Maxwell (1863) equations** couple the **electric field** $\vec{E}$ (2.25a) and **displacement** $\vec{D}$ (2.25b):

$$\nabla \wedge \vec{E} = -\frac{1}{c}\frac{\partial \vec{B}}{\partial t}, \qquad \nabla . \vec{D} = q, \tag{2.25a, b}$$

$$c\nabla \wedge \vec{H} = \vec{J} + \frac{\partial \vec{D}}{\partial t}, \qquad \nabla . \vec{B} = 0, \tag{2.26a, b}$$

and **magnetic field** $\vec{H}$ (2.26a) and **induction** $\vec{B}$ (2.26b) in the unsteady case, with the **electric charge** q and **electric current** $\vec{J}$ densities per unit volume acting as sources and c denoting the speed of light in vacuo. The electric charge and current satisfy the **electric conservation equation** (2.27a):

$$\frac{\partial q}{\partial t} + \nabla . \vec{J} = 0: \qquad \frac{\partial q}{\partial t} = \nabla . \frac{\partial \vec{D}}{\partial t} = -\nabla . \vec{J} - c\nabla . \left(\nabla \wedge \vec{H}\right) = -\nabla . \vec{J}, \tag{2.27a, b}$$

which follows (2.27a) ≡ (2.27b) from (2.25b; 2.26a) since div curl = 0. In a isotropic medium the electric displacement (magnetic induction) is proportional (2.28a) [(2.28b)] to the electric (magnetic) field through the **dielectric permittivity** ε (**magnetic permeability** μ):

$$\vec{D} = \varepsilon \vec{E}, \qquad \vec{B} = \mu \vec{H}; \qquad \vec{J} = \vec{j} + \sigma \vec{E}, \tag{2.28a–c}$$

the total electric current $\vec{J}$ (2.28c) consists of the sum of a **convection (conduction) electric current** $\vec{j}\left(\sigma \vec{E}\right)$ due to the motion of electric charges (proportional to the electric field through the **Ohmic electric conductivity σ**). Thus, the Maxwell equations of the electromagnetic field can be written in terms of the electric field and magnetic induction alone (2.29b, c; 2.30c, d):

$$\varepsilon = const: \qquad \nabla \wedge \vec{E} = -\frac{1}{c}\frac{\partial \vec{B}}{\partial t}, \qquad \nabla . \vec{E} = \frac{q}{\varepsilon}, \tag{2.29a–c}$$

$$\mu, \sigma = const: \qquad \frac{c}{\mu}\nabla \wedge \vec{B} = \vec{j} + \sigma \vec{E} + \varepsilon \frac{\partial \vec{E}}{\partial t}, \qquad \nabla . \vec{B} = 0, \tag{2.30a–d}$$

for a homogeneous medium for which the dielectric permittivity (2.29a), magnetic permeability (2.30a), and Ohmic electrical conductivity (2.30b) are all constant.

2.1.10 Decoupled Electro-Magnetostatic Fields and Potentials

In the steady case (2.31a) in the absence of Ohmic electric conductivity (2.31b), the two pairs of equations decouple [chapter I.24 (I.26)] for the electrostatic (2.31c, d) [magnetostatic (3.32b, c)] field due to electric charges [electric currents (2.32a)]:

$$\frac{\partial q}{\partial t} = 0 = \sigma: \qquad \nabla \wedge \vec{E} = 0, \qquad \nabla . \vec{E} = \frac{q}{\varepsilon}, \tag{2.31a–d}$$

$$\nabla . \vec{j} = 0: \qquad \nabla \wedge \vec{B} = \frac{\mu}{c}\vec{j}, \qquad \nabla . \vec{B} = 0. \tag{2.32a–c}$$

Also (2.31b) [(2.32c)] implies that the electric field (2.33a) [magnetic induction (2.34a)] is minus the gradient (plus the curl) of a **scalar electric (vector magnetic) potential** that satisfies a Poisson equation forced by the electric charge (2.33b) [current (2.34b)]:

$$\vec{E} = -\nabla \Phi_e: \qquad -\frac{q}{\varepsilon} = \nabla . \nabla \Phi_e = \nabla^2 \Phi_e, \tag{2.33a, b}$$

$$\vec{B} = \nabla \wedge \vec{A}: \qquad -\frac{\mu}{c}\vec{j} = -\nabla \wedge \left(\nabla \wedge \vec{A}\right) = \nabla^2 \vec{A}, \qquad \nabla . \vec{A} = 0, \tag{2.34a–c}$$

where a **gauge condition** (2.34c) was used for the vector potential. The solution (III.8.13a) ≡ (2.35a) [(III.8.92) ≡ (2.35b)] of the scalar (vector) Poisson equation (2.33b) [(2.34b)] specifies the electric (magnetic) potential due to a distribution of electric charges (2.35a) [currents (2.35b)] in a region D:

$$\Phi_e(\vec{x}) = \frac{1}{4\pi\varepsilon} \int_D \frac{q(\vec{y})}{|\vec{x}-\vec{y}|} d^3\vec{y}, \qquad \vec{A}(\vec{x}) = \frac{\mu}{4\pi c} \int \frac{\vec{j}(\vec{y})}{(\vec{x}-\vec{y})} d^3\vec{y}. \tag{2.35a, b}$$

From (2.33a, b) [(2.34a, b)] it follows (2.36a) [(2.36b)]:

$$\frac{1}{\varepsilon}\nabla q = -\nabla.(\nabla^2\Phi_e) = -\nabla^2(\nabla\Phi_e) = \nabla^2\vec{E}, \tag{2.36a}$$

$$-\frac{\mu}{c}\nabla\wedge\vec{j} = \nabla\wedge(\nabla^2\vec{A}) = \nabla^2(\nabla\wedge\vec{A}) = \nabla^2\vec{B}, \tag{2.36b}$$

that the electric field (magnetic induction) satisfies a vector Poisson equation forced by the gradient of the electric charge (2.37a) [curl of the electric current (2.37b)]:

$$\nabla^2\vec{E} = \frac{1}{\varepsilon}\nabla q, \qquad \nabla^2\vec{B} = -\frac{\mu}{c}\nabla\wedge\vec{j}. \tag{2.37a, b}$$

These equations no longer hold in the unsteady case (subsection 2.1.11) when the electric field and magnetic induction are coupled by (2.29b) and (2.30c).

2.1.11 Propagation and Diffusion of Electromagnetic Waves

In the unsteady case, the Poisson equation (2.37a) for the electrostatic field is replaced (2.29b, c; 2.30c) by:

$$\begin{aligned}\nabla^2\vec{E} &= -\nabla\wedge(\nabla\wedge\vec{E}) + \nabla(\nabla.\vec{E}) = \frac{1}{c}\frac{\partial}{\partial t}(\nabla\wedge\vec{B}) + \nabla\left(\frac{q}{\varepsilon}\right) \\ &= \frac{\mu}{c^2}\frac{\partial\vec{j}}{\partial t} + \frac{\mu\sigma}{c^2}\frac{\partial\vec{E}}{\partial t} + \frac{\mu\varepsilon}{c^2}\frac{\partial^2\vec{E}}{\partial t^2} + \frac{1}{\varepsilon}\nabla q.\end{aligned} \tag{2.38a}$$

Similarly, in the unsteady case the Poisson equation (2.37b) for the magnetic induction is replaced (2.30c, d; 2.29b) by:

$$\begin{aligned}\nabla^2\vec{B} &= -\nabla\wedge(\nabla\wedge\vec{B}) + \nabla(\nabla.\vec{B}) = -\frac{\mu}{c}\left[\nabla\wedge\vec{j} + \sigma\nabla\wedge\vec{E} + \varepsilon\frac{\partial}{\partial t}(\nabla\wedge\vec{E})\right] \\ &= \frac{\mu\varepsilon}{c^2}\frac{\partial^2\vec{B}}{\partial t^2} + \frac{\mu\sigma}{c^2}\frac{\partial\vec{B}}{\partial t} - \frac{\mu}{c}\nabla\wedge\vec{j}.\end{aligned} \tag{2.38b}$$

In the steady case, (2.38a) [(2.38b)] reduce to the Poisson equation (2.37a) [(2.37b)]. In the unsteady case, both (2.38a) [(2.38b)] are diffusive wave equations (2.39a) [(2.39b)]:

$$\nabla^2 \vec{E} - \frac{1}{c_{em}^2}\frac{\partial^2 \vec{E}}{\partial t^2} - \frac{1}{\alpha_e}\frac{\partial \vec{E}}{\partial t} = \frac{1}{\varepsilon}\nabla q + \frac{\mu}{c^2}\frac{\partial \vec{j}}{\partial t}, \tag{2.39a}$$

$$\nabla^2 \vec{B} - \frac{1}{c_{em}^2}\frac{\partial^2 \vec{E}}{\partial t^2} - \frac{1}{\alpha_e}\frac{\partial \vec{B}}{\partial t} = -\frac{\mu}{c}\nabla \wedge \vec{j}, \tag{2.39b}$$

involving: (i) the **propagation speed** of electromagnetic waves (2.40a); (ii) the **electrical diffusivity** (2.40b):

$$c_{em} = \frac{c}{\sqrt{\varepsilon\mu}}, \qquad \alpha_e = \frac{c^2}{\mu\sigma}; \qquad t - t_0 = \frac{|\vec{x} - \vec{y}|}{c_{em}}, \tag{2.40a–c}$$

the finite speed of propagation of electromagnetic waves (2.40a) implies that a wave emitted at time t_0 by a source at position $\vec{y}$ is received by an observer at position $\vec{x}$ at a time t, increased by the propagation time $t - t_0$, that is equal to the distance $|\vec{x} - \vec{y}|$ divided by the propagation speed c_{em}. The **retarded time** (2.40c) is neglected in the quasi-stationary approximation (subsection 2.1.12).

2.1.12 Retarded Time and Quasi-Stationary Approximation

The electromagnetic propagation speed (2.40a) [Ohmic electric diffusivity (2.40b)] has the dimensions (2.41a) [(2.41b)], where (ℓ, t) are, respectively, the units of length and time:

$$[c_{em}] = \left|\frac{[\partial^2/\partial t^2]}{[\nabla^2]}\right|^{1/2} = \left|\frac{t^{-2}}{\ell^{-2}}\right|^{1/2} = \ell t^{-1}, \quad [\alpha_e] = \left[\frac{\partial/\partial t}{\nabla^2}\right] = \frac{t^{-1}}{\ell^{-2}} = \ell^2 t^{-1}. \tag{2.41a, b}$$

Thus, for an electrical circuit of dimension ℓ the characteristic time for electromagnetic wave propagation (Ohmic electric diffusion) is (2.42a) [(2.42b)]:

$$t_1 \sim \frac{\ell}{c_{em}} = \frac{\ell}{c}\sqrt{\mu\varepsilon} > t_2 \sim \frac{\ell^2}{\alpha_e} = \frac{\ell^2 \mu\sigma}{c^2}; \tag{2.42a, b}$$

for a good insulator with small σ the longer time is that of electromagnetic propagation. For an electrical circuit, the characteristic times are the **period**

of oscillation (2.43a) at the natural frequency (2.23a) [**decay time** (2.43b) associated with damping (2.23b)]:

$$\tau = \frac{2\pi}{\omega_0} = 2\,\pi\sqrt{LC} \quad < \quad \bar{\tau} = \frac{1}{\lambda} = \frac{2L}{R}, \tag{2.43a, b}$$

where for weak damping or low resistance the former is smaller.

The **quasi-stationary approximation** assumes equivalently that: (i) the retarded time (2.40c) can be neglected; (ii) all points of the electrical circuit can be considered at the same time; (iii) the time that electromagnetic waves take to propagate through the circuit (2.42a) is negligible (2.44) compared with the period (2.43a) of natural oscillations:

$$t_2 < \frac{\ell}{c}\sqrt{\mu\varepsilon} \sim t_1 << \tau = 2\pi\sqrt{LC} < \bar{\tau}. \tag{2.44}$$

Since the speed of light in vacuo is large (2.45a):

$$c = 3.0\times 10^8\, ms^{-1}, \quad \ell = 1m, \quad t_1 = \frac{\ell}{c} = 3.3\times 10^{-9}\, s, \quad f_1 = \frac{1}{t_1} = 3.0\times 10^8\, Hz, \tag{2.45a–d}$$

for an electrical circuit with length (2.45b), the time scale being neglected (2.45c) corresponds to a very high-frequency (2.45d). Thus, the quasi-stationary approximation fails for frequencies approaching $f_1/3 = 10^8\, Hz = 100\, MHz$ for a circuit with lengthscale $\ell \sim 1m$, increasing to $10^{10}\, Hz = 10\, GHz$ for a micro-circuit with scale $\ell = 1\ cm$, or $10^{11}\, Hz = 100\, GHz$ for very-large scale integration of circuits with a scale $\ell = 1\ mm$. In the unsteady case, the equation (2.30d) implies the existence of a vector potential (2.34a) that can be substituted in the induction equation (2.25a) leading to (2.46a):

$$0 = \nabla \wedge \left(\vec{E} + \frac{1}{c}\frac{\partial A}{\partial t} \right): \qquad \vec{E} + \frac{1}{c}\frac{\partial \vec{A}}{\partial t} = -\nabla\Phi_e, \tag{2.46a, b}$$

the equation (2.46a) implies the existence of a scalar electric potential (2.46b). The latter equation (2.46b) is valid for the unsteady electromagnetic field and is applied in the quasi-stationary approximation (2.44) to an electrical circuit (subsection 2.1.13) considering the same time at all points.

2.1.13 Electrical Circuit with Electromotive Force or Battery

The equation (2.46b) is integrated along an electrical circuit (2.47b):

$$j = \sigma\vec{E}: \qquad \oint \left(\frac{1}{c}\frac{\partial \vec{A}}{\partial t} + \frac{\vec{j}}{\sigma} + \nabla\Phi_e \right).d\vec{x} = 0, \tag{2.47a, b}$$

where the electric current is related to the electric field (2.47a) through the Ohmic electrical conductivity, which is the second term of (2.28c). In the quasi-stationary approximation (2.44) the electric charge $q(t)$ and current $j(t)$ have the same time dependence at all points of the circuit and the terms in (2.47b) can be interpreted as follows: (i) using the vector potential (2.35b), the first term is proportional to the time derivative of the electric current (2.48a) through the induction corresponding to a self (2.48b):

$$\frac{1}{c}\oint\frac{\partial\vec{A}}{\partial t}.d\vec{x}=\frac{\mu}{4\pi c^2}\frac{d}{dt}\oint\frac{\vec{j}.d\vec{y}}{|\vec{x}-\vec{y}|}=L\frac{dj}{dt}, \qquad L\equiv\frac{\mu}{4\pi c^2}\oint\frac{ds}{|\vec{x}-\vec{y}|}; \tag{2.48a, b}$$

(ii) the second term is the product (2.49a) of the electric current by the resistance (2.49b) obtained integrating the resistivity $1/\sigma$ along the circuit, corresponding to a resistor:

$$\oint\vec{E}.d\vec{x}=\oint\frac{\vec{j}.d\vec{x}}{\sigma}=Rj, \qquad R\equiv\oint\frac{ds}{\sigma}; \tag{2.49a, b}$$

(iii) using the scalar electric potential (2.35a), the third term is proportional to the electric charge (2.50a) through the inverse of the capacity C, corresponding to a capacitor (2.50b):

$$\int_-^+\nabla\Phi_e.d\vec{x}=\frac{1}{4\pi\varepsilon}\oint\frac{q}{|\vec{x}-\vec{y}|}ds=\frac{q}{C}, \qquad \frac{1}{C}=\frac{1}{4\pi\varepsilon}\int_-^+\frac{ds}{|\vec{x}-\vec{y}|}; \tag{2.50a, b}$$

(iv) in (2.50a, b) the potential was taken between the negative and positive pole of a battery, which causes a jump in potential corresponding to an electromotive force (2.51a):

$$F_e(t)=\Phi_+(t)-\Phi_-(t): \qquad \oint\nabla\Phi.d\vec{x}=\int_-^+\nabla\Phi+\Phi_--\Phi_+=\frac{q}{C}-F_e(t), \tag{2.51a, b}$$

and leads to (2.51b) for the change of potential along the whole electrical circuit. Substituting (2.48a; 2.49a; 2.51b) in (2.47b) leads to (2.52b):

$$j=\frac{dq}{dt}\equiv\dot{q}: \qquad L\frac{dj}{dt}+Rj+\frac{q}{C}=F_e(t), \tag{2.52a, b}$$

where the electric charge q and current j are related (2.27a) by (2.52a). Substitution of (2.52a) in (2.52b) leads to (problem 2) *the equation (2.21) for the quasi-stationary electrical circuit, including the definitions of self-induction (2.48b), electrical resistance (2.49b), capacity of a condenser (2.50b), and electromotive force (2.51a).*

2.2 Stable Attractor and Unstable Repeller

The simplest mechanical system consists of a mass and spring, conserving the total energy in the absence of external forcing (subsections 2.2.1); the free motion is an oscillation with constant amplitude around the position of stable equilibrium (subsection 2.2.2). If the parameters of the stable harmonic oscillator vary in time slowly relative to the period, the energy varies in proportion to the natural frequency (subsection 2.2.3). The preceding stable attractor corresponds to a suspended pendulum, whereas an inverted pendulum corresponds to an unstable repeller (subsection 2.2.5), for which the energy increases with time and the free motion is away from the position of unstable equilibrium (subsections 2.2.4).

2.2.1 Harmonic Oscillator: Mass and Spring

The simplest *case I is a mass and a spring without damping (2.53a) or forcing (2.53b), for which (problem 3) the linear equation of motion (2.15) is (2.53c):*

$$\mu = 0 = F_m(t): \qquad m\dot{x} + kx = 0; \tag{2.53a–c}$$

it corresponds to a ***harmonic oscillator*** *(2.54c) with natural frequency (2.54a) and* ***period*** *(2.54b):*

$$\omega_0 \equiv \sqrt{\frac{k}{m}} \equiv \frac{2\pi}{\tau_0} \qquad \ddot{x} + \omega_0^2 x = 0. \tag{2.54a–c}$$

The characteristic polynomial (2.55a) has conjugate imaginary roots (2.55b):

$$P_2(D) = D^2 + \omega_0^2 = (D - \xi_+)(D - \xi_-), \qquad \xi_\pm = \pm i\omega_0, \tag{2.55a, b}$$

corresponding (1.73b, 1.80) in the absence of damping (1.73a) ≡ (2.56a) to the displacement (2.56b) [velocity (2.56c)] that are sinusoidal oscillations with frequency ω_0:

$$\lambda = 0: \quad x(t) = a\cos(\omega_0 t - \alpha), \qquad \dot{x}(t) = -a\omega_0 \sin(\omega_0 t - \alpha); \tag{2.56a–c}$$

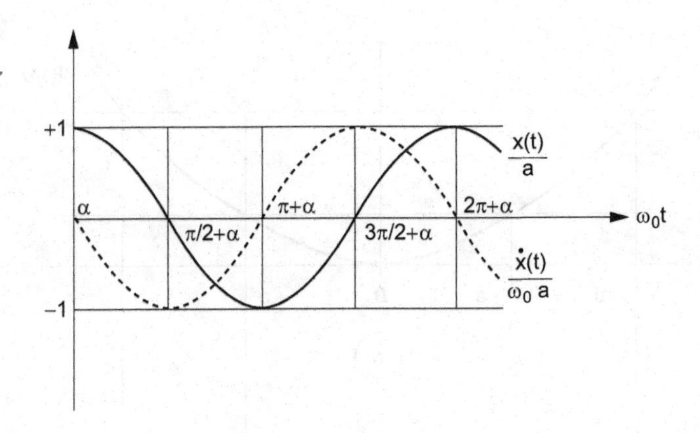

FIGURE 2.4
The linear, undamped, unforced, harmonic oscillator released at initial conditions outside equilibrium performs free oscillations that are sinusoidal with constant amplitude and natural frequency. The velocity has relative to the displacement: (i) an amplitude multiplied by the natural frequency; (ii) a phase lag of one-quarter of the period.

the initial conditions, namely the initial displacement (2.57a) and velocity (2.57b):

$$x_0 \equiv x(0) = a\cos\alpha, \qquad \dot{x}_0 \equiv \dot{x}(0) = a\omega_0 \sin\alpha, \tag{2.57a, b}$$

determine the ***amplitude*** *(2.58a) and the* ***phase*** *(2.58b):*

$$a = \left|(x_0)^2 + \left(\frac{\dot{x}_0}{\omega_0}\right)^2\right|^{1/2}, \qquad \cot\alpha = \frac{\omega_0 x_0}{\dot{x}_0}. \tag{2.58a, b}$$

The free oscillations are illustrated in Figure 2.4, *showing that the velocity (2.56b) is out-of-phase to the displacement (2.56a) by* $\pi/2$:

$$x\left(t+\frac{\tau}{4}\right) = a\cos\left[\omega_0\left(t+\frac{\tau}{4}\right)-\alpha\right] = a\cos\left(\omega_0 t+\frac{\pi}{2}-\alpha\right) = -\sin(\omega_0 t-\alpha) = \frac{\dot{x}(t)}{\omega_0}, \tag{2.59}$$

corresponding to a quarter-period.

2.2.2 Oscillation about a Center of Stable Attraction

The harmonic oscillator corresponds to a potential (2.60a) that is minimum at the origin (Figure 2.5a), *which is the position of stable equilibrium (2.60b–d):*

$$\Phi(x) = \frac{1}{2}kx^2: \qquad \Phi(0) = \Phi'(0) = 0 < \Phi''(0) = k. \tag{2.60a–d}$$

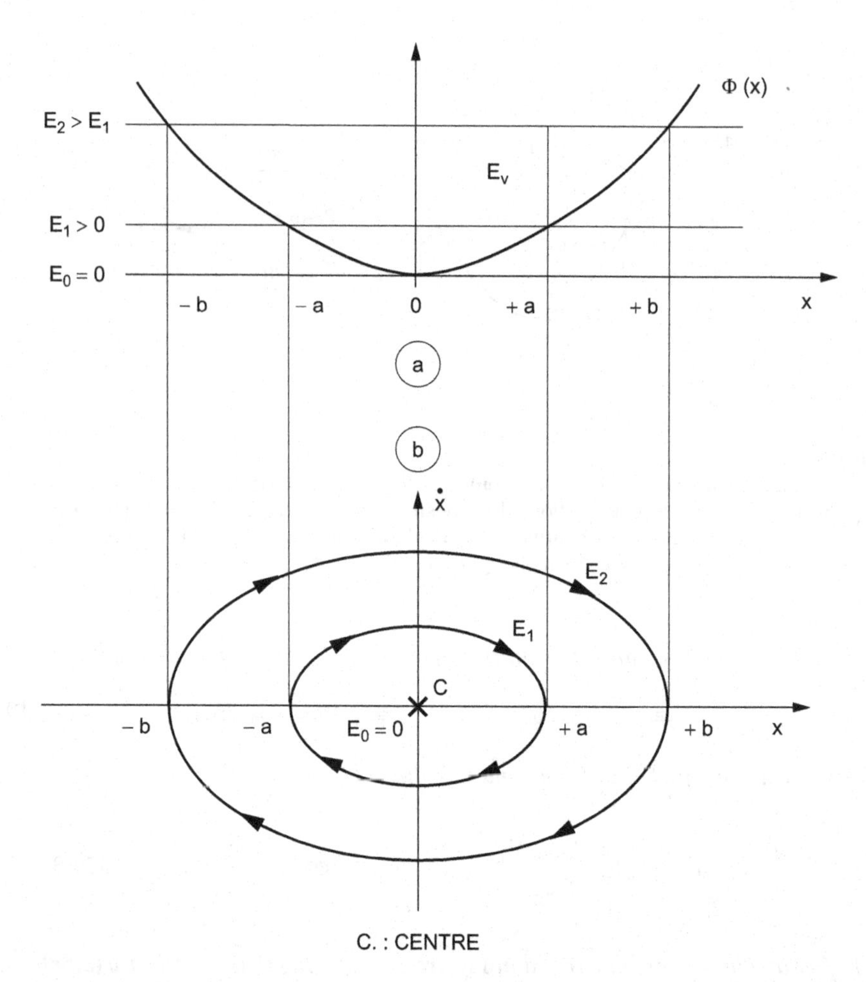

FIGURE 2.5
The free oscillations of the linear harmonic oscillator with neither damping nor forcing (Figure 2.4) corresponds to: (i) a positive quadratic potential (Figure 2.5a) with minimum at the origin that is a positive of stable equilibrium (Figure 2.2a); (ii) the paths in the phase plane of the displacement and the velocity (Figure 2.5b) are ellipses with center at the attractor at the origin.

The potential (2.61a) [kinetic energy (2.61b)] is a quadratic function of the displacement (2.56b) [velocity (2.56c)] multiplied by one-half of the mass (resilience) of the particle (string):

$$\Phi\left(x(t)\right) = \frac{k}{2}\left[x(t)\right]^2 = \frac{k}{2}a^2\cos^2\left(\omega_0 t - \alpha\right), \tag{2.61a}$$

$$E_v\left(\dot{x}(t)\right) = \frac{m}{2}\left[\dot{x}(t)\right]^2 = \frac{m}{2}\omega_0^2 a^2\sin^2\left(\omega_0 t - \alpha\right). \tag{2.61b}$$

Using (2.23a) ≡ (2.62a), it follows that the kinetic energy (2.61b) added to the potential energy (2.61a) leads to a constant total energy (2.62b, c):

$$m\omega_0^2 = k: \qquad E_v + \Phi = \frac{1}{2}ka^2 = \frac{1}{2}m\omega_0^2\,a^2 \equiv E_t = const > 0, \qquad (2.62a\text{–}c)$$

that scales on the square the amplitude.

The motion exchanges potential (2.61a) and kinetic (2.61b) energy to conserve the total energy (2.62b) ≡ (2.62c). In particular, the total energy: (i) reduces to the potential energy only (2.62b) at the maximum displacement equal to the amplitude, when the velocity is zero; (ii) reduces to the kinetic energy (2.62c) at the maximum modulus of the velocity $\omega_0 a$, *which occurs when passing through the equilibrium point, where the potential energy is zero. Eliminating time between the equations (2.56a, b) of the trajectory leads to the* ***path*** *(2.63a) in the* ***phase space****, whose coordinates are the displacement and velocity* (Figure 2.5b)*; the path is an ellipse (2.63a):*

$$x^2 + \left(\frac{\dot{x}}{\omega_0}\right)^2 = a^2 = \frac{2E_t}{k}, \qquad S = \pi\omega_0 a^2 = \frac{2\pi\omega_0 E_t}{k} = \frac{2\pi E_t}{\omega_0 m}, \qquad (2.63a, b)$$

with half-axis a $(\omega_0 a)$ *along the displacement (velocity), so that: (i) the eccentricity increases with frequency; (ii) the half-axis* a *in (2.63b) [area of the ellipse (2.63b)] is proportional to the square root of (to) the energy. The* ***center*** (Figure 2.5a) *is the point of stable equilibrium where the total energy is zero. The* ***stable attractor*** *causes oscillations around the equilibrium position* (Figure 2.5b) *so that the trajectory is* ***closed****, the motion is* ***periodic,*** and *escape to infinity is impossible.*

2.2.3 Adiabatic Invariant for Slow Evolution

Suppose that the natural frequency of the harmonic oscillator varies with time slowly on the scale of a period (2.64a):

$$\frac{1}{\omega_0}\frac{d\omega_0}{dt} << \frac{1}{\tau} = \frac{\omega_0}{2\pi} \quad \Leftrightarrow \quad \frac{d\omega_0}{dt} << \frac{(\omega_0)^2}{2\pi}, \qquad (2.64a, b)$$

corresponding (2.54b) to (2.64b). The **variation** of a path $(x, \dot{x})$ in the phase plane is defined as a **neighboring path** $(x + \delta x, \dot{x} + \delta\dot{x})$, which differs from the original path by first-order infinitesimals, so that the difference (2.65c, d) is a second-order infinitesimal:

$$\varepsilon_1 \neq 0, \infty \neq \varepsilon_2: \qquad \delta x - dx = \varepsilon_1 (dx)^2, \quad \delta v - dv = \varepsilon_2 (dv)^2, \qquad (2.65a\text{–}d)$$

where the coefficients (2.65a, b) are finite and non-zero. The variation of the area (2.66a) enclosed by neighboring paths in the phase plane (Figure 2.5b) is given by (2.66b):

$$S = \oint v\,dx: \qquad \delta S = \oint \left[v\,\delta(dx) + \delta v\,dx \right]. \tag{2.66a, b}$$

The first term on the RHS of (2.66b) is integrated by parts:

$$\oint v\,\delta(dx) = \oint v\,d(\delta x) = [v\,\delta x] - \int \delta x\,dv, \tag{2.67}$$

where the first term on the RHS of (2.67) vanishes because v and δx are the same after one period. Substitution of (2.67) in (2.66b) gives (2.68):

$$\delta\zeta = \oint (\delta v\,dx - \delta x\,dv) = \oint (\varepsilon_2 dv - \varepsilon_1 dx)\,dx\,dv; \tag{2.68}$$

the differences (2.65a–d) are infinitesimals of second-order and hence (2.68) is an infinitesimal of third-order and thus, negligible, implying the conservation of (2.66b) ≡ (2.63b). It has been shown that (problem 4) *if the natural frequency of a harmonic oscillator varies with time slowly in the scale of a period (2.64a) ≡ (2.64b), then there is conservation of an* **adiabatic invariant** *(2.69a), namely the area (2.66a) inside the closed path in the phase plane* (Figure 2.5b):

$$S = const: \qquad \frac{E(t)}{\omega_0(t)} \sim const. \tag{2.69a, b}$$

This implies that: (i) the total energy (2.62b) ≡ (2.62c) varies with time proportionally to the natural frequency (2.69b); (ii)(iii) the half-axis in the direction of the displacement (2.70a) [velocity (2.70b)] of the elliptical path (2.63a) in the phase plane scales (2.63c) as the inverse of (the) square root of the frequency:

$$a(t) \sim \frac{\sqrt{E(t)}}{\omega_0(t)} \sim \frac{1}{\sqrt{\omega_0(t)}}, \qquad b(t) = a(t)\,\omega_0(t) \sim \sqrt{\omega_0(t)}. \tag{2.70a, b}$$

Thus, if the energy increases, so does the natural frequency, implying (Figure 2.6) *that the ellipse is deformed by decreasing (increasing) the maximum displacement (velocity); vice-versa for decreasing energy.* A slow adiabatic variation could apply to the resilience of a spring (subsections 2.2.1–2.2.2) or the length of a pendulum (subsections 2.2.4–2.2.5), since the mass is constant (2.10a).

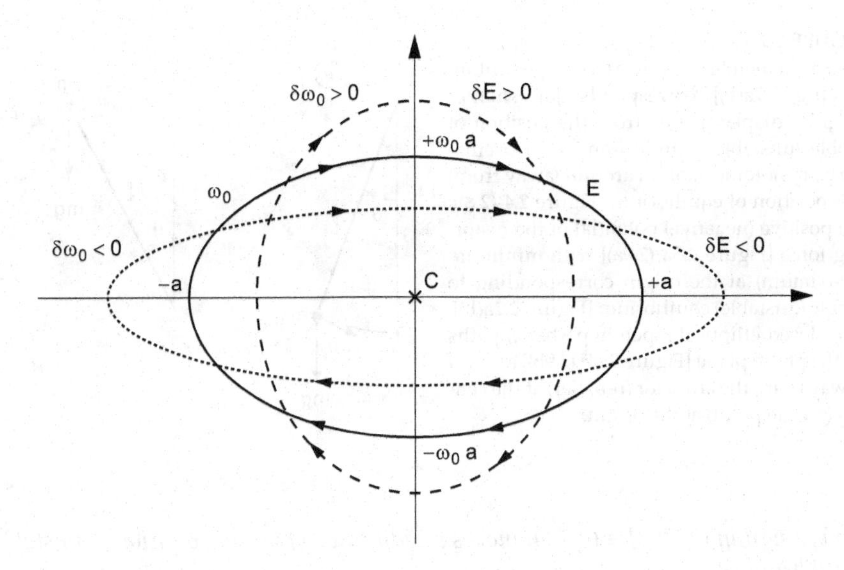

FIGURE 2.6
If the natural frequency of the linear, undamped, unforced oscillator varies slowly on the time scale of a wave period: (i) the oscillations remain sinusoidal with the modified natural frequency (Figure 2.4); (ii) the elliptical paths in the phase plane (Figure 2.5b) are deformed preserving the enclosed area that is an adiabatic invariant; (iii) this implies that the ratio of the total energy to the natural frequency remains constant; (iv) an increasing (decreasing) natural frequency leads to a larger (smaller) total energy, and hence to a smaller (larger) amplitude and a larger (smaller) peak velocity.

2.2.4 Stable (Unstable) Suspended (Inverted) Pendulum

Consider (chapter I.8) a suspended (inverted) pendulum in Figure 2.7a (b), for which the tangential inertia force is balanced by the tangential component of weight (2.71a):

$$m\ell\ddot{\theta} = F_{\mp} = \mp mg\sin\theta = \mp mg\theta\left[1 + O\left(\theta^2\right)\right]; \qquad \text{(2.71a, b)}$$

the linearization of (2.71a) for small angular displacements away from the equilibrium position leads to equation of motion (2.71b) ≡ (2.72b):

$$\omega_0 \equiv \sqrt{\frac{g}{\ell}}: \qquad \ddot{\theta} \pm (\omega_0)^2\,\theta = 0. \qquad \text{(2.72a, b)}$$

showing that: *(i) the (problem 5) suspended pendulum [upper sign in (2.72b)] performs small amplitude oscillations with frequency (2.72a) around the position of stable equilibrium, that is a center; (iii) the (problem 6) inverted pendulum*

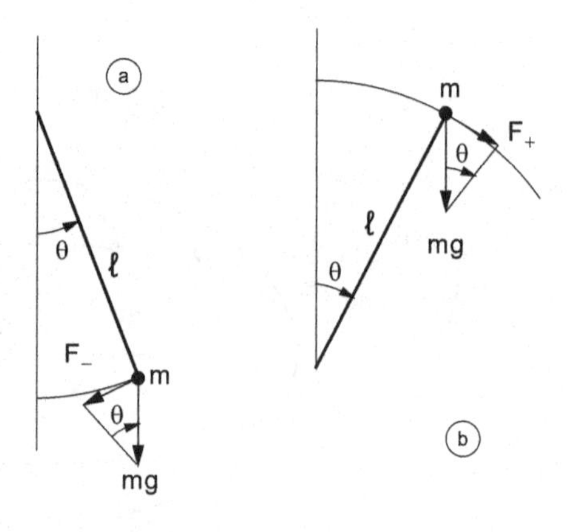

FIGURE 2.7
The suspended (inverted) pendulum [Figure 2.7a(b)] corresponds for smaller angular displacements from the position of stable (unstable) equilibrium to: (i) oscillatory (monotonic) motion around (away from) the position of equilibrium [Figure 2.4 (2.8)]; (ii) positive (negative) potential of the restoring force [Figure 2.5a (2.9a)] with minimum (maximum) at the origin corresponding to stable (unstable) equilibrium [Figure 2.2a(b)]; (iii) closed elliptical (open hyperbolic) paths in the phase plane [Figure 2.6b (2.9b)] around (away from) the attractor (repeller) at the center (saddle point) at the origin.

[lower sign in (2.72b)] ≡ (2.73a) moves steadily away from the position of unstable equilibrium:

$$\ddot{x} - (\omega_0)^2 x = 0: \quad x(t) = a\cosh(\omega_0 t - \alpha), \quad \dot{x}(t) = a\omega_0 \sinh(\omega_0 t - \alpha), \tag{2.73a–c}$$

as shown (1.62a, b; 1.72) by the displacement (2.73b) and velocity (2.73c) increasing monotonically with time (Figure 2.8). *The initial displacement (2.74a) and velocity (2.74b):*

$$x_0 = x(0) = a\cosh\alpha, \qquad \dot{x}_0 = \dot{x}(0) = -a\omega_0 \sinh\alpha, \tag{2.74a, b}$$

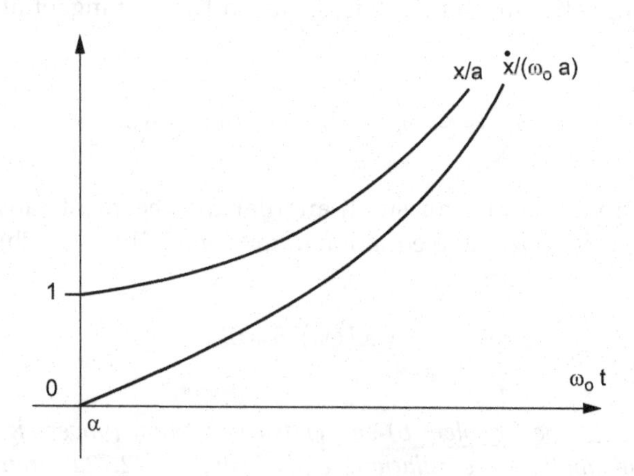

FIGURE 2.8
The linear, undamped, unforced motion due to a repeller at the origin is a monotonic growth of the displacement and the velocity whose ratio is asymptotically constant for large time.

determine the amplitude (2.75a) and phase (2.75b):

$$a \equiv \left| (x_0)^2 - \left(\frac{\dot{x}_0}{\omega_0} \right)^2 \right|^{1/2}, \qquad \coth\alpha = -\frac{\omega_0 x_0}{\dot{x}_0}, \tag{2.75a, b}$$

Thus, *the suspended (inverted) pendulum corresponds [subsections 2.2.1–2.2.3 (2.2.4–2.2.5)] to the case I (II) of stable attractor (**unstable repeller**).* The difference arises from the upper (lower) sign in (2.72b) the equation of motion (2.54c) [(2.73a)] leading to a characteristic polynomial (2.55a) [(2.76a)] with imaginary conjugate (2.55b) [real symmetric (2.76b)] roots:

$$P_2(D) = D^2 - \omega_0^2 = (D - \xi_+)(D - \xi_-), \qquad \xi_\pm = \pm\omega_0, \tag{2.76a, b}$$

and hence, to oscillatory (2.56b, c) [monotonic (2.73b, c)] free motion.

2.2.5 Unstable Repeller and Saddle Point

The potential energy is positive (negative) with minimum (maximum) at the position of equilibrium of the stable attractor (unstable repeller) in Figure 2.5a (2.9a) *with upper (lower) sign in:*

$$F_\mp = \mp kx = -\frac{d\Phi_\mp}{dx}, \qquad \Phi_\mp(x) = \pm\frac{k}{2}x^2. \tag{2.77a, b}$$

The total energy is conserved and positive (2.62b) ≡ (2.62c) [negative (2.78c)] for the stable attractor (unstable repeller):

$$\Phi_+ = -\frac{k}{2}a^2\cosh^2(\omega_0 t - \alpha), \quad E_v = \frac{m}{2}(\omega_0 a)^2 \sinh(\omega_0 t - \alpha), \tag{2.78a, b}$$

$$E_+ = E_v + \Phi_+ = -\frac{k}{2}a^2 = -\frac{m}{2}(\omega_0 a)^2 \equiv const < 0. \tag{2.78c}$$

because: (i) the kinetic energy is always positive (2.61b) [(2.78b)]; (ii) the potential energy is also positive (2.61a) [instead of negative (2.78a) and larger in modulus than the kinetic energy]. A positive (2.62b) ≡ (2.62c) [negative (2.78c)] total energy corresponds to a stable attractor (unstable repeller) because escape to infinity is impossible (not only possible but inevitable). For the unstable repeller (problem 7) for long-time (2.79a) the displacement (2.74a) and velocity (2.74b) are proportional and unbounded (2.79b, c):

$$t \gg \frac{\alpha}{\omega_0}: \qquad \frac{x(t)}{a} \sim \frac{1}{2}e^{\omega_0 t} \sim \frac{\dot{x}(t)}{\omega_0 a}. \tag{2.79a–c}$$

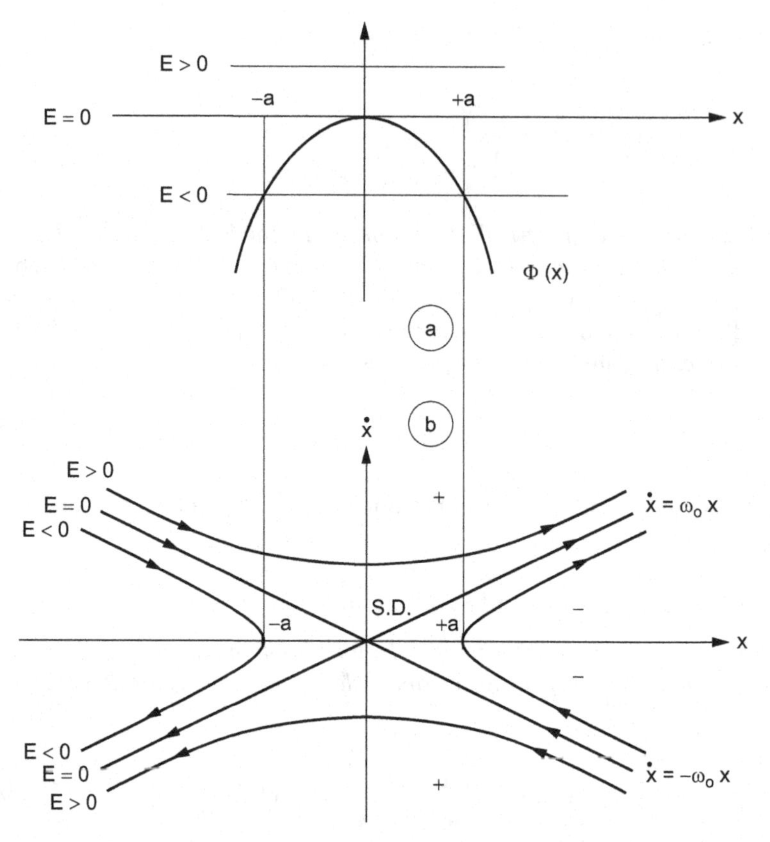

FIGURE 2.9
The negative quadratic potential with maximum at the repeller at the origin (Figure 2.9a), which is a position of unstable equilibrium (Figure 2.7b), corresponds in the phase plane (Figure 2.9b) of the displacement and velocity to: (i) monotonic motion away from the position of unstable equilibrium (Figure 2.8) along hyperbolic paths; (ii) the asymptotes of the hyperbolas have slope specifying the constant asymptotic ratio of the velocity to the displacement; (iii) the asymptotes cross at the saddle point at the repeller at the origin; (iv) the two asymptotes divide the phase plane into four sectors with alternating positive and negative total energy; (*v*) the asymptotes are the lines of zero total energy, that is negative potential energy equal to the modulus of the kinetic energy; (vi) the motion away from the repeller at the origin towards infinity is possible only along the "valleys" of negative total energy.

Eliminating time between the equations of the trajectory (2.73b, c) it follows that the path in phase space for the stable attractor (2.63a) [unstable repeller (2.80a)] is an ellipse (hyperbola) in Figure 2.5b (2.9b):

$$x^2 - \left(\frac{\dot{x}}{\omega_0}\right)^2 = a^2 = -\frac{2E_t}{k}; \qquad \lim_{x\to\infty} \frac{\dot{x}}{x} = \pm\omega_0, \qquad (2.80a, b)$$

for the unstable repeller: (i) the asymptotes of the hyperbolas have slope $\pm\omega_0$ in agreement with (2.79c); (ii) correspond to zero amplitude and energy; (iii) and cross at the point of unstable equilibrium. The point of unstable equilibrium is a **saddle point,** *because: (i) negative energies lead to real amplitudes and possible motion down into the "valleys" for $|\dot{x}| < \omega_0 |x|$; (ii) positive energies would lead to imaginary amplitudes and impossible motion up the "mountains" $|\dot{x}| > \omega_0 |x|$.*

2.3 Free Motion with Critical or Supercritical Damping

The damped oscillator is considered in physical (phase) space in: (i) the case III of critical damping [subsections 2.3.1 (2.3.2)] when the decay to the equilibrium position may be monotonic or have a single extremum; (ii) the case IV of supercritical damping [subsection 2.3.3 (2.3.4)] when the decay to the equilibrium position is always monotonic.

2.3.1 Trajectories of an Oscillator with Critical Damping

In the presence of damping, the free motion of the oscillator (2.22) is specified by the unforced (2.81a) equation (2.81b):

$$f(t) = 0: \qquad 0 = \ddot{x} + 2\lambda\dot{x} + \omega_0^2 x = \left\{ P\left(\frac{d}{dt}\right) \right\} x(t). \qquad \text{(2.81a, b)}$$

The characteristic polynomial (2.82b) of derivatives with regard to time (2.82a):

$$D \equiv \frac{d}{dt}: \qquad P(D) = D^2 + 2\lambda D + \omega_0^2 = (D - \xi_+)(D - \xi_-), \qquad \text{(2.82a, b)}$$

is of the second degree, with roots:

$$\xi_\pm = -\lambda \pm \sqrt{\lambda^2 - \omega_0^2}, \qquad \text{(2.83)}$$

that may be: (i) real and double for $\lambda = \omega_0$; (ii) real and distinct for $\lambda > \omega_0$; (iii) a complex conjugate pair for $\lambda < \omega_0$.

Consider first (i) the case (III) of **critical damping,** equal to the natural frequency, for which the characteristic polynomial (2.82a, b) has a double root:

$$\lambda = \omega_0: \qquad \xi_\pm = -\lambda, \qquad P(D) = (D + \lambda)^2, \qquad \text{(2.84a–c)}$$

and the motion is specified (1.88a; 1.91c) by:

$$\lambda = \omega_0: \quad x(t) = (C_1 + C_2 t)e^{-\lambda t}, \qquad \dot{x}(t) = \frac{dx}{dt} = (C_2 - \lambda C_1 - \lambda C_2 t)e^{-\lambda t}; \tag{2.85a–c}$$

the arbitrary constants of integration (2.86c, d) are determined by the initial conditions (2.86a, b):

$$\{x_0, \dot{x}_0\} \equiv \{x(0), \dot{x}(0)\} = \{C_1, C_2 - \lambda C_1\}: \qquad \{C_1, C_2\} = \{x_0, \dot{x}_0 + \lambda x_0\}. \tag{2.86a, b}$$

Thus, *the displacement (2.87b) and velocity (2.87c) are given by:*

$$\lambda = \omega_0: \quad x(t) = \{x_0 + (\dot{x}_0 + \lambda x_0)t\}e^{-\lambda t}, \quad \dot{x}(t) = \{\dot{x}_0 - \lambda(\dot{x}_0 + \lambda x_0)t\}e^{-\lambda t}, \tag{2.87a–c}$$

for (problem 8) the free motion of an oscillator in the case III of critical damping, (2.87a) showing that an initial linear variation for short time $t << 1/\lambda$, due to the initial conditions, is dominated for long time $t >> 1/\lambda$ by an exponential decay due to damping .

The velocity (2.87c) vanishes (2.88a) at a time (2.88b), corresponding to the maximum displacement in modulus (2.88c):

$$\dot{x}(t_1) = 0, \qquad t_1 = \frac{\dot{x}_0}{\lambda(\dot{x}_0 + \lambda x_0)}, \quad |x|_{max} = |x(t_1)| = \left| x_0 + \frac{\dot{x}_0}{\lambda} \right| \exp(-t_1 \lambda)$$
$$= \left| x_0 + \frac{\dot{x}_0}{\lambda} \right| \exp\left(-\frac{\dot{x}_0}{\dot{x}_0 + \lambda x_0} \right). \tag{2.88a–c}$$

Thus, two cases arise:

$$\frac{x_0 \lambda}{\dot{x}_0} \begin{cases} > -1 \; extremum \quad exists \quad t_1 > 0, & (2.89a) \\ < -1 \; monotonic \quad decay \quad t_1 < 0, & (2.89b) \end{cases}$$

namely (Figure 2.10)*: (i) if the initial displacement and velocity are such that (2.88b) is positive (2.89a), an extremum exists, and the displacement increases in modulus $0 < t < t_1$ to a maximum at time t_1 before decaying to zero $t > t_1$ as $t \to \infty$; (ii) if (2.88b) is negative (2.89b), then the displacement decays monotonically to zero. The latter case occurs if $\lambda x_0 / \dot{x}_0 < -1$; that is possible only if the initial displacement and velocity have opposite signs.*

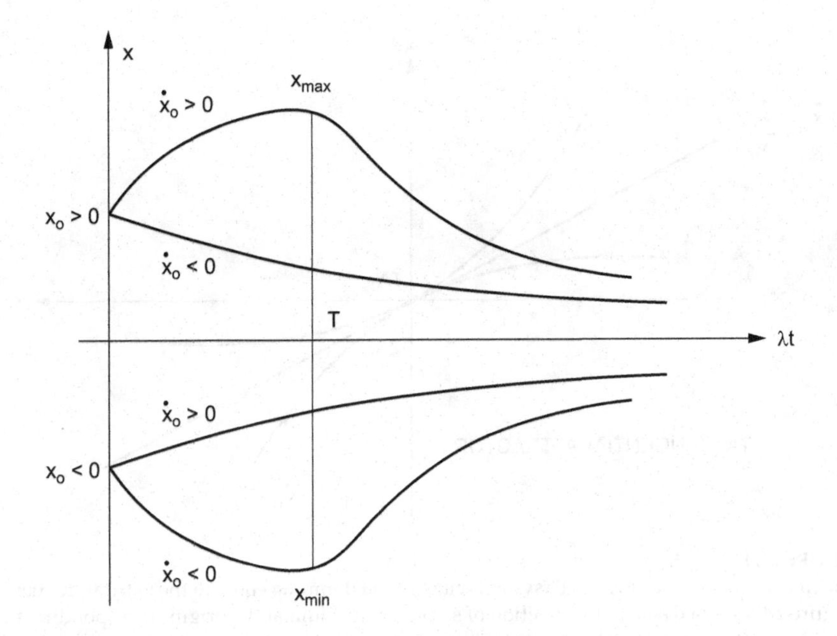

FIGURE 2.10
The linear unforced second-order system with critical damping equal to the natural frequency has: (i) velocity decaying monotonically with time to zero at the equilibrium position, (ii) displacement that ultimately for a long time always decays also monotonically to zero at the equilibrium position; (iii) if the initial velocity has the same sign as the initial displacement there may be an initial increase of the modulus of the displacement before the asymptotic decay (iii); (iv) thus, the decay will be monotonic for all time for the displacement (ii), as it is for the velocity (i), when their initial values have opposite signs.

2.3.2 Critically Damped Oscillator in the Phase Plane

To obtain the paths in the case III of the critical damped oscillator (2.90a) ≡ (2.87a), the time must be eliminated between the displacement (2.87b) and the velocity (2.87c) leading to the identities (2.90b, c):

$$\lambda = \omega_0: \qquad \dot{x}(t) + \lambda x(t) = e^{-\lambda t}\left(\dot{x}_0 + \lambda x_0\right), \tag{2.90a, b}$$

$$\frac{x(t)}{x_0} - \frac{\dot{x}(t)}{\dot{x}_0} = \left(2\lambda + \frac{\dot{x}_0}{x_0} + \lambda^2 \frac{x_0}{\dot{x}_0}\right) t e^{-\lambda t}. \tag{2.90c}$$

The equality (2.90b) is used to define the parameter (2.91a) that appears in (2.90c) ≡ (2.91b):

$$e^{-\lambda t} = \frac{\dot{x}(t) + \lambda x(t)}{\dot{x}_0 + \lambda x_0} \equiv y, \qquad \frac{\dot{x}(t)}{\dot{x}_0} - \frac{x(t)}{x_0} = \left(2 + \frac{\dot{x}_0}{x_0 \lambda} + \frac{x_0 \lambda}{\dot{x}_0}\right) y \log y. \tag{2.91a, b}$$

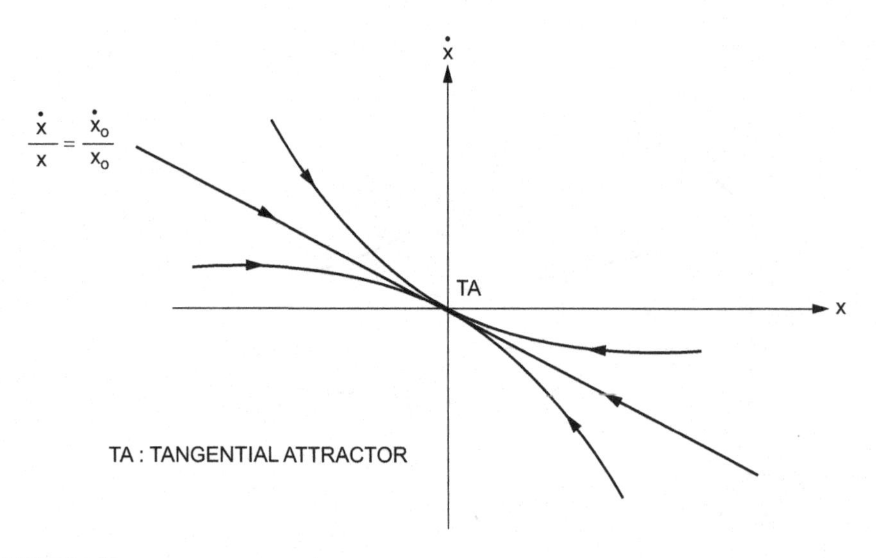

FIGURE 2.11
The linear unforced second-order system with critical damping equal to the natural frequency (Figure 2.10) has a decay to the position of stable equilibrium at the origin corresponding to a tangential attractor in the phase plane (Figure 2.11) since the paths are all tangent to a straight line with slope equal to the ratio of the initial velocity and displacement.

Thus, *the paths of the critically damped oscillator* (2.90a) *are specified in the phase plane by* (2.91b) *involving the parameter (2.91a). The initial conditions* $x/x_0 = 1 = \dot{x}/\dot{x}_0$ *are satisfied* (2.91a) *by* $y = 1$ *in (2.91b). For small* $y << 1$ *the RHS of* (2.91b) *is nearly zero and the paths approach the straight line* $\dot{x}/x = \dot{x}_0/x_0$; *they diverge as y increases, showing that* (Figure 2.11) *for a critically damped oscillator the paths in the phase plane are tangent to the straight line* $\dot{x}/\dot{x}_0 = x/x_0$ *at the equilibrium point, which is a* **tangential attractor**.

2.3.3 Trajectories of an Oscillator with Supercritical Damping

In the case IV of **supercritical damping** (2.92a) the roots (2.83) of the characteristic polynomial (1.82a, b) are (2.92b, c):

$$\lambda > \omega_0: \qquad \xi_\pm = -\lambda \pm \bar{\omega}, \qquad \bar{\omega} \equiv \left|\lambda^2 - \omega_0^2\right|^{1/2} < \lambda; \tag{2.92a–d}$$

the roots for (2.92a) ≡ (2.93a) are real and distinct (2.92b, c), and (2.92d) is satisfied. The roots (problem 9) (2.92b) correspond (1.62a,b; 1.72) to the displacement (2.93b) and velocity (2.93c):

$$\lambda > \omega_0: \qquad x(t) = ae^{-\lambda t}\cosh(\bar{\omega}t - \alpha), \tag{2.93a, b}$$

$$\dot{x}(t) = ae^{-\lambda t}\left\{\bar{\omega}\sinh(\bar{\omega}t - \alpha) - \lambda\cosh(\bar{\omega}t - \alpha)\right\}. \tag{2.93c}$$

The initial conditions (2.94a, b):

$$x_0 \equiv x(0) = a\cosh\alpha, \quad -\dot{x}_0 \equiv -\dot{x}(0) = a(\bar{\omega}\sinh\alpha + \lambda\cosh\alpha) = a\bar{\omega}\sinh\alpha + \lambda x_0, \tag{2.94a, b}$$

determine the amplitude (2.95a) and the phase (2.95b):

$$a = \left|(x_0)^2 - \left(\frac{\dot{x}_0 + x_0\lambda}{\bar{\omega}}\right)^2\right|^{1/2}, \qquad -\tanh\alpha = \frac{\lambda}{\bar{\omega}} + \frac{\dot{x}_0}{x_0\bar{\omega}}. \tag{2.95a, b}$$

that appear in the displacement (2.93b) and the velocity (2.93c). The displacement (2.93b) is the sum of two terms (2.96b):

$$\lambda > \bar{\omega}: \qquad \frac{a}{2}\exp(-\lambda t \pm \bar{\omega}t \mp \alpha) = \frac{a}{2}e^{\mp\alpha}\exp\left[(-\lambda \mp \bar{\omega})t\right], \tag{2.96a–c}$$

and since (2.92a, c) implies (2.92d) ≡ (2.96a), the time dependence in (2.96b) ≡ (2.96c) consists of negative exponentials that decay monotonically to zero as $t \to \infty$. It can be confirmed (2.97a) from (2.93b) that the displacement has the same sign as the amplitude (2.97b) and is smaller for all time, so there is no oscillation or growth, just a monotonic decay:

$$\frac{x(t)}{a} < 1; \qquad \cosh(\bar{\omega}t - \alpha) > \sinh(\bar{\omega}t - \alpha): \qquad \frac{\dot{x}(t)}{a} < 0. \tag{2.97a–c}$$

Also the inequality (2.97b) together with (2.96a) prove (2.97c) that the velocity is negative, confirming a monotonic decay towards the equilibrium position. This is confirmed by the approximations (2.98b, c) for large time (2.98a):

$$t >> \frac{\alpha}{\bar{\omega}}: \qquad x(t) \sim \frac{a}{2}e^{-(\lambda-\bar{\omega})t} \sim \frac{\dot{x}(t)}{\lambda - \bar{\omega}}. \tag{2.98a–c}$$

Thus, *the free motion (2.93b, c) of an oscillator with supercritical damping (2.92a–c), from arbitrary initial conditions (2.95a, b), is a monotonic decay* (Figure 2.12), *towards the equilibrium position $x(t) \to 0$ as $t \to \infty$.*

2.3.4 Supercritically Damped Oscillator in the Phase Plane

In order to eliminate time in the case IV of an oscillator with supercritical damping (2.92a–c), the trajectory may be specified alternatively (1.63a, b) to (2.93a–c), by:

$$\lambda > \omega_0: \qquad \{x(t), \dot{x}(t)\} = a_+\{1, \xi_+\}\exp(\xi_+ t) + a_-\{1, \xi_-\}\exp(\xi_- t); \tag{2.99a–c}$$

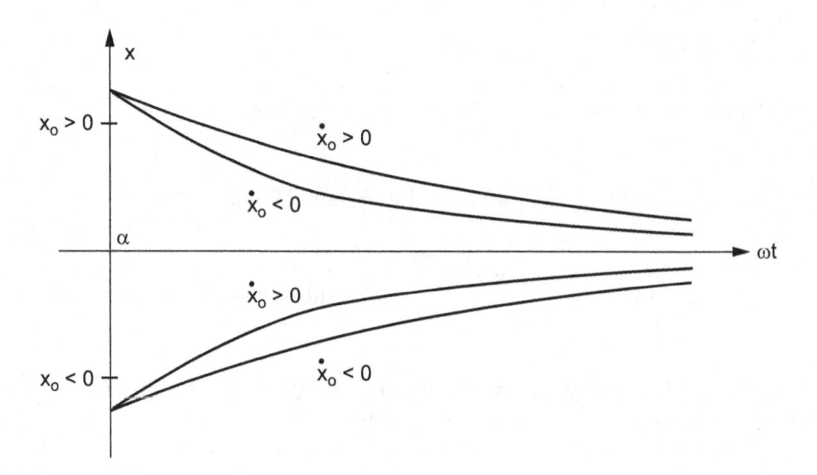

FIGURE 2.12
Linear unforced second-order system with supercritical (critical) damping larger than (equal to) the natural frequency has a decay to the position of stable equilibrium at the origin that is always (not always) monotonic [Figure (2.10)] independent from (depending on) the initial conditions. In the supercritical case, the monotonic decay of the modulus of the displacement towards the equilibrium point at the origin (Figure 2.12) is faster (slower) if the initial displacement and velocity have opposite signs (the same sign).

the amplitudes (2.100c, d) are specified by the initial conditions (2.100a, b):

$$x_0 = a_+ + a_-, \quad \dot{x}_0 = a_+\xi_+ + a_-\xi_-: \quad (\xi_+ - \xi_-)a_\pm = \{\dot{x}_0 - \xi_- x_0, \xi_+ x_0 - \dot{x}_0\}. \tag{2.100a–d}$$

From (2.99b, c) follow (2.101a, b), where the RHS are constants and can be evaluated at time $t = 0$:

$$(\xi_+ x - \dot{x})\exp(-\xi_- t) = a_-(\xi_+ - \xi_-) = \xi_+ x_0 - \dot{x}_0, \tag{2.101a}$$

$$(\xi_- x - \dot{x})\exp(-\xi_+ t) = a_+(\xi_- - \xi_+) = \xi_- x_0 - \dot{x}_0. \tag{2.101b}$$

Time appears in (2.101a, b) as a common factor (2.102a, b):

$$\left(\frac{\xi_+ x - \dot{x}}{\xi_+ x_0 - \dot{x}_0}\right)^{1/\xi_-} = e^t = \left(\frac{\xi_- x - \dot{x}}{\xi_- x_0 - \dot{x}_0}\right)^{1/\xi_+}; \tag{2.102a, b}$$

time is eliminated between (2.102a, b) leading to (2.102c):

$$\frac{\dot{x} - \xi_+ x}{\dot{x}_0 - \xi_+ x_0} = \left(\frac{\dot{x} - \xi_- x}{\dot{x}_0 - \xi_- x_0}\right)^{\xi_-/\xi_+}. \tag{2.102c}$$

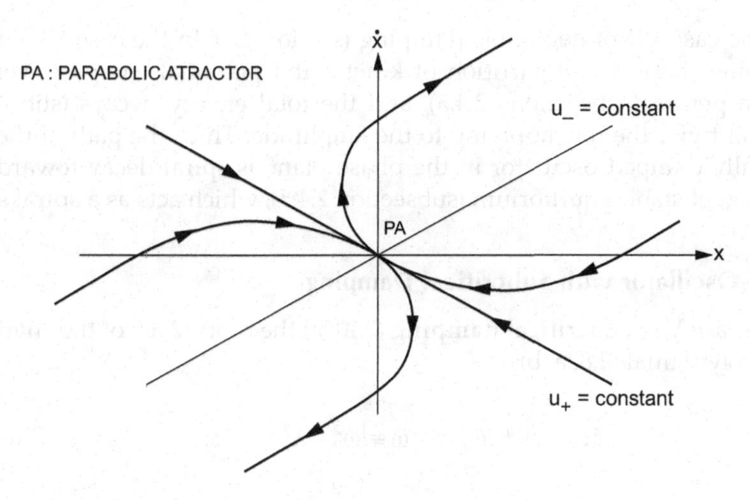

FIGURE 2.13
The linear unforced second-order system with supercritical damping larger than the natural frequency has a monotonic decay towards the position of stable equilibrium at the origin (Figure 2.12) corresponding to a tangential attractor since all paths are power-law parabolas with u_--axis of "symmetry" and tangent to the u_+-axis.

Thus, *the paths of an oscillator (2.81b) with supercritical damping (2.82a, b; 2.92a–d) in the phase plane are parabolas (2.103a) with axis (2.103b, c):*

$$u_+ = (u_-)^{\vartheta}, \qquad u_\pm \equiv \frac{\dot{x} - \xi_\pm x}{\dot{x}_0 - \xi_\pm x_0}, \tag{2.103a–c}$$

and exponent (2.104b):

$$\lambda > \omega: \qquad \vartheta \equiv \frac{\xi_-}{\xi_+} = \frac{\lambda + \omega}{\lambda - \omega} > 1, \tag{2.104a, b}$$

that all pass through the position of stable equilibrium (Figure 2.13), *which is a* **parabolic attractor.**

2.4 Free Oscillations with Strong, Weak, or No Damping

There are three instances of a damped oscillator, namely critical (case III: subsections 2.3.1–2.3.2), supercritical (case IV: subsections 2.3.3–2.3.4) and subcritical damping (section 2.4). The latter, subcritically damped oscillator (section 2.4), splits into three subcases: (i) case V of strong subcritical damping (subsection 2.4.1); (ii) the case VI of weak damping (subsection 2.4.2);

(iii) the case VII of negligible damping (section 2.2). In the case VI of weak damping there is equipartition of kinetic and potential energies averaged over a period (subsections 2.4.3), and the total energy decays (subsection 2.4.4) at twice the rate applying to the amplitude. Thus, the path of the sub-critically damped oscillator in the phase plane is spiral decay towards the position of stable equilibrium (subsection 2.4.5), which acts as a spiral sink.

2.4.1 Oscillator with Subcritical Damping

In the case V of **subcritical damping** (2.105a) the roots (2.83) of the characteristic polynomial (2.82a, b):

$$\lambda < \omega_0: \qquad \xi_\pm = -\lambda \pm i\bar{\omega}, \qquad \bar{\omega} \equiv \left|\omega_0^2 - \lambda^2\right|^{1/2} < \omega_0, \tag{2.105a–d}$$

are a complex conjugate pair (2.105b, c); the imaginary part (2.105c) is the **oscillation frequency** that coincides with (2.92c) the real term with ± sign in (2.92b), and satisfies a different inequality (2.105d) ≠ (2.92d). *The oscillation frequency:*

$$\bar{\omega}\begin{cases} = \omega_0 & \text{if} \quad \lambda = 0, & (2.105\text{e}) \\ < \omega_0 & \text{if} \quad 0 < \lambda < \omega_0, & (2.105\text{f}) \\ = 0 & \text{if} \quad \lambda = \omega_0, & (2.105\text{g}) \end{cases}$$

is: (i) equal to the natural frequency (2.23a) ≡ (2.54a) in the absence of damping (2.105e); (ii) is reduced (2.105f) by subcritical damping; (iii) is zero for critical damping (2.105g) when there is no oscillation. The free motion (1.73a, b; 1.80) involves both damping at the exponential rate λ and oscillation at the oscillation frequency $\bar{\omega}$:

$$\lambda < \omega_0: \qquad x(t) = ae^{-\lambda t}\cos(\bar{\omega}t - \alpha), \tag{2.106a, b}$$

$$\dot{x}(t) = -ae^{-\lambda t}\left\{\bar{\omega}\sin(\bar{\omega}t - \alpha) + \lambda\cos(\bar{\omega}t - \alpha)\right\}, \tag{2.106c}$$

involving an **amplitude** a and a **phase** α. The initial conditions (2.107a, b):

$$x_0 \equiv x(0) = a\cos\alpha, \quad \dot{x}_0 \equiv \dot{x}(0) = a(\bar{\omega}\sin\alpha - \lambda\cos\alpha) = a\bar{\omega}\sin\alpha - \lambda x_0, \tag{2.107a, b}$$

specify the amplitude (2.108a) and the phase (2.108b):

$$a = \left|(x_0)^2 + \left(\frac{\dot{x}_0 + x_0\lambda}{\bar{\omega}}\right)^2\right|^{1/2}, \qquad \tan\alpha = \frac{\lambda}{\bar{\omega}} + \frac{\dot{x}_0}{x_0\bar{\omega}}, \tag{2.108a, b}$$

The constants a, α in the case of subcritical damping (2.108a, b) are similar to the case of overcritical damping (2.95a, b), changing one sign in the first formula, and exchanging hyperbolic for circular tangent in the second formula.

2.4.2 Strong, Weak, or Negligible Damping

The displacement (2.106b) in the case V of ***strong subcritical damping*** *(2.106a) corresponds* (Figure 2.14) *to (problem 10): (i) a sinusoidal oscillation of frequency $\bar{\omega} < \omega_0$ in (2.105f) less than the natural frequency ω_0 with a phase shift (2.108b); (ii) an amplitude decaying rapidly at the exponential rate λ from an initial amplitude.* Thus, *the displacement becomes (2.106a, b) ≡ (2.109a, b):*

$$\lambda < \omega_0: \qquad x(t) = a e^{-\lambda t} \cos\{2\pi(t - \tau_0)/\bar{\tau}\}; \tag{2.109a, b}$$

with phase shift (2.110b) relative to the period of oscillation (2.110a):

$$\bar{\tau} = \frac{2\pi}{\bar{\omega}} = 2\pi\left|\omega_0^2 - \lambda^2\right|^{-1/2}, \qquad \tau_0 = \frac{\alpha}{\bar{\omega}} = \frac{\alpha\bar{\tau}}{2\pi}. \tag{2.110a, b}$$

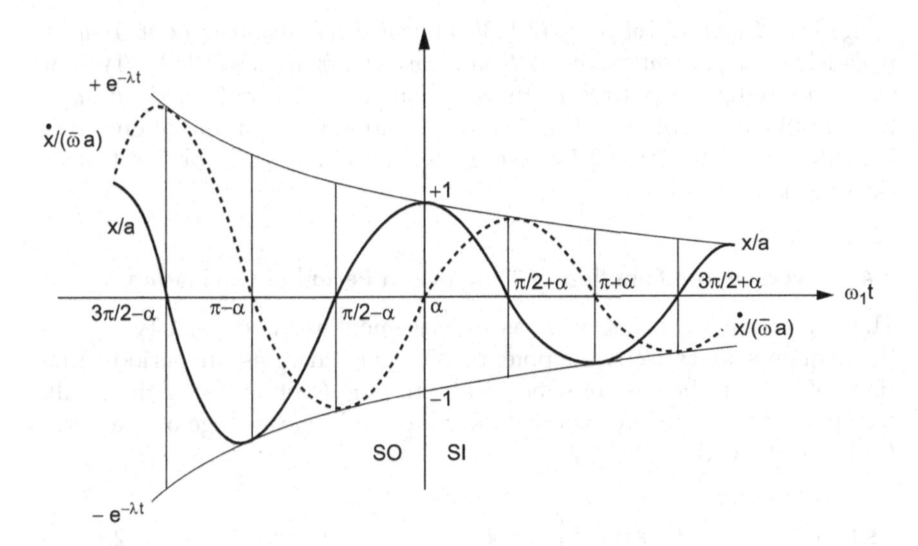

FIGURE 2.14
The linear unforced second-order system with subcritical damping smaller than the natural frequency: (i) has an oscillatory decay towards the position of equilibrium at the origin with exponentially decreasing amplitude; (ii) the frequency of oscillation is equal to the natural frequency for weak damping and smaller for strong damping; (iii) the velocity has relative to the displacement an amplitude multiplied by the oscillation frequency and a phase lag of one-quarter of the period.

In the limit $\lambda \to \omega_0$ of critical damping, the period diverges $\tau_1 \to \infty$, and the frequency vanishes $\bar{\omega} \to 0$, so that the oscillation ceases (Figure 2.10) *apart from a possible single maximum or minimum, which cannot exist for overcritical damping* (Figure 2.12). *In (problem 11) the opposite (or the case VI) limit of* ***weak damping*** *(2.111a):*

$$\lambda^2 << \omega_0^2: \qquad \bar{\omega} = \omega_0, \qquad \bar{\tau} = \frac{2\pi}{\bar{\omega}} = \frac{2\pi}{\omega_0} = \tau_0, \qquad (2.111a–c)$$

the: (i) frequency (2.111b) and period (2.111c) of oscillation corresponds to the natural frequency, as in the undamped case (2.56b, c); (ii) the amplitude decay is slow (2.112a–c):

$$\theta = \omega_0 t - \alpha: \qquad x(t) = ae^{-\lambda t}\cos\theta, \qquad \dot{x}(t) = -ae^{-\lambda t}\left(\lambda\cos\theta + \omega_0\sin\theta\right). \qquad (2.112a–c)$$

In case I of ***negligible damping*** *(problem 3), the amplitude is constant* (Figure 2.4):

$$\lambda << \omega_0: \qquad x(t) = a\cos(\omega_0 t - \alpha), \qquad \dot{x}(t) = -a\omega\sin(\omega_0 t - \alpha). \qquad (2.113a–c)$$

in agreement with (2.56b, c) ≡ (2.113b, c), where zero damping (2.56a) may be replaced by damping much smaller than the natural frequency (2.113a). The constant (decaying) amplitude in the undamped (2.113a–c) [weakly damped (2.112a–c)] free oscillation, implies conservation (dissipation) of energy, as is confirmed (subsection 2.4.4) using averages over a wave period (subsection 2.4.3).

2.4.3 Average of a Function of Time over a Period of Oscillation

The oscillation variables, such as displacement $x(t)$ and velocity $\dot{x}(t)$ and their squares, that specify the potential Φ and E_v energies, are periodic functions of time in the case of subcritical damping (section 2.4) of the oscillatory motion, and may be averaged over a period. The average over a period (2.114a) is defined by (2.114b):

$$0 \le t < \tau: \qquad \langle f(\omega t)\rangle \equiv \frac{1}{\tau}\int_0^\tau f(\omega t)\,dt = \frac{1}{2\pi}\int_0^{2\pi} f(\theta)\,d\theta, \qquad (2.114a–c)$$

and becomes a circular average (2.114c), using the change of variable:

$$\theta = \omega t = \frac{2\pi}{\tau}t, \qquad dt = \frac{d\theta}{\omega} = \frac{\tau}{2\pi}d\theta. \qquad (2.115a, b)$$

The examples of the calculation of time averages over a period of oscillation include:

$$\langle\cos(\omega t)\rangle = \langle\sin(\omega t)\rangle = 0 = \langle\cos(\omega t)\sin(\omega t)\rangle, \qquad (2.116\text{a–c})$$

$$\langle\cos^2(\omega t)\rangle = \frac{1}{2} = \langle\sin^2(\omega t)\rangle, \qquad (2.117\text{a, b})$$

(i) the average of a cosine or sine is zero (2.116a, b); (ii) also for the cross-product (2.116c), that consists of factors out-of-phase by $\pi/2$; (iii) the square of sine or cosine has factors in phase, leading to a non-zero mean value 1/2 in (2.117a, b). The results (2.116a–c; 2.117a, b) can be proved as follows: (i) the sine and cosine have (2.116a, b) zero mean value:

$$2\pi\langle\cos(\omega t)\rangle = \int_0^{2\pi}\cos\theta\, d\theta = 0 = \int_0^{2\pi}\sin\theta\, d\theta = 2\pi\langle\sin(\omega t)\rangle; \qquad (2.118\text{a, b})$$

(ii) the product of sine and cosine (2.116c) is proportional to a sine of double argument, and has zero mean value by (2.118c):

$$\langle\sin(\omega t)\cos(\omega t)\rangle = \frac{1}{2}\langle\sin(2\theta)\rangle = 0; \qquad (2.118\text{c})$$

(iii) the square of sine and cosine (2.117a, b) have mean value one-half:

$$\langle\cos^2(\omega t)\rangle, \langle\sin^2(\omega t)\rangle = \langle\cos^2\theta\rangle, \langle\sin^2\theta\rangle = \left\langle\frac{1\pm\cos(2\theta)}{2}\right\rangle = \frac{1}{2}, \qquad (2.119\text{a, b})$$

apart from a cosine of double argument, which has zero mean value.

2.4.4 Equipartition, Conservation, and Dissipation of Energy

The kinetic, potential, and total energies and their average over a period of oscillation are calculated in Examples 10.4.1–10.4.2 for strong subcritical damping. The case I of negligible damping has already been considered (section 2.2), and the case VI of weak damping is considered next. In the case of a free damped oscillation, the total energy must decay by dissipation, but the equipartition of kinetic and potential energies still holds, in the case of weak damping, as shown next. In the case of weak damping (2.111a–c), the decay of amplitude occurs on a time scale $1/\lambda >> 1/\omega_0 \sim \tau_0/2\pi$ much larger than the period, so that time averages are not applied to the exponential amplitude **envelope**, but only to the sinusoidal **waveform**. The displacement (2.112b) [velocity (2.112c)] has zero mean value over a period (2.120b) [(2.120c)] as follows from (2.116a) [(2.116b)] using the phase function (2.120a):

$$\theta \equiv \omega_0 t - \alpha: \qquad \langle x(t)\rangle = a\langle\cos\theta\rangle = 0, \qquad \langle\dot{x}(t)\rangle = \omega_0 a\langle\sin\theta\rangle = 0. \qquad (2.120\text{a–c})$$

The potential (2.5b) [kinetic (2.10b)] energy follows from (2.112b) [(2.112c)] as a function of time (2.121a) [(2.121b)]:

$$\Phi_m(t) = \frac{1}{2}k\left[x(t)\right]^2 = \frac{k}{2}a^2 e^{-2\lambda t}\cos^2\theta, \tag{2.121a}$$

$$E_v(t) = \frac{1}{2}m\left[\dot{x}(t)\right]^2 = \frac{m}{2}a^2 e^{-2\lambda t}\left(\omega_0\sin\theta + \lambda\cos\theta\right)^2. \tag{2.121b}$$

The average over a period of the square of the velocity in (2.121b) is given by:

$$\begin{aligned} e^{2\lambda t}\left\langle\left[\dot{x}(t)\right]^2\right\rangle &= a^2\left[\omega_0^2\left\langle\sin^2\theta\right\rangle + 2\lambda\omega_0\left\langle\sin\theta\cos\theta\right\rangle + \lambda^2\left\langle\cos^2\theta\right\rangle\right] \\ &= \frac{a^2}{2}\left(\omega_0^2 + \lambda^2\right) = \frac{\omega_0^2 a^2}{2}\left[1 + O\left(\frac{\lambda}{\omega_0}\right)^2\right], \end{aligned} \tag{2.122}$$

where: (i) the middle term on the RHS is zero by (2.116c); (ii) using (2.117a, b) leads to (2.122) where the third term is negligible compared with the first in the weak damping approximation (2.111a).

The average over a period is given for: (i) the potential energy (2.121a) exactly by (2.123a):

$$\left\langle\Phi_m(t)\right\rangle = \frac{k}{4}a^2 e^{-2\lambda t}; \qquad \omega_0^2 >> \lambda^2: \qquad \left\langle E_v(t)\right\rangle = \frac{m}{4}a^2\omega_0^2 e^{-2\lambda t}, \tag{2.123a–c}$$

(ii) for the kinetic energy (2.121b) by (2.123c) using (2.122) the weak damping approximation (2.123b). It follows that the sum of potential (2.121a) and kinetic (2.121b) energies, that is, the total energy, is given by (2.124b) using (2.23a) ≡ (2.124a):

$$m\omega_0^2 = k: \quad E_t(t) = \Phi_m(t) + E_v(t) = \frac{k}{2}a^2 e^{-2\lambda t}\left[1 + \frac{2\lambda}{\omega_0}\cos\theta\sin\theta + \left(\frac{\lambda}{\omega_0}\right)^2\sin^2\theta\right]. \tag{2.124a, b}$$

For weak damping (2.125a) the average over a period of the potential (2.123a) and kinetic (2.123c) energy is the same (2.125b), and the ***equipartion of energies*** *implies that the average of the total energy over a period is (2.125c), twice either of them:*

$$\omega_0^2 >> \lambda^2: \qquad 2\left\langle\Phi_m(t)\right\rangle = 2\left\langle E_v(t)\right\rangle = E_t(t) = -\frac{k}{2}a^2 e^{-2\lambda t} = \frac{m}{2}\omega_0^2 a^2 e^{-2\lambda t}, \tag{2.125a–c}$$

and they all decay exponentially with time on twice the damping rate. The rate of decay with time of the total energy averaged over a period equals minus the dissipation:

$$\frac{d}{dt}(\langle E_t \rangle) = -k\lambda a^2 e^{-2\lambda t} = -\Psi_m, \tag{2.126}$$

as can be confirmed from:

$$\langle \Psi_m(t) \rangle = \mu \left\langle \left[\dot{x}(t) \right]^2 \right\rangle = m\lambda a^2 \omega_0^2 e^{-2\lambda t} = k\lambda a^2 e^{-2\lambda t}, \tag{2.127}$$

where were used (2.8b; 2.23b, 2.122; 2.23a).

2.4.5 Oscillator with Subcritical Damping in the Phase Plane

From (2.106b, c) in the form (2.128a) follows (2.128b):

$$\dot{x} + \lambda x = -a\bar{\omega}e^{-\lambda t}\sin(\bar{\omega}t - \alpha): \qquad x^2 + \left(\frac{\dot{x} + \lambda x}{\bar{\omega}}\right)^2 = a^2 e^{-2\lambda t}. \tag{2.128a, b}$$

In the case of negligible damping $\lambda = 0, \omega = \omega_0$ this corresponds (2.128b) ≡ (2.63a) to an elliptic path (Figure 2.5b) in the phase plane around the position of stable equilibrium at the center. In the case of weak damping, the path (2.128b) is an ellipse whose half-axis decay $e^{-\lambda t}$ is like the amplitude and whose area decays $e^{-2\lambda t}$ like the energy so that the path is not exactly closed and resembles an elliptic spiral decaying towards the center. Strictly a path in the phase space cannot involve time, and the preceding approximate interpretation does not extend to strong damping.

In the case V of strong subcritical damping, time is completely eliminated from (2.128b) by: (i) using (2.106b) and (2.128a) to obtain (2.129a):

$$-\tan(\bar{\omega}t - \alpha) = \frac{\lambda}{\bar{\omega}} + \frac{\dot{x}}{\bar{\omega}x}; \quad x^2 + \left(\frac{\dot{x} + \lambda x}{\bar{\omega}}\right)^2 = a^2 \exp\left\{-\frac{2\lambda}{\bar{\omega}}\left[\alpha - \arctan\left(\frac{\lambda}{\bar{\omega}} + \frac{\dot{x}}{\bar{\omega}x}\right)\right]\right\}. \tag{2.129a, b}$$

(ii) substituting (2.129a) in (2.128b) to obtain (2.129b). Introducing the complex variable (2.130a) with modulus (2.130b) and phase (2.130c):

$$z \equiv x + i\frac{\dot{x} + \lambda x}{\bar{\omega}} \equiv re^{i\phi}, \quad r \equiv |z| = \left| x^2 + \left(\frac{\dot{x} + \lambda x}{\omega}\right)^2 \right|^{1/2}, \qquad \tan\phi \equiv \frac{\lambda}{\bar{\omega}} + \frac{\dot{x}}{\bar{\omega}x}:$$

$$r = a\exp\left[-\frac{\lambda}{\bar{\omega}}(\alpha - \phi)\right]. \tag{2.130a–d}$$

the path (2.129b) in the phase plane is a logarithmic spiral (2.130d).

Thus, the path of a subcritical oscillator in the phase plane (2.129b) ≡ (2.130a–d) is a decay along a logarithmic spiral (Figure 2.15b) *towards the position of stable equilibrium, which acts as a* ***spiral sink*** *(SI) consistent with a positive potential with a minimum* (Figure 2.15a). *The same path taken in the opposite direction would correspond to a* ***spiral source*** *(SO) and would apply to* ***amplified*** *motion away from a position of unstable equilibrium (section 2.5).*

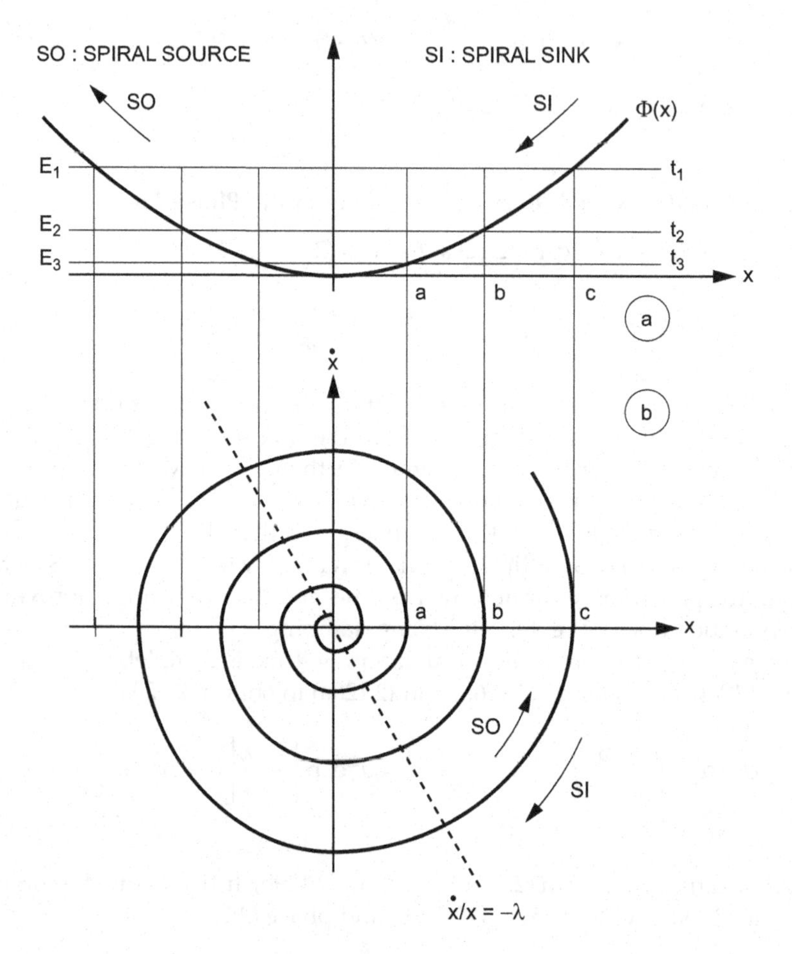

FIGURE 2.15
The linear unforced second-order system with subcritical damping smaller than the natural frequency has an oscillatory decay towards the position of stable equilibrium at the origin (Figure 2.14) corresponding in the phase plane of the displacement and velocity to a logarithmic spiral toward the spiral sink at the center (Figure 2.15b); this replaces the ellipses (Figure 2.5) for undamped oscillations by a spiral decay towards the center for the same positive quadratic potential (Figure 2.15a ≡ 2.5a) corresponding to stable equilibrium (Figure 2.2a). The logarithmic spiral path may be described in opposite directions for a sink (source) at the attractor (repeller) at the center corresponding to a decaying (growing) oscillation [Figure 2.14 (2.18)] that is a case of damped (amplified) motion [Figure 2.9–2.15 (2.16–2.21)].

2.5 Mechanical and Electrical Amplified Oscillations

The latter case VIII of amplification (subsection 2.5.3) or reduced damping (subsection 2.5.2) corresponding to "negative" damping is possible for simple mechanical systems, for example: (i) a mass and a spring on a rolling belt with friction (subsection 2.5.1); (ii) the Froude pendulum suspended from a rotating cam causing a friction torque (subsection 2.5.4). An electrical analogue (iii) is a self-capacitor circuit with a valve (subsection 2.5.5).

2.5.1 Amplified Mechanical Circuit

The basic mechanical circuit consists (Figure 2.1) of a mass m and spring k, with a damper μ; if (problem 12) the mass is placed on a rolling carpet (Figure 2.16) with velocity u, the equation of motion (2.22) has an extra term:

$$m\ddot{x} + \mu\dot{x} + kx = H(u - \dot{x}), \tag{2.131}$$

namely, the forcing by an **applied friction force** that depends on the difference of velocity between the belt u and the mass $\dot{x}$. The dependence of the friction force on the velocity (Figure 2.17) has: (i) an initial value (2.132a) corresponding to **static friction**; (ii) it then reduces for small velocity (2.132b); (iii) it eventually increases for larger velocities. For small velocity $\dot{x}$ of the mass, the linear approximation to the friction force between the mass and the belt is given by the first two terms of the Taylor series (I.23.32b) ≡ (2.132c) around the belt velocity x:

$$h_0 \equiv H(u), h_1 = -\frac{dH}{du} > 0: \quad H(u - \dot{x}) = H(u) - \dot{x}\frac{dH}{du} + O(\dot{x}^2) = h_0 + h_1\dot{x} + O(\dot{x}^2). \tag{2.132a–c}$$

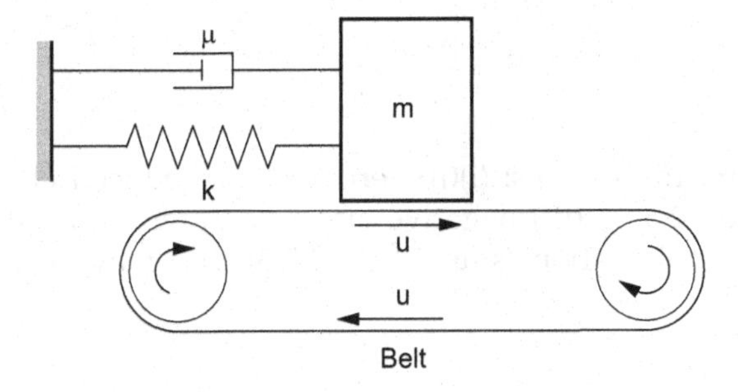

FIGURE 2.16
The unforced mechanical system consisting of a mass, damper and a spring (Figure 2.1) when placed in a conveyor belt with friction (Figure 2.16) has an effective damping that may be: (i) zero leading to oscillations with constant amplitude (Figure 2.4); (ii) positive effective damping in the critical (Figure 2.10), supercritical (Figure 2.12) and subcritical (Figure 2.14) damping cases; (iii) negative effective damping leading to amplified motion (Figure 2.18) that may also be monotonic or oscillatory.

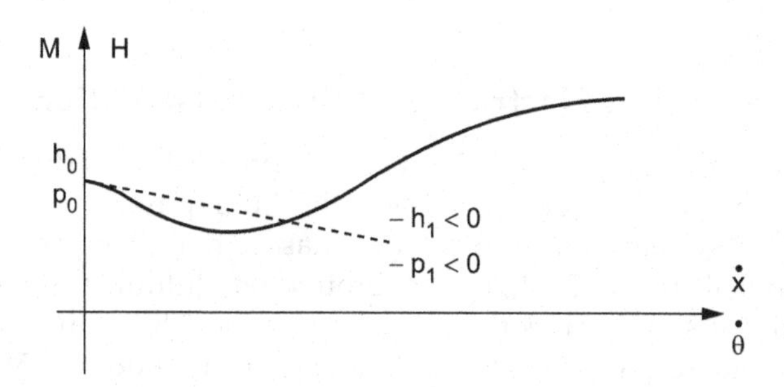

FIGURE 2.17
The friction force H: (i) has a finite value h_0 for zero velocity corresponding to static friction; (ii) for small velocity the friction force initial decreases with slope $-h_1$ where $h_1 > 0$; (iii) for larger velocity the kinematic friction increases again.

Substitution of (2.132c) in the equation of motion (2.131) leads to (2.133a):

$$m\ddot{x} + (\mu - h_1)\dot{x} + kx = h_0; \qquad x_1 = \frac{h_0}{k}, \tag{2.133a, b}$$

the particular integral (2.133b) of the forced equation (2.133a) shows that the static friction (2.132a) shifts the equilibrium position to (2.133b). Relative to the new equilibrium position (2.133b), the relative displacement (2.134a) satisfies the equation of motion (2.134b):

$$\bar{x}(t) = x(t) - x_1: \qquad \ddot{\bar{x}} + 2\bar{\lambda}\dot{\bar{x}} + \omega_0^2 \bar{x} = 0, \tag{2.134a, b}$$

where the **effective damping** (2.135b) is the difference between the damping (2.23b) and the **amplification factor** (2.235a):

$$\nu \equiv \frac{h_1}{2m}: \qquad \bar{\lambda} = \frac{\mu - h_1}{2m} = \lambda - v. \tag{2.135a, b}$$

Thus, there are three cases: (i)(ii) zero $\bar{\lambda} = 0$ or reduced effective damping (subsection 2.5.2); (iii) negative effective damping $\bar{\lambda} < 0$, which corresponds to amplification (subsection 2.5.3) that may be monotonic or oscillatory.

2.5.2 Zero or Reduced Effective Damping

Thus, for a mechanical system consisting of a spring, mass, and damper (2.131) subject to an applied friction force (2.132c) there are (2.134b) five cases without amplification $\bar{\lambda} \geq 0$ in (1.135b) as for the harmonic oscillator (sections 2.2–2.4). In (problem 13) the case VII of **zero effective damping** (2.136a), which is when the amplification exactly balances the damping (2.136b), the oscillation has constant amplitude (2.56b) ≡ (2.136c) with unchanged natural frequency (Figure 2.4):

$$\bar{\lambda} = 0: \qquad \lambda = \nu, \qquad \bar{x}(t) = a\cos(\omega_0 t - \alpha). \tag{2.136a–c}$$

The case VIII (problem 14) of **critical effective damping** (2.137a) corresponds to the damping (2.137b) and leads (2.87b) ≡ (2.137c) to a monotonic decay (2.137d) with possible initial growth (Figure 2.10):

$$\bar{\lambda} = \omega_0: \quad \lambda = \omega_0 + \nu, \qquad \bar{x}(t) = e^{-\bar{\lambda}t}\left[\bar{x}_0 + \left(\dot{\bar{x}}_0 + \bar{\lambda}\bar{x}_0\right)t\right]$$
$$= \left\{\bar{x}_0 + \left[\dot{\bar{x}}_0 + (\lambda - \nu)\bar{x}_0\right]t\right\}\exp(-\omega_0 t). \tag{2.137a–d}$$

The case IX of **supercritical effective damping** (2.138a) corresponds (problem 15) to the damping (2.138b) and leads (2.93b) ≡ (2.138c) to (2.92c) monotonic (2.138d) decay (Figure 2.12):

$$\bar{\lambda} > \omega_0: \quad \lambda > \omega_0 + \nu, \quad \bar{x}(t) = ae^{-\bar{\lambda}t}\cosh\left(t\sqrt{\bar{\lambda}^2 - \omega_0^2} - \alpha\right)$$
$$= a\exp\left[-(\lambda - \nu)t\right]\cosh\left(t\sqrt{\lambda^2 + v^2 - 2\lambda v - \omega_0^2} - \alpha\right). \tag{2.138a–d}$$

The case X of **strong subcritical effective damping** (2.139a) corresponds (problem 16) to the damping (2.139b) and leads (2.106b) ≡ (2.139c) to (2.105c) a damped (2.139c) oscillation (Figure 2.14) with modified frequency (2.139d):

$$\bar{\lambda} < \omega_0: \quad \lambda < \omega_0 + \nu, \quad \bar{x}(t) = ae^{-\bar{\lambda}t}\cos\left(t\sqrt{\omega_0^2 - \bar{\lambda}^2} - \alpha\right)$$
$$= a\exp\left[-(\lambda - \nu)t\right]\cos\left(t\sqrt{\omega_0^2 + 2v\lambda - \nu^2 - \lambda^2} - \alpha\right). \tag{2.139a–d}$$

The case XI of **weak subcritical effective damping** (2.140a) corresponds (problem 17) to the damping (2.140b) and leads (2.112b) ≡ (2.140c) to a damped oscillation at the natural frequency:

$$\bar{\lambda}^2 << \omega_0^2: \quad \lambda(\lambda - 2\nu) << \omega_0^2 - \nu^2,$$
$$\bar{x}(t) = ae^{-\bar{\lambda}t}\cos(\omega_0 t - \alpha) = a\exp\left[-(\lambda - \nu)t\right]\cos(\omega_0 t - \alpha). \tag{2.140a–d}$$

There are three more cases, XII to XV, of negative effective damping corresponding to amplification (subsection 2.5.3).

2.5.3 Monotonic or Oscillatory Amplification and Overstability

For a negative effective damping corresponding to amplification, there are cases of critical (XII), supercritical (XIII), and subcritical (XIV) amplification (Figure 2.18).

The **critical amplification** (case XII) corresponds (problem 18) to negative effective damping, equal to minus the natural frequency (2.141a), leading (2.135b) to (2.141b) the displacement (2.87b) ≡ (2.141c), which is a monotonic growth with possible initial decay:

$$\bar{\lambda} = -\omega_0: \quad \lambda = \nu - \omega_0, \qquad \bar{x}(t) = \left[\bar{x}_0 + \left(\dot{\bar{x}}_0 + \bar{\lambda}\bar{x}_0\right)t\right]e^{-\bar{\lambda}t}$$

$$= \left\{\bar{x}_0 + \left[\dot{\bar{x}}_0 - (\nu + \omega_0)\bar{x}_0\right]t\right\}\exp(\omega_0 t). \tag{2.141a–d}$$

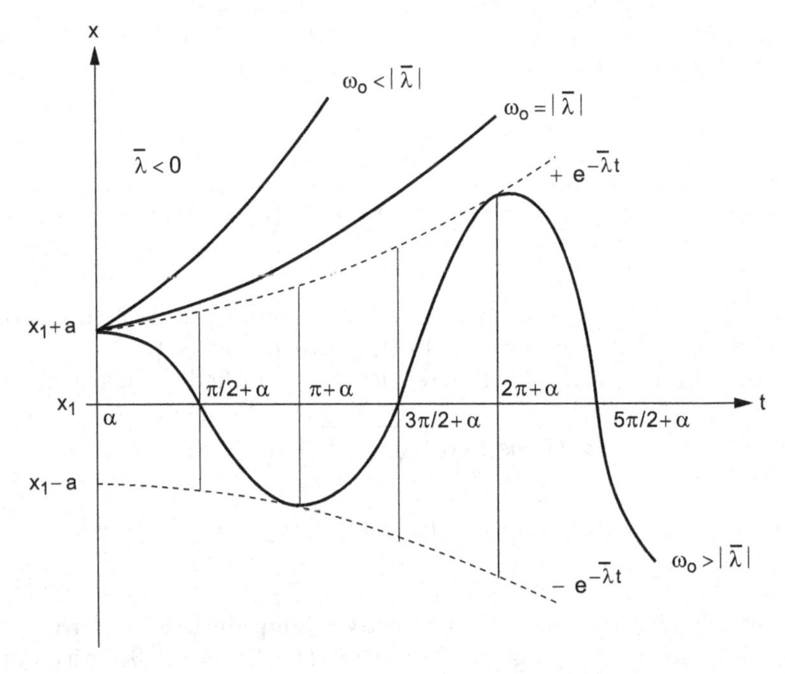

FIGURE 2.18
The unforced mechanical system placed in a conveyor belt (Figure 2.16) in the case of kinematic friction (Figure 2.17) larger than the damping, that is negative effective damping leads to an unstable motion away from equilibrium, that may be of three types: (i) monotonic growth for negative effective damping larger in modulus than the natural frequency, corresponding to supercritical amplification; (ii) for critical amplification, that is negative effective damping equal in modulus to the natural frequency, the ultimate asymptotic growth is slower than in the case of supercritical amplification (i), and there may be an initial decay if the velocity is negative; (iii) for subcritical amplification, that is negative effective damping smaller in modulus than the natural frequency, the growth is oscillatory, corresponding to overstability. In all cases amplified (i)(iii) or damped the static friction displaces the equilibrium position from the origin to x_1.

The **supercritical amplification** (case XIII) corresponds (problem 19) to negative effective damping, larger in modulus than the natural frequency (2.142a), leading (2.142b) to a displacement (2.93b) ≡ (2.142c), with monotonic (2.92b) growth (2.142d):

$$\omega_0 < -\bar{\lambda}: \quad \lambda < \nu - \omega_0, \quad \bar{x}(t) = a e^{-\bar{\lambda} t} \cosh\left(t\sqrt{\bar{\lambda}^2 - \omega_0^2} - \alpha\right)$$

$$= a \exp\left[(\nu - \lambda)t\right] \cosh\left(t\sqrt{\lambda^2 + \nu^2 - 2\lambda\nu - \omega_0^2} - \alpha\right). \tag{2.142a–d}$$

The **subcritical amplification** (case XIV) corresponds (problem 20) to negative effective damping, with modulus smaller than the natural frequency (2.143a), leading (2.143b) to a displacement (2.106b) ≡ (2.143c), with (2.105c) modified frequency and monotonically increasing amplitude (2.143d):

$$\omega_0 > -\bar{\lambda}: \quad \lambda > \nu - \omega_0, \quad \bar{x}(t) = a e^{-\bar{\lambda} t} \cos\left(t\sqrt{\omega_0^2 - \bar{\lambda}^2} - \alpha\right)$$

$$= a \exp\left[(\nu - \lambda)t\right] \cos\left(t\sqrt{\omega_0^2 + 2\lambda\nu - \lambda^2 - \nu^2} - \alpha\right). \tag{2.143a–d}$$

The oscillation with increasing amplitude may be designated **overstability**.

2.5.4 Pendulum Supported on a Cam with Friction (Froude Pendulum)

Another example of mechanical amplified oscillator is (problem 21), the **Froude pendulum** (Figure 2.19), which is suspended from a cam rotating at an angular velocity Ω, and causing an **applied friction torque** that depends on the difference from the angular velocity of the pendulum:

$$m\ell\ddot{\theta} + \mu\ell\dot{\theta} + mg\sin\theta = M\left(\Omega - \dot{\theta}\right), \tag{2.144}$$

where μ is the friction coefficient due to air resistance. The applied frictional torque (2.145a–c) [force (2.132a–c)] have (Figure 2.17) a similar dependence for small deviations of angular velocity:

$$p_0 \equiv M(\Omega), p_1 \equiv -\frac{dM}{d\Omega} > 0: \qquad M\left(\Omega - \dot{\theta}\right) = M(\Omega) - \theta\frac{dM}{d\Omega} + O\left(\dot{\theta}^2\right)$$

$$= p_0 + p_1\dot{\theta} + O\left(\dot{\theta}^2\right); \tag{2.145a–c}$$

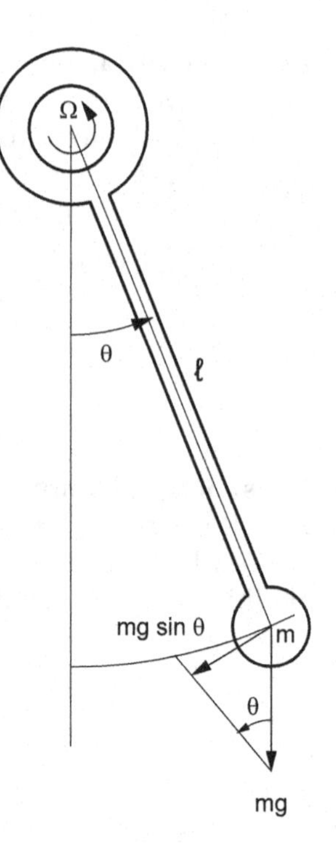

FIGURE 2.19
A mechanical system analogous tto he mass-damper-spring on a conveyor belt (Figure 2.16) is a suspended pendulum supported on a cam that causes friction opposing the motion, and leads to a similar motion including monotonic instability and oscillatory instability or overstability (Figure 2.18). It is assumed that the friction moment, as the friction force, involves (Figure 2.17): (i) a static friction moment p_0; (ii) an initial decrease with slope $-p_1 > 0$ with $p_1 > 0$ for small angular velocity; (iii) the friction moment may increase again for large angular velocity.

for small amplitude oscillations of the pendulum (2.146a), the equation of motion (2.144) becomes (2.146b):

$$\theta^2 << 1: \qquad m\ddot{\theta} + \left(\mu - \frac{p_1}{\ell}\right)\dot{\theta} + \frac{mg}{\ell}\theta = \frac{p_0}{\ell}, \qquad \theta_1 = \frac{p_0}{mg}, \tag{2.146a–c}$$

implying that the position of equilibrium is shifted to (2.146c). The deviation from the equilibrium position (2.147a) satisfies (2.147b):

$$\bar{\theta}(t) \equiv \theta(t) - \theta_1: \qquad m\ddot{\bar{\theta}} + \left(\mu - \frac{p_1}{\ell}\right)\dot{\bar{\theta}} + \frac{mg}{\ell}\bar{\theta} = 0, \tag{2.147a, b}$$

which is similar to (2.134b) with: (i) the natural frequency (2.23a) ≡ (2.72a) ≡ (2.148a) of the suspended pendulum:

$$\omega_0 = \sqrt{\frac{g}{\ell}}; \qquad \bar{\lambda} = \frac{\mu}{2m} - \frac{p_1}{2m\ell} = \lambda - \bar{p}, \qquad \bar{p} = \frac{p_1}{2m\ell}, \tag{2.148a–c}$$

(ii) the effective damping (2.148b) involving the amplification factor (2.148c) and leading to the same eight cases, VII to XV, as before (subsections 2.5.2–2.5.3).

2.5.5 Electrical Circuit with a Valve

The mass on a rolling belt (subsection 2.5.1) and Froude pendulum (subsection 2.5.4) are mechanical amplified oscillators, that have as analogue (problem 22) an electrical circuit with (Figure 2.20) a **valve, a diode, a transistor,** or other **device** that appears in (2.21) as an applied electromotive force corresponding to a resistance R_a associated with the electric current $\dot{q}_a$ from an external circuit:

$$L\ddot{q} + R\dot{q} + \frac{q}{C} = R_a\dot{q}_a. \tag{2.149}$$

The external applied current is related to the current in the electric circuit (2.150a):

$$\dot{q}_a \equiv \frac{dq_a}{dt} = \frac{\partial q_a}{\partial q}\frac{dq}{dt} = s\dot{q}, \qquad s \equiv \frac{\partial q_a}{\partial q} > 0, \tag{2.150a, b}$$

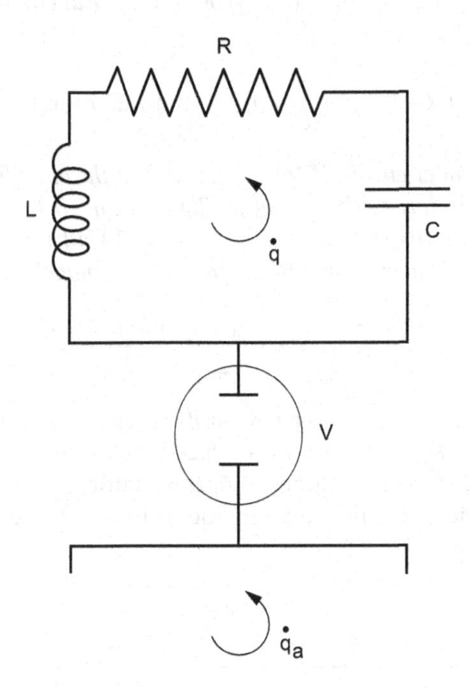

FIGURE 2.20
An electrical circuit that can have monotonic or oscillatory instability (Figure 2.18) as the translational (rotational) mechanical system (Figure 2.16 (2.19)], consists of the basic electrical circuit with self, resistor, and capacitor (Figure 2.3) with battery replaced by another device like a valve (Figure 2.20) that supplies an external electric current $\dot{q}_a$ depending on the electric current $\dot{q}$ in the circuit (Figure 2.21).

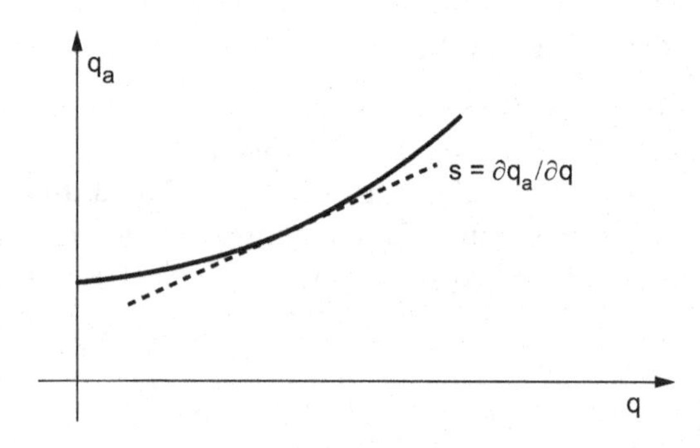

FIGURE 2.21
In the case of the amplified electrical circuit (Figure 2.20), analogous to the translational (rotational) amplified mechanical system [Figure 2.16 (2.19)] the friction force (moment) as a function of the linear (angular) velocity (Figure 2.17), is replaced by the characteristic of the valve (Figure 2.21), that supplies an increasing external electric current for an increasing electric current in the circuit. This may lead to a negative effective electrical resistance, implying monotonic or oscillatory instability (Figure 2.18).

through the ***characteristic*** *of the device that generally has positive slope* (Figure 2.21) *in (2.150b). The equation (2.149) of the electrical circuit (2.150a) becomes (2.151a):*

$$L\ddot{q}+(R-R_a s)\dot{q}+\frac{q}{C}=0; \qquad \ddot{q}+2\bar{\lambda}\dot{q}+\omega_0^2 q=0, \qquad (2.151\text{a, b})$$

the amplified electrical circuit (2.151b) corresponds to the amplified mechanical displacement (2.134b) [rotational (2.147b)] oscillator with: (i) the deviation from the position of equilibrium as the variable (2.134a) [(2.147a)] replaced by the electric charge q; (ii) natural frequencies (2.152a) [effective dampings (2.152b)]:

$$\omega_0 \equiv \sqrt{\frac{k}{m}},\sqrt{\frac{g}{\ell}},\frac{1}{\sqrt{LC}}, \qquad \bar{\lambda} \equiv \frac{\mu-h_1}{2m},\frac{\mu-p_1/\ell}{2m},\frac{R-R_a s}{2L}. \qquad (2.152\text{a, b})$$

The effective damping (2.152b) can be zero/positive/negative leading to the same eight cases, VII to XIV, as before (subsections 2.5.2–2.5.3). The 14 preceding cases, I to XIV, of damped/amplified monotonic/oscillatory motion (response) of a mechanical (electrical circuit are all included in the damped/amplified free response (subsections 2.5.2–2.5.3).

2.6 Comparison of Zero with Small Mass

The differential equation of motion is (subsection 2.6.1) of the first (second) order for zero (small) mass [cases XV–XVI (XIX)] leading to a comparison involving also initial conditions, to confirm if the two distinct solutions remain close over time (subsection 2.6.2). The intermediate degenerate cases XVII (XVIII) correspond to rest (uniform motion).

2.6.1 Uniform, Damped, or Amplified Motion

If the mass is zero (2.153a) the free motion of a mechanical circuit (2.15) leads to (2.153b):

$$m = 0: \qquad \mu\dot{\tilde{x}} + k\tilde{x} = 0, \qquad \tilde{x}(t) = x_0 \exp\left(-\frac{kt}{\mu}\right), \tag{2.153a–c}$$

whose solution (2.153c) is an exponential growth (decay) in the case XV (XVI) of positive $\mu > 0$ (negative $\mu < 0$) damping [problem 23 (24)]; in both cases the velocity (2.154a) is related to the displacement (2.153c) by (2.154b), implying that the initial condition for the velocity is determined by the initial displacement:

$$\dot{\tilde{x}}(t) = -\frac{kx_0}{\mu}\exp\left(-\frac{kt}{\mu}\right), \qquad \dot{\tilde{x}}_0 = -\frac{k}{m}\tilde{x}_0, \tag{2.154a, b}$$

as appropriate for a first-order differential equation. The case XVII of zero mass (2.155a) and damping (2.155b) implies (problem 25) remaining in the position of equilibrium (2.155c) for all time (2.155d):

$$m = 0 = \mu: \qquad \tilde{x}(t) = 0 = \dot{\tilde{x}}(t). \tag{2.155a–d}$$

The case XVIII of no spring (2.156a) and no damper (2.156b) would lead (problem 26) to (2.156c–e) uniform motion:

$$k = 0 = \mu: \qquad \ddot{x} = 0, \qquad \dot{x}(t) = \dot{x}_0, \qquad x(t) = x_0 + \dot{x}_0 t. \tag{2.156a–e}$$

If the mass is not zero (2.157a), the solution of the equation of motion (2.15) is (2.99b, c; 2.100c, d) ≡ (2.157b):

$$m \neq 0: \qquad (\xi_+ - \xi_-)x(t) = (\xi_+ x_0 - \dot{x}_0)\exp(\xi_- t) - (\xi_- x_0 - \dot{x}_0)\exp(\xi_+ t), \tag{2.157a, b}$$

which is valid for arbitrary mass; it involves the roots (2.83; 2.23a, b) of the characteristic polynomial (2.82a, b):

$$\begin{aligned} \xi_\pm &\equiv -\frac{\mu}{2m} \pm \left|\left(\frac{\mu}{2m}\right)^2 - \frac{k}{m}\right|^{1/2} = -\frac{\mu}{2m}\left\{1 \pm \left|1 - \frac{4mk}{\mu^2}\right|^{1/2}\right\} \\ &= -\frac{\mu}{2m}\left\{1 \pm \left[1 - \frac{2mk}{\mu^2} + O\left(\frac{m^2k^2}{\mu^4}\right)\right]\right\}; \end{aligned} \tag{2.158}$$

these simplify (problem 27) for small mass (2.159a) to (2.159b–c):

$$1 >> \frac{mk}{\mu^2} = \frac{\xi_-}{\xi_+}: \qquad \xi_+ = -\frac{\mu}{m}, \qquad \xi_- = -\frac{k}{\mu}, \qquad \xi_+ - \xi_- = -\frac{\mu}{m}. \tag{2.159a–d}$$

leading to (2.159d) because $|\xi_+| >> |\xi_-|$. This allows comparison of the two cases of zero (2.153a–c) and small (2.159a–d) mass.

2.6.2 Proximity of Initial Conditions and Condition of Small Mass

Substitution of (2.159b–d) for small (2.159a) mass in (2.157b) leads to:

$$\frac{\mu}{m} x(t) = -\left(\dot{x}_0 + \frac{k}{\mu} x_0 \right) \exp\left(-\frac{\mu}{m} t \right) + \left(\dot{x}_0 + \frac{\mu}{m} x_0 \right) \exp\left(-\frac{k}{\mu} t \right), \tag{2.160}$$

which is the solution of the second-order equation of motion for small mass; subtracting the solution (2.153c) of the first-order equation of motion (2.153b) for zero mass leads to:

$$x(t) - \tilde{x}(t) = -\frac{m}{\mu} \left(\dot{x}_0 + \frac{k}{\mu} x_0 \right) \exp\left(-\frac{\mu}{m} t \right) + \frac{m}{\mu} \dot{x}_0 \exp\left(-\frac{k}{\mu} t \right). \tag{2.161}$$

The second-order equation of motion (2.15) has a unique solution specified by two independent initial conditions $(x_0, \dot{x}_0)$; the first-order equation of motion (2.153b) has only one initial condition $\tilde{x}_0$, which specifies the initial velocity (2.154b). Thus, the two solutions can be compared only for close initial conditions (2.162a):

$$\left| \dot{x}_0 + x_0 \frac{k}{\mu} \right| < \varepsilon: \qquad \left| \frac{m}{\mu} \left(x_0 + \frac{k}{\mu} \dot{x}_0 \right) \exp\left(-\frac{\mu}{m} t \right) \right| < \varepsilon, \tag{2.162a, b}$$

implying that the first term on the RHS of (2.161) is negligible for all times (2.162b); it would vanish as $m \to 0$ both on account of the amplitude factor m and the term $-m^{-1}$ in the exponential. The remaining second-order term on the RHS of (2.161) shows that the difference of displacements (2.163a) simplifies to (2.163b) in the approximation (2.162a) ~ (2.154b) thus, leading (2.153c) to (2.163c):

$$x(t) - \tilde{x}(t) = \frac{m}{\mu} \dot{x}_0 \exp\left(-\frac{k}{m} t \right) = -\frac{km}{\mu^2} x_0 \exp\left(-\frac{k}{m} t \right) = -\frac{km}{\mu^2} \tilde{x}(t); \tag{2.163a–c}$$

the condition (2.159a) ≡ (2.164a) of small mass shows that for initial conditions satisfying (2.162a) the solutions of the first-order (2.153b, c) and second-order (2.81b; 2.160) differential equations remain close for all times (2.164a):

$$m << \frac{\mu^2}{k}: \qquad \left| \frac{x(t) - \tilde{x}(t)}{\tilde{x}(t)} \right| < \frac{km}{\mu^2} << 1. \tag{2.164a, b}$$

Thus, *the solution (2.153c) of the first-order equation of motion (2.153b) for (cases XV–XVI) zero mass (2.153a), remains (problem 27) for all time close (2.164b) to the solution (2.160) of the second-order equation of motion (2.81b) for the case XIX of small mass (2.164a), provided that the initial conditions (2.162a) are compatible.* This addresses the delicate question of taking a limit $m \to 0$ in the coefficients of a differential equation (2.15) in a case when it depresses its order from two to one in (2.153b).

2.7 Forced Oscillations, Resonance, and Beats

Besides the 19 cases, I to XIX, of free motion (sections 2.2–2.6) the cases XX to XXX of forced motion are examined in the sequel (sections 2.7–2.9, notes 2.2–2.7). Starting with sinusoidal forcing at an applied frequency, in the absence of damping, there are three cases: (i) in the case XV of applied frequency, distinct from the natural frequency (subsection 2.7.1), the amplitude is constant because the applied force is out-of-phase with the velocity, and the average work over a period is zero (subsection 2.7.2); (ii) in the case XVI of coincident applied and natural frequencies (subsection 2.7.3), there is undamped resonance, that is the amplitude (energy) grows linearly (quadratically) with time, because the applied force is in phase with the velocity, and accumulates net work over each period (subsection 2.7.4); (iii) the intermediate case XVII of close but not coincident applied and natural frequencies leads to beats (subsection 2.7.5), that is oscillations whose amplitude "envelope" and energy oscillate at a low "modulation" frequency, because the work done by the applied forces is partially in phase with the velocity (subsection 2.7.6).

2.7.1 Applied Frequency Distinct from Natural Frequency

The total motion consists of the free motion (sections 2.2–2.6) plus the forced motion. The latter is considered first (sections 2.7–2.8) as the motion (2.165b) due to sinusoidal external forcing, with amplitude f_a and **applied frequency** ω_a:

$$\lambda = 0: \qquad \ddot{x} + \omega_0^2 x = f(t) = f_a \cos(\omega_a t) = f_a \ \mathrm{Re}\left\{e^{i\omega_a t}\right\}, \qquad (2.165\text{a, b})$$

in the absence of damping (2.165a). The solution of (2.165b) is sought as a **forced oscillation**, with the same applied frequency ω_a, and generally distinct amplitude b:

$$x_*(t) = b\cos(\omega_a t) = \mathrm{Re}\left\{b e^{i\omega_a t}\right\}, \qquad (2.166)$$

which is determined by substitution in the equation of motion (2.165b) leading to:

$$f_a e^{i\omega_a t} = \left\{ \frac{d^2}{dt^2} + \omega_0^2 \right\} b e^{i\omega_a t} = \left(\omega_0^2 - \omega_a^2\right) b e^{i\omega_a t} = \left(\omega_0^2 - \omega_a^2\right) x_*(t). \quad (2.167)$$

If the case XX, the applied frequency ω_a of the external forcing (2.165b), is distinct (2.168a) from the natural frequency ω_0 of the oscillator, then (2.167) can be solved for the forced motion:

$$\omega_a \neq \omega_0: \quad \left\{x_*(t), \dot{x}_*(t)\right\} = \frac{f_a}{\omega_0^2 - \omega_a^2} \operatorname{Re}\left\{e^{i\omega_a t}, i\omega_a e^{i\omega_a t}\right\} = \frac{f_a}{\omega_0^2 - \omega_a^2}\left\{\cos(\omega_a t), -\omega_a \sin(\omega_a t)\right\}, \quad (2.168a\text{–}c)$$

specifying (problem 28) the displacement (2.168b) and the velocity (2.168c) with constant amplitudes. This implies that the work of the applied force over a period must be zero, as is checked next (subsection 2.7.2).

2.7.2 Forced Oscillations with Constant Amplitude and Energy

The potential (2.5b; 2.168b) [kinetic (2.10b; 2.168c)] energy of the forced undamped oscillator (2.169a) [(2.170a)]:

$$\Phi_m(t) = \frac{k f_a^2}{2\left(\omega_0^2 - \omega_a^2\right)} \cos^2(\omega_a t), \qquad \langle \Phi_m(t) \rangle = \frac{k f_a^2}{4\left(\omega_0^2 - \omega_a^2\right)^2}, \quad (2.169a, b)$$

$$E_v(t) = \frac{m\omega_a^2 f_a^2}{2\left(\omega_0^2 - \omega_a^2\right)^2} \sin^2(\omega_a t), \qquad \langle E_v(t) \rangle = \frac{m\omega_a^2 f_a^2}{4\left(\omega_0^2 - \omega_a^2\right)^2}, \quad (2.170a, b)$$

have different averages (2.169b) [(2.170b)] over a period $\tau_a = 2\pi/\omega_a$ of the applied frequency outside resonance (2.168a) because $k = m\omega_0^2 \neq m\omega_a^2$. The sum of the potential (2.169a) and kinetic (2.170a) energies, that is the total energy (2.171a):

$$E_t(t) = E_r(t) + \Phi_m(t) = \frac{f_a^2}{2\left(\omega_0^2 - \omega_a^2\right)^2}\left\{k\cos^2(\omega_a t) + m\omega_a^2 \sin^2(\omega_a t)\right\}, \quad (2.171a)$$

$$\langle E_t \rangle = \frac{f_a^2}{4\left(\omega_0^2 - \omega_a^2\right)^2}\left\{k + m\omega_a^2\right\} = \frac{m f_a^2}{4} \frac{\omega_0^2 + \omega_a^2}{\left(\omega_0^2 - \omega_a^2\right)^2}, \quad (2.171b)$$

whose mean value over a period is (2.171b). In the absence of dissipation $\Psi = 0$, this implies $d\left[\langle E_t \rangle\right]/dt = 0$ that (2.12) the activity of external forcing is zero on the mean $\langle A \rangle = 0$. This can be confirmed by noting that the external force (2.165b) is in phase with the displacement (2.168b), and hence out-of-phase by $\pi/2$ with the velocity (2.168c), so that the activity (2.172a):

$$A(t) = F(t)\dot{x}_*(t) = -\frac{mf_a^2\omega_a}{2\left(\omega_0^2 - \omega_a^2\right)}\sin(2\omega_a t), \quad \langle A(t) \rangle = 0, \tag{2.172a, b}$$

has zero mean (2.172b) over a period of oscillation (2.116c). It follows that a *forced, undamped (2.165a) oscillation at (case XX) applied frequency distinct from the natural frequency (2.168a) leads (problem 28) to constant amplitude* (Figure 2.22a) *and mean potential (2.169a, b), kinetic (2.170a, b,) and total (2.171a, b) energies because the external force (2.165b) is in phase (out-of-phase by $\pi/2$) with the displacement (2.168b) [velocity (2.168c)], implying that the activity (2.172a) has zero mean (2.172b) over a period of oscillation.*

2.7.3 Applied Frequency Equal to the Natural Frequency

If (case XXI) the applied frequency equals the natural frequency $\omega_a = \omega_0$, it should not be concluded from (2.168b) that the amplitude is "infinite," because: (i) mathematically (2.168b) was obtained from (2.167) dividing by $\omega_a^2 - \omega_0^2 = 0$ and division by zero is not permissible; (ii) physically an infinite amplitude implies an infinite energy, and there is no way a finite force (2.165b) can do infinite work in a finite time. Thus, the solution (2.168b, c) breaks down in the case XXI of **resonance** (1.138a–c), when the applied frequency coincides with the natural frequency, that is both are a simple root of the characteristic polynomial. This suggests differentiating (2.167) once with regards to ω_a:

$$itf_a e^{i\omega_a t} = \left(\omega_0^2 - \omega_a^2\right) itbe^{i\omega_a t} - 2\omega_a be^{i\omega_a t}, \tag{2.173}$$

and then setting $\omega_a = \omega_C$ in (2.173) leading to (2.174a):

$$itf_a e^{i\omega_0 t} = -2\omega_0 x_*(t): \qquad x_*(t) = -\frac{f_a}{2\omega_0}\operatorname{Re}\left\{ie^{i\omega_0 t}\right\}, \tag{2.174a, b}$$

which is equivalent to (2.174a) ≡ (2.174b). It follows that (problem 29) *the undamped oscillation (2.165a) forced (2.165b) ≡ (2.175b) at the natural frequency (2.175a):*

$$\omega_a = \omega_0: \qquad \ddot{x} + \omega_0^2 x = f_a\cos(\omega_0 t) = \operatorname{Re}\left(f_a e^{i\omega_0 t}\right), \tag{2.175a, b}$$

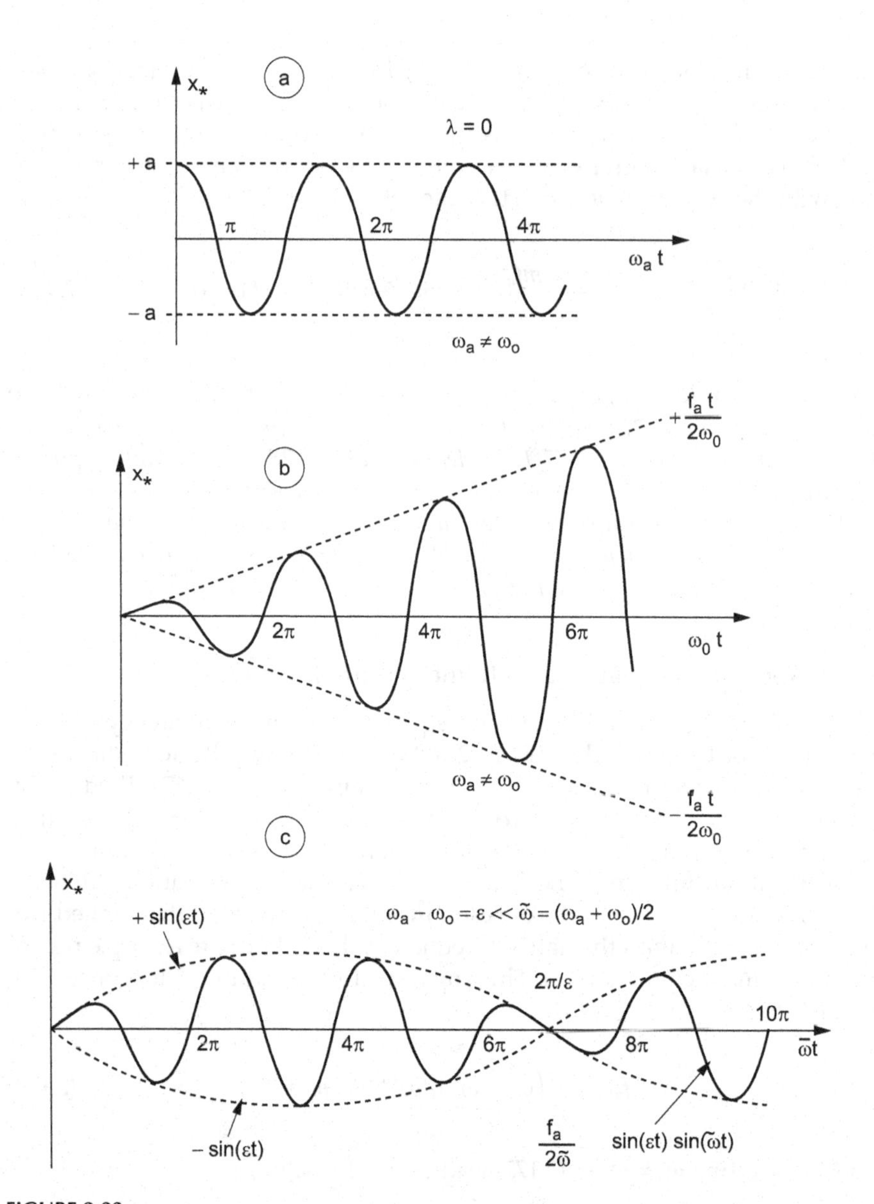

FIGURE 2.22
A linear undamped second-order system with constant coefficients and natural frequency ω_0 when forced sinusoidally at an applied frequency ω_a: (i) performs in-phase oscillations with constant amplitude at the applied frequency (Figure 2.22a) in the non-resonant case when it is different from the natural frequency; (ii) in the resonant case of applied frequency equal to the natural frequency, the oscillations have an amplitude linearly increasing with time (Figure 2.22b) and have a phase lead of one-quarter of a period relative to the forcing; (iii) the transition between the (i) non-resonant and the (ii) resonant cases, that is the case of close natural and applied frequencies, there are beats (Figure 2.22c) that are sinusoidal oscillations at the arithmetic mean of frequencies, with a sinusoidal amplitude modulation specified by the small difference of frequencies, and hence on a much longer period.

leads to **resonance**, *specified by the displacement (2.174b) ≡ (2.176b) and velocity (2.176c):*

$$\omega_a = \omega_0: \quad x_*(t) = \frac{f_a}{2\omega_0} t \sin(\omega_0 t), \quad \dot{x}_*(t) = \frac{f_a}{2\omega_0}\{\sin(\omega_0 t) + \omega_0 t \cos(\omega_0 t)\}. \tag{2.176a–c}$$

The *displacement (2.176b) [(2.168b)] for a resonant (2.176a) [non-resonant (2.168a)] forced [case XXI (XX)], undamped (2.165a) oscillation, has (Figure 2.22b) an amplitude growing linearly in time (constant amplitude), and is out-of-phase by $\pi/2$ (exactly in phase) relative to the external force (2.175b) [(2.165b)]. This implies that the external applied forced does (does no) work over a period of oscillation [subsection 2.7.4 (2.7.2)].*

2.7.4 Undamped Resonance with Growing Amplitude and Energy

The amplitude of the undamped (2.165a) resonant (2.176a) oscillator increases linearly with time for the displacement (2.176b) [velocity (2.176c)] and leads (2.5a) [(2.10b)] to the potential (2.177a) [kinetic (2.177b)] energy:

$$\Phi_m(t) = \frac{f_a^2 k}{8\,\omega_0^2} t^2 \sin^2(\omega_0 t), \tag{2.177a}$$

$$E_v(t) = \frac{f_a^2 m}{8\,\omega_0^2}\left[\sin(\omega_0 t) + \omega_0 t \cos(\omega_0 t)\right]^2, \tag{2.177b}$$

$$E_t(t) = \frac{f_a^2}{8\,\omega_0^2}\left[\left(m + kt^2\right)\sin^2(\omega_0 t) + m\omega_0 t \sin(2\omega_0 t) + m\omega_0^2 t^2 \cos^2(\omega_0 t)\right], \tag{2.177c}$$

whose sum is the total energy (2.177c). The exact values of the potential energy (2.177a), the kinetic energy (2.177b), and the total energy (2.177c) averaged over a period of oscillation are indicated in example 10.4.3. Assuming that the amplitude variation is small over a period of oscillation, the time average is taken only over the terms (2.116c; 1.117a, b) in the potential (2.178a), kinetic (2.178b), and total (2.178c) energies:

$$\langle \Phi_m(t)\rangle = k\left(\frac{f_a}{4\omega_0}\right)^2 t^2 = \frac{m}{16} f_a^2 t^2, \tag{2.178a}$$

$$\langle E_r(t)\rangle = m\left(\frac{f_a}{4\omega_0}\right)^2 \left(1 + \omega_0^2 t^2\right) \sim \frac{m}{16} f_a^2 t^2, \tag{2.178b}$$

$$\langle E_t(t)\rangle \left(\frac{f_a}{4\omega_0}\right)^2 \left(m + 2\omega_0^2 t^2\right) \sim \frac{m}{8} f_a^2 t^2. \tag{2.178c}$$

In (2.178b,c) only the term growing faster $O(t^2)$ with time was retained because of the approximation of slow amplitude variation over a wave period; the calculation of contributions of lower order $O(1)$ to the energy requires an exact calculation of time averages over a wave period (Example 10.4.3). Thus, in the case of undamped resonance the dominant term in the total energy over time (2.178c) grows like the square of time, implying (2.12) in the absence of dissipation (2.179a) that the activity of the applied forced must grow linearly with time (2.179b):

$$\Psi(\dot{x})=0: \qquad \frac{d}{dt}\left[\langle E_t(t)\rangle\right]=\frac{m}{4}f_a^2 t=\langle A(t)\rangle. \tag{2.179a,b}$$

The latter result (2.179b) is confirmed calculating the average (2.180b) of the activity of the applied force (2.180a) over a wave period:

$$A(t)=mf(t)\dot{x}_*(t)=\frac{mf_a^2}{4\omega_0}\sin(2\omega_0 t)+\frac{mf_a^2}{2}t\cos^2(\omega_0 t),\langle A(t)\rangle=\frac{m}{4}f_a^2 t, \tag{2.180a, b}$$

in agreement with (2.179b) ≡ (2.180b). It has been shown *that an undamped (2.165a), resonant (2.176a) oscillation (2.175b) at the natural frequency (2.23a), has linearly growing amplitude (2.176b), because the displacement is out-of-phase to the external force by $\pi/2$; hence the velocity (2.176c) has a term in phase, leading to an activity (2.180a) averaged over a period (2.180b), that grows linearly in time, implying that the potential (2.177a), kinetic (2.177b), and total (2.178c) energies averaged over a period grow quadratically in time (2.178a–c) in the absence of dissipation (2.179a).*

2.7.5 Beats for Close Applied and Natural Frequencies

The question arises on how the transition is made between constant (linearly growing) amplitude in Figure 2.22a(b), for undamped forcing at an applied frequency distinct $\omega_a \neq \omega_0$ (equal $\omega_a = \omega_0$) to the natural frequency. In order to explain this transition, consider the forced oscillation (2.168b) at the applied frequency ω_a, together with an undamped free oscillation (2.113b) at the natural frequency ω_0, with the same amplitude and out-of-phase by π, that is opposite signs:

$$x_*(t)=\frac{f_a}{\omega_0^2-\omega_a^2}\left\{\cos(\omega_a t)-\cos(\omega_0 t)\right\}. \tag{2.181}$$

Since (2.168b) is a solution of the forced equation, it is permissible to add in (2.181) a free oscillation that satisfies the unforced equation. Consider (problem 30) a condition approaching resonance, which is an applied frequency (2.182c) close to (2.182a) to the natural frequency (2.182b), so that the arithmetic average of frequencies is (2.182e) and their difference is (2.182d):

$$\varepsilon^2 \ll \tilde{\omega}^2: \quad \omega_0 = \tilde{\omega} + \varepsilon, \quad \omega_a = \tilde{\omega} - \varepsilon, \quad \omega_0 - \omega_a = 2\varepsilon, \qquad \tilde{\omega} = \frac{\omega_0 + \omega_a}{2}. \tag{2.182a–e}$$

It follows (2.182a) ≡ (2.183a) that:

$$(\omega_0 - \omega_a)^2 \ll (\omega_0 + \omega_a)^2: \qquad \omega_0^2 - \omega_a^2 = (\omega_0 - \omega_a)(\omega_0 + \omega_a) = 4\tilde{\omega}\varepsilon, \tag{2.183a, b}$$

$$\cos(\omega_a t) - \cos(\omega_0 t) = \cos\{(\tilde{\omega} - \varepsilon)t\} - \cos\{(\tilde{\omega} + \varepsilon)t\} = 2\sin(\varepsilon t)\sin(\tilde{\omega} t), \tag{2.183c}$$

leads to the displacement:

$$x_*(t) = \frac{f_a}{2\tilde{\omega}\varepsilon}\sin(\varepsilon t)\sin(\tilde{\omega} t), \tag{2.184}$$

exhibiting the phenomenon of **beats**: *as the applied frequency ω_a approaches the natural frequency ω_0, an oscillation occurs (case XXII) at the average frequency:*

$$x_*(t) = \frac{f_a}{\omega_0^2 - \omega_a^2}\sin\left(\frac{\omega_0 - \omega_a}{2}t\right)\sin\left(\frac{\omega_0 + \omega_a}{2}t\right), \tag{2.185}$$

with a sinusoidal envelope at half the difference frequency, that is (2.182a) with a long-time scale (Figure 2.22c). *If the applied frequency ω_a moves away from the natural frequency ω_0, the beats* (Figure 2.22c) *become oscillations with nearly constant amplitude* (Figure 2.22a). *Conversely, in the case of resonance, when the applied frequency coincides with the natural frequency the displacement (2.184):*

$$\lim_{\omega_a \to \omega_0} x_*(t) = \frac{f_a t}{2}\lim_{\tilde{\omega} \to \omega_0}\frac{\sin(\tilde{\omega} t)}{\tilde{\omega}}\lim_{\varepsilon \to 0}\frac{\sin(\varepsilon t)}{\varepsilon t} = \frac{f_a t}{2\omega_0}\sin(\omega_0 t), \tag{2.186}$$

acquires an amplitude growing linearly in (2.186) time and a $\pi/2$ phase shift (Figure 2.22b).

The preceding argument, leading to an undamped resonant oscillation (2.186) in agreement with (2.176b), justifies how the resonant displacement

(2.176b) may be obtained from the non-resonant displacement (2.168b): (i) either using (2.185) the limit (2.186) ≡ (2.187):

$$\lim_{\varepsilon\to 0} x_*(t) = \lim_{\omega_a\to\omega_0} \frac{2f_a}{\omega_0+\omega_a}\frac{\sin\left[(\omega_0-\omega_a)t/2\right]}{\omega_0-\omega_a}\sin\left(\frac{\omega_0+\omega_a}{2}t\right) = \frac{f_a}{2\,\omega_0}t\sin(\omega_0 t); \tag{2.187}$$

(ii) or using the *l'Hôspital* rule (I.19.35) ≡ (1.139) to lift the 0: 0 indeterminacy in (2.181) in the limit $\omega_0 \to \omega_a$:

$$\lim_{\omega_a\to\omega_0} \frac{d\left\{f_a\cos(\omega_a t)\right\}/d\omega_a}{d\left\{\left(\omega_0^2-\omega_a^2\right)\right\}/d\omega_a} = \lim_{\omega_a\to\omega_0}\frac{f_a t\sin(\omega_a t)}{2\omega_a} = \frac{f_a}{2\omega_0}t\sin(\omega_0 t), \tag{2.188}$$

by differentiating the numerator and denominator with regards to ω_a, and then setting $\omega_a = \omega_0$, leading to (2.188) ≡ (2.186).

2.7.6 Low-Frequency Envelope and Energy Modulation for Beats

In the case of beats, the displacement (2.184) leads to the velocity:

$$\dot{x}_*(t) = \frac{f_0}{2\tilde{\omega}\varepsilon}\left[\tilde{\omega}\sin(\varepsilon t)\cos(\tilde{\omega}t) + \varepsilon\cos(\varepsilon t)\sin(\tilde{\omega}t)\right] \tag{2.189}$$

where the second term in square brackets is small but not negligible. The potential (2.5b) [kinetic (2.10b)] energy corresponding to the displacement (2.184) [velocity (2.189)] are (2.190a) [(2.190b)] not equal:

$$\Phi_m(t) = \frac{k}{8}\left(\frac{f_a}{\tilde{\omega}\varepsilon}\right)^2 \sin^2(\varepsilon t)\sin^2(\tilde{\omega}t), \tag{2.190a}$$

$$E_v(t) = \frac{m}{8}\left(\frac{f_a}{\tilde{\omega}\varepsilon}\right)^2 \tilde{\omega}\sin(\varepsilon t)\cos(\tilde{\omega}t)\left\{\tilde{\omega}\sin(\varepsilon t)\cos(\tilde{\omega}t) + 2\varepsilon\cos(\varepsilon t)\sin(\tilde{\omega}t) + O\left(\varepsilon^2\right)\right\}; \tag{2.190b}$$

$$E_t(t) = \frac{k}{8}\left(\frac{f_a}{\tilde{\omega}\varepsilon}\right)^2\left[\sin^2(\varepsilon t) + \frac{\varepsilon}{\tilde{\omega}}\sin(\varepsilon t)\cos(\varepsilon t)\sin(2\tilde{\omega}t) + O\left(\frac{\varepsilon^2}{\tilde{\omega}^2}\right)\right], \tag{2.190c}$$

where a term $O\left(\varepsilon^2/\tilde{\omega}^2\right)$ was omitted both in the kinetic (2.190b) and total (2.190c) energies. The exact values of the average over an oscillation period of the potential (2.190a), kinetic (2.190b), and total (2.190c) energies associated with beats are indicated in Example 10.4.3. Since the period $2\pi/\varepsilon >> 2\pi/\tilde{\omega}$ of the amplitude modulation is much longer than the period of the oscillation, the average in time applies only to the $\cos, \sin(\bar{\omega}t)$ terms, implying that *on average, there is equipartition of kinetic and potential energy:*

$$\langle \Phi_m \rangle = k\left(\frac{f_a}{4\tilde{\omega}\varepsilon}\right)^2 \sin^2(\varepsilon t) = m\left(\frac{f}{4\varepsilon}\right)^2 \sin^2(\varepsilon t) = \langle E_v \rangle = \frac{\langle E_t \rangle}{2}, \quad (2.191\text{a–c})$$

and the total energy oscillates at the square of the modulation amplitude.

2.8 Damped Resonance for the Frequency and Decay

The sinusoidal forcing can be considered both in the absence (presence) [section 2.7 (2.8)] of damping, both in the non-resonant [case XX (XXIII)] and the resonant [case XXI (XXIV)] situations of distinct (coincident) applied and natural frequencies (subsection 2.8.1). The amplitude and phase of the oscillation are constant (subsection 2.8.2) and such that the work of the applied force is exactly balanced by energy dissipation (subsection 2.8.3). If the applied force has (case XXV) both an applied frequency and an applied temporal decay (subsection 2.8.4) resonance occurs (case XXX) only if both coincide with the respective oscillation frequency and damping (subsection 2.8.6); in all cases (XXV–XXX) the linear growth of amplitude is dominated by the exponential decay in time (subsection 2.8.5).

2.8.1 Sinusoidal Forcing in the Presence of Damping

The linear growth of amplitude, for undamped resonance (Figure 2.22b), would be limited by non-linear effects in the restoring force (2.3), once the displacement becomes large (chapter 4). As the displacement increases, the velocity also does and with it the friction force, so that dissipation may limit amplitude growth in the case of linear damped forced oscillations. To consider this case (XXIII), return (problem 31) to the damped oscillator (2.22), with sinusoidal forcing (2.165b) at the applied frequency (2.192a):

$$\ddot{x} + 2\lambda\dot{x} + \omega_0^2 x = f_a e^{i\omega_a t}, \qquad x_*(t) = b e^{i\omega_a t}, \quad (2.192\text{a, b})$$

and seek a forced oscillation (2.192b), with the same frequency ω_a, and generally distinct amplitude b, determined by substitution into the equation of motion:

$$\begin{aligned} f_a e^{i\omega_a t} &= \left\{\frac{d^2}{dt^2} + 2\lambda\frac{d}{dt} + \omega_0^2\right\} b e^{i\omega_a t} \\ &= \left(\omega_0^2 + 2i\lambda\omega_a - \omega_a^2\right) b e^{i\omega_a t} = \left(\omega_0^2 - \omega_a^2 + 2i\lambda\omega_a\right) x_*(t). \end{aligned} \quad (2.193)$$

Since in the presence of dissipation $\lambda \neq 0$, the coefficient on the RHS of (2.193) is complex, it does not vanish, even at resonance $\omega_a = \omega_0$, and it is always possible to divide by it, leading to a displacement:

$$x_*(t) = \text{Re}\left\{be^{i\omega at}\right\} = \text{Re}\left\{\frac{f_a e^{i\omega_a t}}{\omega_0^2 - \omega_a^2 + 2i\omega_a\lambda}\right\} = \text{Re}\left\{\frac{f_a}{c}\exp\left[i(\omega_a t - \beta)\right]\right\}, \quad (2.194)$$

where the denominator is a complex number:

$$\omega_0^2 - \omega_a^2 + 2i\omega_a\lambda = ce^{i\beta}, \quad (2.195)$$

with modulus (2.196a) and phase (2.196b):

$$c = \left|\left(\omega_0^2 - \omega_a^2\right)^2 + 4\omega_a^2\lambda^2\right|^{1/2}, \qquad \tan\beta = \frac{2\omega_a\lambda}{\omega_0^2 - \omega_a^2}, \quad (2.196a, b)$$

satisfying (2.195) ≡ (2.197a, b):

$$c\cos\beta = \omega_0^2 - \omega_a^2, \qquad c\sin\beta = 2\omega_a\lambda. \quad (2.197a, b)$$

The displacement (2.198a) and the velocity (2.198b)]:

$$\begin{aligned} x_*(t) &= \frac{f_a}{c}\cos(\omega_a t - \beta) = \frac{f_a}{c}\left[\cos(\omega_a t)\cos\beta - \sin(\omega_a t)\sin\beta\right] \\ &= f_a\frac{\left(\omega_0^2 - \omega_a^2\right)\cos(\omega_a t) + 2\omega_a\lambda\sin(\omega_a t)}{\left(\omega_0^2 - \omega_a^2\right)^2 + 4\lambda^2\omega_a^2}, \end{aligned} \quad (2.198a)$$

$$\begin{aligned} \dot{x}_*(t) &= \text{Re}\left\{\frac{i\omega_a f_a}{c}e^{i(\omega_a t - \beta)}\right\} = -\frac{f_a\omega_a}{c}\sin(\omega_a t - \beta) \\ &= -\frac{f_a}{c}\omega_a\left[\sin(\omega_a t)\cos\beta - \cos(\omega_a t)\sin\beta\right] \\ &= -f_a\,\omega_a\frac{2\omega_a\lambda\cos(\omega_a t) - \left(\omega_0^2 - \omega_a^2\right)\sin(\omega_a t)}{\left(\omega_0^2 - \omega_a^2\right) + 4\lambda^2\omega_a^2}, \end{aligned} \quad (2.198b)$$

have terms both in phase (the first) and out-of-phase (the second) with the force.

2.8.2 Amplitude and Phase of Forced Oscillations

Thus, *a linear damped oscillator with sinusoidal forcing (2.192a) has displacement (2.198a) [velocity (2.198b)] with amplitude (2.198a;2.196a) ≡ (2.199a) [multiplied by ω_a in (2.198b)]:*

$$b = \frac{f_a}{c} = f_a\left|\left(\omega_0^2 - \omega_a^2\right)^2 + 4\omega_a^2\lambda^2\right|^{-1/2}, \quad (2.199a, b)$$

and phase $\beta(\beta+\pi/2)$ in (2.196b). In the absence of damping (2.200a) the displacement is in phase with the force (2.200c) and the amplitude is constant (2.200d) leading to (2.200e) ≡ (2.168b):

$$\lambda=0, \quad \omega_0 \neq \omega_a: \quad \beta=0, \quad b=\frac{f_a}{\omega_0^2-\omega_a^2}, \quad x_*(t)=\frac{f_a}{\omega_0^2-\omega_a^2}\cos(\omega_a t), \qquad \text{(2.200a–e)}$$

outside resonance (2.200b). In (problem 32) the case XXIV of resonance (2.201b) in the presence of damping (2.201a), the displacement is out-of-phase to the force (2.201c) and the amplitude is maximum (2.201d) leading to (2.201e):

$$\lambda \neq 0, \quad \omega_0=\omega_a: \quad \beta=\frac{\pi}{2}, \quad b=\frac{f_a}{2\omega_0\lambda}, \qquad x_*(t)=\frac{f_a}{2\omega_0\lambda}\sin(\omega_a t). \qquad \text{(2.201a–e)}$$

In the case of undamped (2.202a) resonance (2.202b), neither (2.200e) nor (2.201e) hold, and the constant amplitude is replaced (2.176b) ≡ (2.202c–e) by an amplitude growing linearly with time:

$$\lambda=0, \quad \omega_0=\omega_a: \quad \beta=\frac{\pi}{2}, \quad b=\frac{f_a t}{2\omega_0}, \qquad x_*(t)=\frac{f_a t}{2\omega_0}\sin(\omega_a t). \qquad \text{(2.202a–e)}$$

Thus, *the amplitude* (Figure 2.23a): *(i) decays as the applied frequency ω_a is farther from the natural frequency; (ii) increases as the damping reduces. The phase* (Figure 2.23b) *is $\pi/2$ at resonance, with a steeper slope for smaller damping λ, and is zero (π) in the absence of damping for $\omega_0 > \omega_a$ $(\omega_a > \omega_0)$.* The constant amplitude implies constant energy, and thus, the phase shift must be such that the activity of the applied force balances the dissipation; this is confirmed next (subsection 2.8.3).

2.8.3 Constant Amplitude and Balance of Activity and Damping

The displacement (2.198a) [velocity (2.198b)] of the linear damped sinusoidally forced oscillator (2.192a) imply the potential (2.156a) [kinetic (2.156b)]:

$$\Phi_m(t)=\frac{1}{2}k\left[x_*(t)\right]^2=\frac{1}{2}kb^2\cos^2(\omega_a t-\beta), \qquad \text{(2.203a)}$$

$$E_v(t)=\frac{1}{2}m\left[\dot{x}_*(t)\right]^2=\frac{1}{2}m\omega_a^2\, b^2\sin^2(\omega_a t-\beta). \qquad \text{(2.203b)}$$

The average over a period of the potential (2.203a) [kinetic (2.203b)] energy (2.204a) [(2.204b)]:

$$\langle\Phi_m(t)\rangle = \frac{kb^2}{4}=\frac{mb^2}{4}\omega_0^2, \qquad \langle E_v(t)\rangle = \frac{mb^2}{4}\omega_a^2, \qquad \text{(2.204a, b)}$$

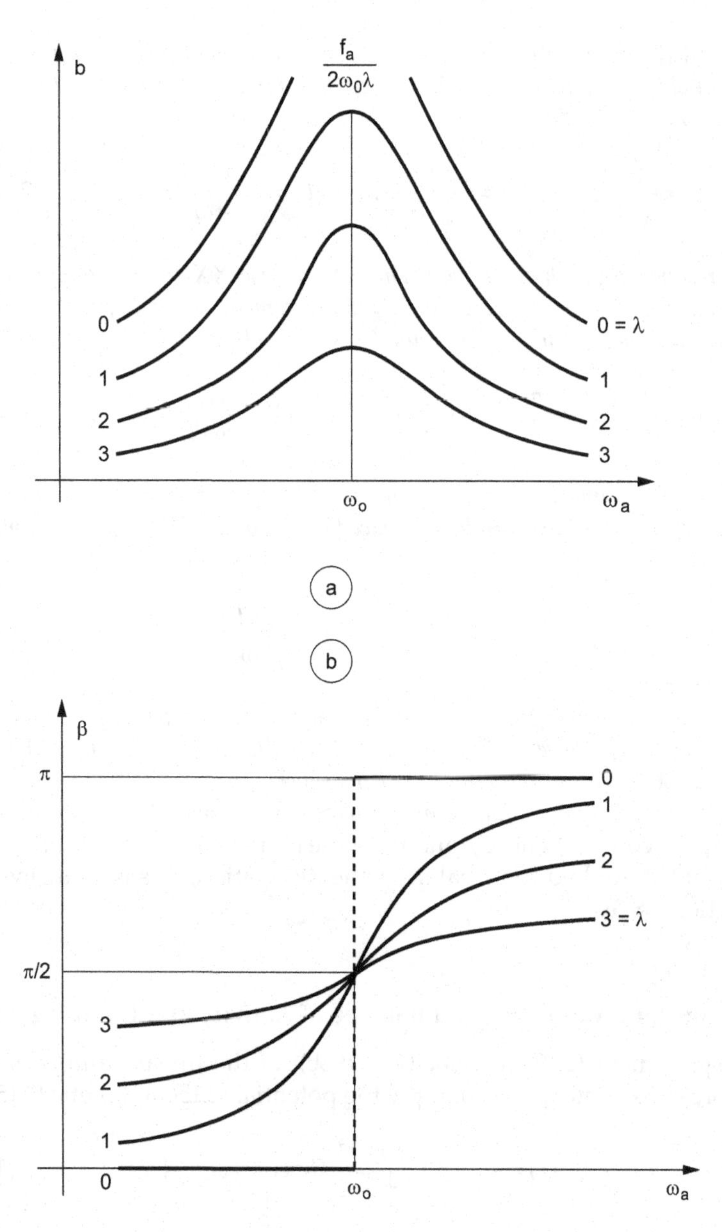

FIGURE 2.23
In the contrast with the undamped case (Figure 2.22) a damped second-order system with constant coefficients subject to sinusoidal forcing at an applied frequency always oscillates at this frequency with constant amplitude: (i) for a given damping the maximum amplitude is in the resonant condition of applied equal to the natural frequency (Figure 2.23a) and the maximum amplitude increases with decreasing non-zero damping; (ii) the phase difference between the forcing and the displacement is one-quarter period for all dampings at the resonance condition of equal natural and applied frequencies, with slope increasing for smaller damping, and becoming a phase jump of half-a-period for zero damping.

is equal at resonance and not equal outside resonance. The total energy averaged over a period is constant (2.205a):

$$\langle E_t(t)\rangle = \langle \Phi_m(t)\rangle + \langle E_v(t)\rangle = \frac{mb^2}{4}\left(\omega_0^2 + \omega_a^2\right), \tag{2.205a}$$

$$\frac{d}{dt}\{\langle E(t)\rangle\} = 0: \qquad \langle \Psi(t)\rangle = \langle A(t)\rangle, \tag{2.205b, c}$$

and thus, (2.205b) the average over a period of the dissipation and activity of the applied force must be equal (2.205c). This can be checked from: (i) the dissipation (2.206a) [activity of the applied force (2.206b)]:

$$\Psi(t) = \mu\left[\dot{x}_*(t)\right]^2 = 2\lambda m b^2 \omega_a^2 \sin^2(\omega_a t - \beta), \tag{2.206a}$$

$$A(t) = F(t)\dot{x}_*(t) = -m f_a b \omega_a \cos(\omega_a t)\sin(\omega_a t - \beta); \tag{2.206b}$$

(ii) the average dissipation (2.207a) [activity (2.207b)] during a period:

$$\langle \Psi(t)\rangle = m\lambda b^2 \omega_a^2, \qquad \langle A(t)\rangle = \frac{1}{2} m f_a \omega_a b \sin\beta; \tag{2.207a, b}$$

(iii) the two expressions coincide (2.205c) if (2.208a) holds:

$$b = \frac{f_a \sin\beta}{2\omega_a \lambda} = \frac{f_a}{c}, \tag{2.208a, b}$$

implying (2.208b) by (2.197b), in agreement with (2.199a). Thus, the phase difference β between the displacement (2.194) and the force (2.192a), is such that the activity (2.207b) balances (2.205c) the dissipation (2.207a) when averaged over a period. In the passage from (2.206a) [(2.206b)] to (2.207a) [(2.207b)] were used (2.208c) [(2.208d)]:

$$\langle \cos(\omega_a t)\sin(\omega_a t - \beta)\rangle = \cos\beta\langle \cos(\omega_a t)\sin(\omega_a t)\rangle - \sin\beta\langle \cos^2(\omega_a t)\rangle = -\frac{\sin\beta}{2}, \tag{2.208c}$$

$$\begin{aligned}\langle \sin^2(\omega_a t - \beta)\rangle &= \left\langle \left[\sin(\omega_a t)\cos\beta - \sin\beta\cos(\omega_a t)\right]^2\right\rangle \\ &= \cos^2\beta\langle \sin^2(\omega_a t)\rangle + \sin^2\beta\langle \cos^2(\omega_a t)\rangle - \cos\beta\sin\beta\langle \sin(2\omega_a t)\rangle \\ &= \frac{\cos^2\beta + \sin^2\beta}{2} = \frac{1}{2}.\end{aligned} \tag{2.208d}$$

A linear damped oscillator with forcing (2.192a) has potential (2.203a) [kinetic (2.203b)] energies, whose averages over a period (2.204a) [(2.204b)]: (i) are the same at resonance (2.209b); (ii/iii) outside resonance the kinetic energy is larger (smaller) than the potential energy for applied frequency larger (smaller) than the natural frequency (2.209c) [(2.209a)]:

$$\frac{\langle E_v \rangle}{\langle \Phi_m \rangle} = \left(\frac{\omega_a}{\omega_0} \right)^2 \begin{cases} <1 & \text{if} \quad \omega_a < \omega_0, \\ =1 & \text{if} \quad \omega_a = \omega_0, \\ >1 & \text{if} \quad \omega_a > \omega_0. \end{cases} \tag{2.209a, b, c}$$

Their sum is a constant average total energy over a period (2.205a) in agreement with the dissipation function (2.206a) [activity of the applied force (2.206b)] having the same (2.205c) average over a period (2.207a) [(2.207b)].

2.8.4 Simultaneous Forcing in Frequency and Damping

The calculation of the response of a damped oscillator, to an external force may concern both [subsections 2.8.1–2.8.3 (2.8.4–2.8.6)] the cases XX–XXIV (XXV–XXX) of an applied frequency ω_a (and an exponential decay rate λ_a):

$$\ddot{x} + 2\lambda\dot{x} + \omega_0^2 x = f_a e^{-\lambda_a t} \cos(\omega_a t) = \operatorname{Re}\left\{ f_a e^{-\lambda_a t + i\omega_a t} \right\}. \tag{2.210a}$$

The particular integral of (2.210a) is (1.129b) the displacement response (2.210c):

$$P_2(i\omega_a - \lambda_a) \neq 0: \qquad x_*(t) = \operatorname{Re}\left\{ \frac{f_a e^{i\omega_a t - \lambda_a t}}{P_2(-\lambda_a + i\omega_a)} \right\}, \tag{2.210b, c}$$

in the non-resonant case of the non-vanishing (2.210b) characteristic polynomial (2.211a):

$$\begin{aligned} P_2(i\omega_a - \lambda_a) &= (i\omega_a - \lambda_a)^2 + 2\lambda(i\omega_a - \lambda_a) + \omega_0^2 \\ &= \omega_0^2 - \omega_a^2 + \lambda_a^2 - 2\lambda_a\lambda + i2\omega_a(\lambda - \lambda_a). \end{aligned} \tag{2.211a}$$

In the presence of subcritical damping, (2.105a) ≡ (2.111b), the natural frequency (2.23a) differs from the oscillation frequency (2.105d), which is introduced in the characteristic polynomial (2.211a) leading to (2.211c):

$$\begin{aligned} \lambda < \omega_0: \quad P_2(i\omega_a - \lambda_a) &= \bar{\omega}^2 - \omega_a^2 + \lambda^2 + \lambda_a^2 - 2\lambda_a\lambda + i2\omega_a(\lambda - \lambda_a) \\ &= \bar{\omega}^2 - \omega_a^2 + (\lambda - \lambda_a)(\lambda - \lambda_a + 2i\omega_a) \equiv c e^{i\beta}. \end{aligned} \tag{2.211b, c}$$

The characteristic polynomial (2.211c) is complex with modulus (2.212a) and phase (2.212b):

$$c = \left|P_2(i\omega_a - \lambda_a)\right| = \left|\left[\bar{\omega}^2 - \omega_a^2 + (\lambda - \lambda_a)^2\right]^2 + 4\omega_a^2(\lambda - \lambda_a)^2\right|^{1/2}, \tag{2.212a}$$

$$\tan\beta = \frac{\operatorname{Im}\left[P_2(i\omega_a - \lambda_a)\right]}{\operatorname{Re}\left[P_2(i\omega_a - \lambda_a)\right]} = \frac{2\omega_a(\lambda - \lambda_a)}{\bar{\omega}^2 - \omega_a^2 + (\lambda - \lambda_a)^2}. \tag{2.212b}$$

Substituting (2.211c) in (2.210c):

$$x_*(t) = \operatorname{Re}\left\{\frac{f_a}{c}\exp(-\lambda_a t)\exp(i\omega_a t - \beta)\right\}, \tag{2.213}$$

specifies (problem 33) *the displacement (2.214b) and the velocity (2.214c) of the damped oscillator (2.210a) forced by an applied frequency ω_a (and decay λ_a) in the general case XXV of subcritical damping (2.211b) when (2.214a) they do not both coincide with the oscillation frequency ω (damping λ):*

$$\{\omega_a, \lambda_a\} \neq \{\bar{\omega}, \lambda\}: \qquad x_*(t) = \frac{f_a}{c}\exp(-\lambda_a t)\cos(\omega_a t - \beta), \tag{2.214a, b}$$

$$\dot{x}(t) = -\frac{f_a}{c}\exp(-\lambda_a t)\left[\omega_a \sin(\omega_a t - \beta) + \lambda_a \cos(\omega_a t - \beta)\right]. \tag{2.214c}$$

In the case of sinusoidal forcing $\omega_a \neq 0 = \lambda_a$ the amplitude (2.212a) [phase (2.212b)] simplify to (2.196a) [(2.196b)], using (2.105d); in (problem 34) the opposite case XXVI of monotonically decaying external force (2.215a):

$$\omega_a = 0: \qquad x_*(t) = \frac{f_a}{\bar{\omega}^2 + (\lambda - \lambda_a)^2}\exp(-\lambda_a t), \tag{2.215a,b}$$

$$\dot{x}_*(t) = -\frac{f_a \lambda_a}{\bar{\omega}^2 + (\lambda - \lambda_a)^2}\exp(-\lambda_a t), \tag{2.215c}$$

the displacement (2.215b) [velocity (2.215c)] is also monotonic.

2.8.5 Coincidence of One or Both of Frequency and Decay

Returning to the general case XXV of decaying sinusoidal $\lambda_a \neq 0 \neq \omega_a$ external force (2.210a), there is no resonance if: (i) the (problem 35) applied frequency equals the oscillation frequency (2.216a), but the applied decay is distinct from the natural *damping (2.216b) simplifying (case XXVII) the amplitude factor (2.212a) [phase (2.212b)] to (2.216c) [(2.216d)]:*

$$\omega_a - \bar{\omega} = 0 \neq \lambda - \lambda_a: \quad c = (\lambda - \lambda_a)\left|(\lambda - \lambda_a)^2 + 4\omega_a^2\right|^{1/2}, \quad \tan\beta = \frac{2\omega_a}{\lambda - \lambda_a}, \tag{2.216a–d}$$

in the displacement (2.214b) and the velocity (2.214c); (ii) in (problem 36) the case XXVIII when the applied decay equals the natural damping (2.217a) but the applied and oscillation frequencies do not coincide (2.217b):

$$\lambda_a - \lambda = 0 \neq \omega_a - \bar{\omega}: \qquad x_*(t) = \frac{f_a}{\bar{\omega}^2 - \omega_a^2} e^{-\lambda t} \cos(\omega_a t), \tag{2.217a–c}$$

$$\dot{x}_*(t) = -\frac{f_a}{\bar{\omega}^2 - \omega_a^2} e^{-\lambda t}\left[\omega_a \sin(\omega_a t) + \lambda \cos(\omega_a t)\right]; \tag{2.217d}$$

(iii) in (problem 37) the case XIX when the applied and natural frequencies coincide (2.218a) and the applied decay and damping also coincide (2.218b) leading to the displacement (2.218c) and the velocity (2.218d):

$$\omega_a - \omega_0 = 0 = \lambda_a - \lambda: \quad x_*(t) = \frac{f_a}{\bar{\omega}^2 - \omega_0^2} \operatorname{Re}\left\{e^{(i\omega_a - \lambda_a)t}\right\} = -\frac{f_a}{\lambda^2} e^{-\lambda t} \cos(\omega_0 t), \tag{2.218a–c}$$

$$\dot{x}_*(t) = \frac{f_a}{\lambda} e^{-\lambda t}\left[\cos(\omega_0 t) + \frac{\omega_0}{\lambda} \sin(\omega_0 t)\right]. \tag{2.218d}$$

The resonance occurs only in the case XXX opposite to (2.214a), that is, only if the applied decay equals the natural damping and the applied frequency equals the oscillation frequency modified by damping that is distinct from the natural frequency (subsection 2.8.6).

2.8.6 Resonance with Damping and Decaying Forcings

The forcing (2.210a) with an applied frequency ω_a (decay λ_a) leads to resonance (problem 38) when the characteristic polynomial, (2.211a) ≡ (2.211b), has a simple root (2.219a, b) in which case the displacement is given (1.134a, b) by (2.219c):

$$P_2(i\omega_a - \lambda_a) = 0 \neq P_2'(i\omega_a - \lambda_a): \qquad x(t) = \operatorname{Re}\left\{f_a t \frac{e^{-\lambda t + i\bar{\omega} t}}{P_2'(i\bar{\omega} - \lambda)}\right\}; \tag{2.219a–c}$$

involving the derivative (2.220a) of the characteristic polynomial (2.82b) evaluated (2.220b) at $i\omega - \lambda$:

$$P_2' = 2(D+\lambda), \qquad P_2'(i\bar{\omega} - \lambda) = 2i\bar{\omega}. \qquad (2.220a, b)$$

Substitution of (2.220b) in (2.219c) specifies:

$$\omega_a - \bar{\omega} = 0 = \lambda_a - \lambda: \quad x_*(t) = \frac{f_a}{2\bar{\omega}} te^{-\lambda t} \operatorname{Re}\left(-ie^{i\bar{\omega}t}\right) = \frac{f_a}{2\bar{\omega}} te^{-\lambda t} \sin(\bar{\omega}t), \qquad (2.221a–c)$$

$$\dot{x}_*(t) = \frac{f_a}{2\bar{\omega}} e^{-\lambda t}\left[(1-\lambda t)\sin(\bar{\omega}t) + \bar{\omega}t\cos(\bar{\omega}t)\right], \qquad (2.221d)$$

the displacement (2.221a) [velocity (2.221d)] of a damped oscillator (2.210a) forced resonantly (case XXX) by an applied decay equal to the natural damping (2.221a) and an applied frequency equal to the oscillation frequency (2.221b). The linear amplitude growth with time due to resonance is dominated by the exponential decay in (2.221c, d), except in the absence of damping $\lambda = 0$ when undamped resonance is regained (2.176b, c). Three more distinct forcings of the undamped (damped) harmonic oscillator (problems 39–44) are considered [cases XXXI–XXXIII (XXXIV–XXXVI)] in the Example 10.3.

2.9 Arbitrary, Bounded, and Exponential Forcings

The displacement of a linear damped or amplified oscillator with arbitrary forcing can be addressed by the method of variation of parameters (section 2.9) distinguishing the cases of non-critical (critical) damping or amplification [subsection 2.9.1 (2.9.2)]. This leads to four cases of forcing by an arbitrary function of time (subsection 2.9.3), namely: (i) critical damping or amplification (case XXXVII); (ii) no damping or amplification (case XXXVIII); (iii)(iv) super(sub)critical damping or amplification [case XXXIX (XL)]. The forcing function may have any dependence on time that leads to convergent integrals, for example, a sinusoid with exponentially decaying amplitude (subsection 2.9.4). The simplest case of constant forcing (case XLI) supplies an upper bound (case XLII) for the displacement by a finite forcing function (subsection 2.9.5).

2.9.1 Response to an Integrable Forcing Function

The response of the circuit to arbitrary forcing can be obtained (notes 1.1–1.4) by the **method of variation of parameters**, as the free response (2.99b) with the coefficients not constants $a_\pm$ but arbitrary functions $A_\pm(t)$ of time:

$$x(t) = A_+(t)\exp(\xi_+ t) + A_-(t)\exp(\xi_- t). \qquad (2.222)$$

The functions $A_\pm(t)$ are specified by requiring (2.222) to satisfy the equation of motion (2.22) plus one other compatible and independent condition chosen at will. The second condition is chosen to be (2.223a):

$$\dot{A}_+ \exp(\xi_+ t) + \dot{A}_- \exp(\xi_- t) = 0: \quad \dot{x}(t) = A_+ \xi_+ \exp(\xi_+ t) + A_- \xi_- \exp(\xi_- t), \tag{2.223a, b}$$

so that the displacement (2.222) implies a velocity (2.223b) that does not involve derivatives of $A_\pm$; thus, in the acceleration:

$$\ddot{x}(t) = \xi_+ \left(\dot{A}_+ + \xi_+ A_+\right) \exp(\xi_+ t) + \xi_- \left(\dot{A}_- + \xi_- A_-\right) \exp(\xi_- t), \tag{2.224}$$

appear only in first-order derivatives $\dot{A}_\pm$ of $A_\pm$.

Substituting (2.222; 2.223b; 2.224) in the equation of motion (2.22) yields (2.225):

$$\begin{aligned} &f(t) - \xi_+ \dot{A}_+ \exp(\xi_+ t) - \xi_- \dot{A}_- \exp(-\xi_- t) \\ &\quad = \exp(\xi_+ t) A_+ \left(\omega_0^2 + 2\lambda\xi_+ + \xi_+^2\right) + \exp(\xi_- t) A_- \left(\omega_0^2 + 2\lambda\xi_- + \xi_-^2\right) = 0, \end{aligned} \tag{2.225}$$

where the RHS vanishes because $\xi_\pm$ are roots of the characteristic polynomial (2.82b), that is, $\exp\pm(\xi_\pm t)$ are free motions satisfying the unforced equation of motion. The coefficients $\dot{A}_\pm$ may be eliminated between (2.225) and (2.223a), leading to (2.226):

$$f(t) = \pm(\xi_+ - \xi_-)\ \dot{A}_\pm(t)\ \exp(\xi_\pm t); \tag{2.226}$$

the latter is a simple first-order differential equation (2.226) for $\dot{A}_\pm$, whose solution is (2.227b) where $a_\pm$ are arbitrary constants:

$$f(s) \in \mathcal{E}(|R): \qquad A_\pm(t) = a_\pm \pm (\xi_+ - \xi_-)^{-1} \int^t f(s) \exp(-\xi_\pm s)\, ds, \tag{2.227a, b}$$

and the forcing function is integrable on the real line (2.227a). Substituting (2.227b) in (2.222) leads to:

$$\xi_+ \neq \xi_-: \qquad x(t) = a_+ \exp(\xi_+ t) + a_- \exp(\xi_- t) + x_*(t), \tag{2.228a, b}$$

$$\begin{aligned} (\xi_+ - \xi_-) x_*(t) &= \exp(\xi_+ t) \int^t f(s) \exp(-\xi_+ s)\, ds - \exp(\xi_- t) \int^t f(s) \exp(-\xi_- s)\, ds, \\ &= \int^t f(s) \left\{\exp\left[\xi_+ (t-s)\right] - \exp\left[\xi_- (t-s)\right]\right\} ds, \end{aligned} \tag{2.228c,d}$$

showing that *the response of a circuit to arbitrary forcing (2.22) by a function integrable on the real line (2.227a) consists of the free motion (2.228b) ≡ (2.99b) plus the forced motion (2.228c) ≡ (2.228d); the solution (2.228b–d) applies in all cases XXVIII–XLI of forcing, except for critical damping (2.228a)*; the case XXXVI of critical damping is considered next (subsection 2.9.2).

2.9.2 Method of Variation of Parameters for Forcing

The case of critical damping, when the characteristic polynomial (2.84a–c) has a double root (2.229a), is excluded from (2.228a–d); in this case, the solution (2.222) is replaced (2.85b) by (2.229b):

$$\xi_+ = \xi_- \equiv \xi = -\lambda = -\omega_0: \qquad x(t) = \left[A_0(t) + tA_1(t)\right] e^{\xi t}. \tag{2.229a, b}$$

Upon the arbitrary functions $A(t), B(t)$ is imposed the condition (2.230a) simplifying the velocity (2.230b):

$$\dot{A}_0 + t\dot{A}_1 = 0: \qquad \dot{x}(t) = \left(\xi A_0 + A_1 + \xi t A_1\right) e^{\xi t}, \tag{2.230a, b}$$

and also the acceleration (2.231):

$$\ddot{x}(t) = \left(\xi \dot{A}_0 + \dot{A}_1 + \xi A_1 + \xi t \dot{A}_1 + \xi^2 A_0 + \xi A_1 + \xi^2 t A_1\right) e^{\xi t}. \tag{2.231}$$

Substitution in the equation (2.22) of motion (2.232b) for critical damping (2.232a):

$$\xi_\pm = \xi = -\omega_0 = -\lambda: \qquad \ddot{x} - 2\xi\dot{x} + \xi^2 x = f(t), \tag{2.232a, b}$$

of (2.229b; 2.230b; 2.231) leads to (2.233a):

$$f(t) e^{-\xi t} = \xi \dot{A}_0 + \dot{A}_1 + \xi t \dot{A}_1 = \dot{A}_1 = -\frac{\dot{A}_0}{t}, \tag{2.233a–c}$$

where (2.230a) was used, leading to (2.233b) ≡ (2.233c). From (2.233b, c) follow the coefficients (2.234b, c):

$$f \in \mathcal{E}(|R): \quad A_1(t) = a_1 + \int^t f(s) e^{-\xi s}\, ds, \quad A_0(t) = a_0 - \int^t f(s) e^{-\xi s} s\, ds, \tag{2.234a–c}$$

where (a_0, a_1) are arbitrary constants and the forcing function is integrable on the real line (2.234a). Substituting (2.234b, c) in the solution (2.229b) yields:

$$\xi_\pm = \xi = -\lambda = -\omega_0: \quad x(t) = a_0 + a_1 t + x_*(t), \quad x_*(t) = e^{\xi t} \int^t f(s) e^{-\xi s} (t-s) ds. \tag{2.235a–c}$$

Thus, *the response of a mechanical system (2.235a) [(2.22)] to forcing by a function integrable over time (2.234a) [≡ (2.227a)] in the case(s) XXXVII (XXXVIII–XLI) of critical (non-critical) damping consists of the sum of the: (i) free motion, (2.235b) ≡ (2.85b) [(2.228b) ≡ (2.99b)]; (ii) forced motion, (2.235c) [(2.228c) ≡ (2.228d)]. The case XXXVII of critical damping (2.235c) can be obtained from the general cases XXXVIII–XLI of non-critical damping (2.228c) by taking the coincidence limit (2.236a) of the two roots of the characteristic polynomial:*

$$\xi_+ - \xi_- = \varepsilon \to 0:$$

$$\begin{aligned} \lim_{\xi_+ \to \xi_-} x_*(t) &= \lim_{\varepsilon \to 0} \frac{1}{\varepsilon} \exp(\xi_+ t) \int^t \exp(-\xi_+ s) f(s) \left\{ 1 - \exp\left[-\varepsilon(t-s) \right] \right\} ds \\ &= \lim_{\varepsilon \to 0} \exp(\xi t) \int^t e^{-\xi s} \lim_{\varepsilon \to 0} \left[t - s + O(\varepsilon) \right] f(s) ds \\ &= e^{\xi t} \int^t e^{-\xi s} (t-s) f(s) ds, \end{aligned} \tag{2.236a, b}$$

leading to (2.236b), which coincides with (2.235c) ≡ (2.236b).

2.9.3 Arbitrary Forcing with Critical or Non-Critical Damping

There are four cases of forcing by an integrable function of time for a linear or harmonic damped or amplified oscillator or linear second-order system or circuit, namely the same four cases as for free oscillations (sections 2.1–2.5). The method of variation of parameters leads: (i) to (2.235a–c) for (problem 45) critical damping or amplification (case XXXVII):

$$\lambda = \omega_0: \qquad \ddot{x} + 2\lambda \dot{x} + \lambda^2 x = f(t), \quad x_*(t) = \int^t f(s) e^{-\lambda(t-s)} (t-s) ds, \tag{2.237a–c}$$

and to (2.228a–d) otherwise. The latter has three subcases, namely, (ii) no damping or amplification and (iii)(iv) super (sub)critical damping or amplification. In the case (ii) of (problem 46) no damping or amplification (2.238a) the characteristic polynomial (2.55a) has roots (2.55b) leading (2.228d) to the forced displacement (2.238b):

$$\ddot{x} + \omega_0^2 x = f(t): \qquad x_*(t) = \int^t f(s) e^{-\lambda(t-s)} \frac{e^{i\omega_0(t-s)} - e^{-i\omega_0(t-s)}}{2i\omega_0} ds, \qquad (2.238\text{a, b})$$

which simplifies to (2.239b):

$$\lambda = 0: \qquad x_*(t) = \int^t f(s) \frac{\sin\left[\omega_0(t-s)\right]}{\omega_0} ds. \qquad (2.239\text{a, b})$$

that applies (case XXXVIII) without damping (2.239a).

In (problem 47) the case (iii) of supercritical damping, (2.92a) ≡ (2.240a), the roots (2.92b, c) of the characteristic polynomial imply (2.228d) the forced displacement (2.240b):

$$\lambda > \omega_0: \qquad x_*(t) = \int^t e^{-\lambda(t-s)} f(s) \frac{e^{\overline{\omega}(t-s)} - e^{-\overline{\omega}(t-s)}}{2\overline{\omega}} ds, \qquad (2.240\text{a, b})$$

this simplifies to (2.241b):

$$\lambda > \omega_0: \qquad x_*(t) = \int^t f(s) e^{-\lambda(t-s)} \frac{\sinh\left[\overline{\omega}(t-s)\right]}{\overline{\omega}} ds, \qquad (2.241\text{a, b})$$

in the case XXXIX for supercritical damping or amplification (2.241a). In the remaining case (iv) of (problem 48) subcritical damping, (2.105a) ≡ (2.242a), the roots (2.105b, c) lead (2.228d) to the forced displacement (2.242b):

$$\lambda > \omega_0: \qquad x_*(t) = \int^t f(s) e^{-\lambda(t-s)} \frac{e^{i\overline{\omega}(t-s)} - e^{-i\overline{\omega}(t-s)}}{2i\overline{\omega}} ds; \qquad (2.242\text{a,b})$$

this simplifies to (2.243b).

$$\lambda < \omega_0: \qquad x_*(t) = \int^t f(s) e^{-\lambda(t-s)} \frac{\sin\left[\overline{\omega}(t-s)\right]}{\overline{\omega}} ds. \qquad (2.243\text{a, b})$$

In the case XL of subcritical damping or amplification (2.243b), it has been shown that *the forcing by an integrable function of time leads to a displacement specified: (i) by (2.239b) in the case XXXVIII of absence of damping or amplification (2.239a); (ii) in the presence of critical damping or amplification (2.237b) by (2.237c) valid for (2.237a); (iii)(iv) for (2.15) super(sub)critical damping (2.241a) [(2.242a)] by (2.241b) [(2.242b)]. In all cases, the forcing is by an arbitrary function of time, such that the integrals converge, namely, (2.237c)/(2.239b)/(2.241b)/(2.243b), respectively, in the cases (i)/(ii)/(iii)/(iv).* This is applied next to three cases of (subsection 2.9.4) forcing function: (a) sinusoidal oscillation with exponentially decaying amplitude (subsection 2.9.4) as a check to compare with preceding results (subsection 2.8.4); (b) the simplest case of constant forcing that leads to forcing by a bounded function of time (subsection 2.9.5).

2.9.4 Cases of Exponential and Constant Forcing

The response of a circuit to arbitrary forcing (2.228c) can be used in particular when considering (case XXV) the forcing (2.210a) ≡ (2.22; 2.244b) with applied frequency ω_a and decay λ_a, not both coincident with the unforced values (2.214a) ≡ (2.244a):

$$\{\lambda_a, \omega_a\} \neq \{\lambda, \bar{\omega}\}: \qquad f(t) = \mathrm{Re}\left\{f_a \exp\left[(i\omega_a - \lambda_a)t\right]\right\} = f_a e^{-\lambda_a t}\cos(\omega_a t), \tag{2.244a, b}$$

leading (2.105b, c) to:

$$\begin{aligned} x_*(t) &= \mathrm{Re}\left\{\frac{f_a}{\xi_+ - \xi_-}\left[\exp(\xi_+ t)\int^t \exp\left[(-\xi_+ - \lambda_a + i\omega_a)s\right]ds\right.\right. \\ &\qquad \left.\left. - \exp(\xi_- t)\int^t \exp\left[(-\xi_- - \lambda_a + i\omega_a)s\right]ds\right]\right\} \\ &= \mathrm{Re}\left\{\frac{f_a}{2i\bar{\omega}}\left[\exp(\xi_+ t)\frac{\exp\left[(-\xi_+ - \lambda_a + i\omega_a)t\right]}{-\xi_+ - \lambda_a + i\omega_a}\right.\right. \\ &\qquad \left.\left. - \exp(\xi_- t)\frac{\exp\left[(-\xi_- - \lambda_a + i\omega_a)t\right]}{-\xi_- - \lambda_a + i\omega_a}\right]\right\} \\ &= \mathrm{Re}\left\{\frac{f_a}{2i\bar{\omega}}\exp(-\lambda_a t + i\omega_a t)\left[\frac{1}{\lambda - \lambda_a + i(\omega_a - \bar{\omega})} - \frac{1}{\lambda - \lambda_a + i(\omega_a + \bar{\omega})}\right]\right\} \\ &= \mathrm{Re}\left\{\frac{f_a \exp\left[(-\lambda_a + i\omega_a)t\right]}{(\lambda - \lambda_a)^2 + \bar{\omega}^2 - \omega_a^2 + i2\omega_a(\lambda - \lambda_a)}\right\}, \end{aligned} \tag{2.245}$$

that agrees with (2.210c; 2.211c) ≡ (2.245).

The (problem 49) case XLII of uniform forcing (2.192a) with non-critical damping (2.228c) leads to (2.202b):

$$\begin{aligned} f(t) = f_0: \qquad x_*(t) &= \frac{f_0}{\xi_+ - \xi_-}\left[e^{\xi_+ t}\int^t e^{-\xi_+ s}\,ds - e^{\xi_- t}\int^t e^{-\xi_- s}\,ds\right] \\ &= \frac{f_0}{\xi_+ - \xi_-}\left(\frac{1}{\xi_-} - \frac{1}{\xi_+}\right) = \frac{f_0}{\xi_+\xi_-} = \frac{f_0}{\omega_0^2}, \end{aligned} \tag{2.246a, b}$$

noting that $\xi_+\xi_- = \omega_0^2$ from (2.82b). The same result is obtained (2.247b) in the case (2.247a) of critical damping (2.235c):

$$\xi \equiv \xi_\pm = -\lambda \equiv -\omega_0: \quad x_*(t) = f_0 e^{\xi t} \int^t e^{-\xi s}(t-s)\,ds = f_0 e^{\xi t}\left(t + \frac{\partial}{\partial \xi}\right)\int^t e^{-\xi s}\,d\xi$$

$$= f_0 e^{\xi t}\left(t + \frac{\partial}{\partial \xi}\right)\frac{e^{-\xi t}}{-\xi} = \frac{f_0}{\xi^2} = \frac{f_0}{\omega_0^2}. \tag{2.247a, b}$$

The response (2.246b) ≡ (2.247b) in the case XLI of (Problem 49) constant forcing (2.246a) follows immediately from (2.22) or (2.238a) or (2.237b), and is the same in all cases because it is determined by the spring alone. The displacement for constant forcing, (2.246b) ≡ (2.247b), also supplies an upper bound for the displacement forced by a finite function of time (subsection 2.9.5).

2.9.5 Upper Bound for the Displacement Due to Finite Forcing

In the case of (problem 50) bounded forcing (2.248a) with critical damping or amplification (2.237c), the displacement has an upper bound (2.248b):

$$|f(t)| \le \frac{F_{max}}{m}: \qquad |x_*(t)| \le \frac{F_{max}}{m}\left|\int^t e^{-\lambda(t-s)}(t-s)\,ds\right|; \tag{2.248a, b}$$

the evaluation of the integral is similar to (2.247b) yielding:

$$\lambda = \omega_0: \qquad |x_*(t)| \le \frac{F_{max}}{m\lambda^2} = \frac{F_{max}}{m\omega_0^2} = \frac{F_{max}}{k}. \tag{2.249a, b}$$

The upper bound for the forced displacement is determined by the spring alone since only its resilience k appears in (2.249b). In the case of non-critical damping or amplification (2.250a), the upper bound for the displacement (2.228d) under finite forcing (2.248a) is (2.250b):

$$\lambda \ne \omega_0: \qquad |x_*(t)| \le \frac{F_{max}}{m}\left|\int^t \frac{e^{\xi_+(t-s)} - e^{\xi_-(t-s)}}{\xi_+ - \xi_-}\,ds\right|; \tag{2.250a, b}$$

the integral (2.250b) is evaluated as (2.246b) leading to (2.251b):

$$\lambda \ne \omega_0: \qquad |x_*(t)| \le \frac{F_{max}}{m\omega_0^2} = \frac{F_{max}}{k}, \tag{2.251a, b}$$

that is the same result, (2.251b) ≡ (2.249b), with non-critical (2.251a) or critical (2.249a) damping or amplification. In (2.246b) and (2.250b), the *product (2.252a) was used of roots of the characteristic polynomial (2.82a, b), which like the sum of roots (2.252b):*

$$\xi_+\xi_- = \omega_0^2, \qquad \xi_+ + \xi_- = -2\lambda, \tag{2.252a, b}$$

follows from:

$$P_2(D) = D^2 + 2\lambda D + \omega_0^2 = (D - \xi_+)(D - \xi_-) = D^2 - (\xi_+ + \xi_-)D + \xi_+\xi_-. \tag{2.253}$$

It has been shown that *a harmonic oscillator (2.22) with critical (2.249a) or non-critical (2.251a) damping subject (case XLII) to (problem 50) arbitrary bounded forcing (2.148a) ≡ (2.254a):*

$$|f(t)| \le F_{max}: \qquad |x_*(t)| \le \frac{F_{max}}{k}, \tag{2.254a, b}$$

has in both cases, (2.249b) ≡ (2.251b) ≡ (2.254b), an upper bound for the forced component of the displacement due to the spring acting alone; the total displacement is the sum of the free (and forced) displacements [sections 2.2–2.6 (sections 2.7–2.9 and notes 2.4–2.10)].

NOTE 2.1: 52 Cases of Linear One-Dimensional Oscillations

The harmonic oscillator is the simplest case in Table 3.1 that balances the inertia force associated with the mass against the restoring force exerted by a spring, which in a linear approximation is proportional to the distance; this is the case I that corresponds to a pendulum suspended in the gravity field, performing small amplitude oscillations about the equilibrium position; in the case II of an inverted pendulum the force is repulsive instead of attractive, leading to a monotonic motion away from the position of equilibrium that is an unstable repeller. Adding to the linear attractive force, a linear friction force opposite to the velocity leads to the damped oscillator, with four cases: (case III) critical damping leading to a decay to the equilibrium position that is monotonic or has a single extremum; (case IV) supercritical damping for which the decay is always monotonic; (case V) subcritical damping for which the decay is oscillatory; (case VI) weak damping that is a particular case of subcritical damping for which the oscillatory decay takes place at the natural frequency. In all the damped cases (cases III–VI), the equilibrium position is a stable attractor. The equilibrium position is unstable if the damping is replaced by amplification away from an unstable repeller, and also leads to eight cases: (case VII) zero effective damping; (case VIII) critical effective damping; (case IX) supercritical effective damping; (cases

X–XI) strong (weak) subcritical effective damping; (case XII) critical amplification; (cases XIII–XIV) super(sub)critical amplification. A particular simplification of all damped (cases III–VI) and amplified (cases VII–XIV) cases, is the case XIX of small mass, which includes exponential growth (case XV) or decay (case XVI); the other "degenerate" case is uniform motion (case XVIII) and rest (case XVII).

In the presence of forcing and in the absence of damping there are three cases, depending on whether the applied and natural frequencies are: (case XX) distinct leading to a forced non-resonant oscillation with constant amplitude; (case XXI) coincident, leading to undamped resonance, corresponding to an oscillation with an amplitude increasing linearly with time; (case XXII) close but not coincident, leading to the intermediate case of beats, which is oscillations with a slow modulation of amplitude. For sinusoidal forcing in the presence of damping, the amplitude of oscillation is always constant, both in the non-resonant (resonant) case XXIII (XXIV) of distinct (coincident) applied and natural frequencies. In the case of a sinusoidal applied force with exponential decay, there is no resonance in general (case XXV); "resonance" occurs only if the applied decay equals the natural damping and the applied frequency equals the oscillation frequency (case XXX) and the oscillation still decays in time. The oscillation frequency differs from the natural frequency in the presence of damping and thus, there is no resonance: (i) if the applied frequency is zero (case XXVI); (ii–iii) if the applied and oscillation frequencies coincide but the applied decay and natural damping do not coincide (case XXVII) or vice-versa (case XXVIII); (iv) if the applied decay coincides with the natural damping and the applied frequency coincides with the natural frequency but not with the oscillation frequency (case XXIX). In all cases, XXV–XXX, the exponential amplitude decay is dominant relative to the constant (linearly growing) amplitude in the non-resonant cases XXV–XXIX (resonant case XXX). Resonances do not occur for forcing without (with) damping involving a power of time [case XXXI (XXIV)], also multiplied by an exponential decay [case XXXII (XXXV)] and a sinusoidal oscillation [case XXXIII (XXXVI)].

Of the preceding 36 cases, the first 24 cases (cases I–XXIV) demonstrate essential properties of the "harmonic oscillator" whereas the remaining 12 cases (cases XXV–XXXVI) are various particular cases of forcing. The forcing by arbitrary functions of time corresponds to the remaining 14 cases (cases XXXVII–L) for which five methods can be used (Table 2.2). The first method A is the method of variation of parameters that distinguishes the case XXXVII of critical damping and cases XXXIX (XL) of super(sub)critical damping, besides the case of no damping (case XXXVIII). The presence or absence of damping does not affect constant forcing (case XLI) and leads to the same result for bounded forcing (case XLII). The second method B concerns forcing by discrete spectra represented by the Fourier series and distinguishes the non-resonant (resonant) cases without [case XLIII (XLIV)] and with [case XLV (XLVI)] damping. The third method C concerns forcing by a continuous spectrum represented by a Fourier integral and distinguishes the case XLVII of no damping, from critical damping [case XLVIII) and super(sub)critical damping [case XLIX (L)]. They are applied to two Gaussian forcings (cases LI–LII). The fourth (fifth) methods D(E) use the influence function (Laplace transform) and are discussed in the note 2.3. Before proceeding to forcing by arbitrary functions of time (notes 2.3–2.10) a brief reference is made to generalized oscillators or systems (note 2.2).

NOTE 2.2: Non-Linear Multidimensional Vibrations

The 52 cases in the Table 2.1 concern the linear second-order ordinary differential equation with constant coefficients that allows (Diagram 2.1) several variations: (i) positive (negative) restoring force for an attractor to stable (repeller from unstable) equilibrium, and neither for indifferent equilibrium; (ii) positive (negative) damping for a decaying (amplified) motion, with an intermediate case of constant amplitude; (iii) no forcing or resonant (non-resonant) forcing at the natural parameters; (iv) no mass, small mass, or non-negligible mass as regards the inertia force. The designation harmonic oscillator strictly applies to the case of linear restoring versus inertia force without damping, amplification, or forcing, or more broadly to linear second-order differential equations cases with constant coefficients.

The 52 cases in the Table 2.1 and $3^4 = 81$ combinations of the harmonic oscillator in Diagram 2.2 involve seven restrictions (i) to (viii), which will

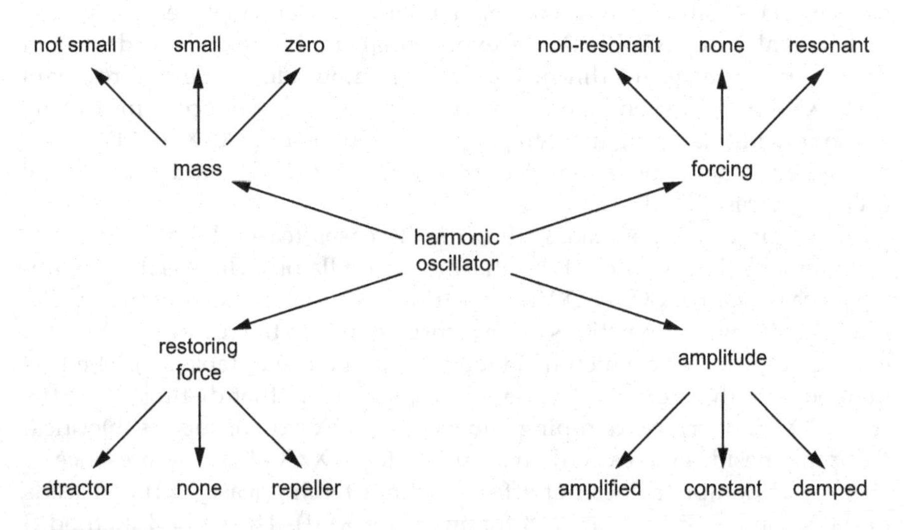

DIAGRAM 2.1
The harmonic oscillator (2.22) may be an attractor or repeller free or forced in the presence or absence of damping or amplification, and is specified by the general linear second-order forced ordinary differential equation with constant coefficients.

TABLE 2.1
52 Cases of the Linear Oscillator

Case	Conditions	Damping Amplification	Attractor or Repeller	Forcing Resonance	Section	Figure	Phase Plane	Displacement Velocity	Amplitude Phase	Energies Activity Dissipation	Time Average
I	$\omega_0^2 > 0 = \lambda = F$	no	attractor	no-no	2.2.1–2.2.4	2.4	2.5	(2.56b, c)	(2.58a, b)	(2.61a, b; 2.62b, c; 2.63b)	—
II	$\omega_0^2 < 0 = \lambda = F$	no	repeller	no-no	2.2.4–2.2.5	2.8	2.9	(2.73b, c)	(2.75a, b)	(2.77a–b; 2.78a–c)	—
III	$\lambda = \omega_0 > 0 = F$	critical damping	attractor	no-no	2.3.1–2.3.2	2.10	2.11	(2.85b, c)	(2.87b, c)	—	—
IV	$\lambda > \omega_0 > 0 = F$	supercritical damping	attractor	no-no	2.3.3–2.3.4	2.12	2.13	(2.93b, c; 2.92c)	(2.95a, b)	—	(10. ?)
V	$\omega_0 > \lambda > 0 = F$	subcritical damping	attractor	no-no	2.4	2.14	2.15	(2.106b, c; 2.105c)	(2.108a, b)	(10.15 a–d)	(10.19a–d)
VI	$\omega_0^2 > \lambda^2 > 0 = F$	weak damping	attractor	no-no	2.4.2	2.14	2.15	(2.112a–c)	(2.108a, b)	(2.121a, b; 2.124b) (2.127)	(2.123a, c; 2.125a–c) (2.127)
VII	$\lambda - \nu = 0 = F$	zero effective damping	attractor	no-no	2.5.2	2.4	2.5	(2.136a–c)	—	—	—
VIII	$\lambda - \omega_0 - \nu = 0 = F$	critical effective damping	attractor	no-no	2.5.2	2.10	2.11	(2.137a–d)	—	—	—
IX	$\lambda - \omega_0 - \nu > 0 = F$	supercritical effective damping	attractor	no-no	2.5.2	2.12	2.13	(2.138a–d)	—	—	—
X	$\lambda - \omega_0 - \nu < 0 = F$	strong subcritical effective damping	attractor	no-no	2.5.2	2.14	2.15	(2.139a–d)	—	—	—
XI	$\omega_0^2 >> (\lambda - \nu)^2 > 0 = F$	weak subcritical effective damping	attractor	no-no	2.5.2	2.14	2.15	(2.140a–d)	—	—	—

(Continued)

TABLE 2.1 *(Continued)*

Case	Conditions	Damping Amplification	Attractor or Repeller	Forcing Resonance	Section	Figure	Phase Plane	Displacement Velocity	Amplitude Phase	Energies Activity Dissipation	Time Average
XII	$\lambda - \nu + \omega_0 = 0 = F$	critical amplification	attractor	no-no	2.5.3	2.18	—	(2.141a–d)	—	—	—
XIII	$\lambda + \omega_0 - \nu < 0 = F$	supercritical amplitude	attractor	no-no	2.5.3	2.18	—	(2.142a–d)	—	—	—
XIV	$\omega_0 > \nu > 0 = F$	subcritical amplification	repeller	no-no	2.5.3	2.18	—	(2.143a–d)	—	—	—
XV	$\mu, k > 0 = m = F$	damping	attractor	no-no	2.6.1	—	—	(2.153a–c)	(2.154a, b)	—	—
XVI	$\mu < 0 < k, m = 0 = F$	amplification	repeller	no-no	2.6.1	—	—	(2.153a–c)	(2.154a, b)	—	—
XVII	$m = \mu = 0 = F$	rest	either	no-no	2.6.1	—	—	(2.155c, d)	—	—	—
XVIII	$k = \mu = F = 0 \neq m$	uniform motion	neither	no-no	2.6.1	—	—	(2.156d, e)	—	—	—
XIX	$k > 0 = F \neq \mu$ $mk << \mu^2$	no	neither	no-no	2.6.1–2.6.2	—	—	(2.160)	—	—	—
XX	$\lambda \neq 0 \neq \omega_0 = \omega_a$ $f \sim \exp(i\omega_a t)$	no	attractor	yes-no	2.7.1–2.7.2	2.22a	—	(2.168b, c)	—	(2.169a, 2.170a, 2.171a; 2.172a)	(2.169b, 2.170b, 2.171b; 2.172b)
XXI	$\lambda = 0 = \omega_0 \neq \omega_a$ $f \sim \exp(i\omega_a t)$	no	attractor	yes-yes	2.7.3–2.7.4	2.22b	—	(2.176b, c)	—	(2.177a–c; 2.180a)	(2.178a–c; 2.180b; 2.179a,b)
XXII	$\lambda = 0 \neq \omega_0 = \omega_a - 2\varepsilon$ $f \sim \exp(i\omega_a t)$	yes	attractor	yes almost	2.7.5–2.7.6	2.22c	—	(2.184; 2.189)	—	(2.190a–c)	(2.191a–c)
XXIII	$\lambda \neq 0 \neq \omega_0 \neq \omega_a$ $f \sim \exp(i\omega_a t)$	yes	attractor	yes-no	2.8.1–2.8.3	2.23a, b	—	(2.198a, b)	(2.197a, b)	(2.203a, b; 2.206a, b)	(2.204a, b, 2.205a–c, 2.209a–c; 2.207a, b)
XXIV	$\lambda \neq 0 \neq \omega_0 = \omega_a$ $f \sim \exp(i\omega_a t)$	yes	neither	yes-no	2.8.1–2.8.3	2.23a, b	—	(2.201e)	(2.201c, d)	(2.203a, b; 2.206a, b)	(2.204a, b, 2.205a–c, 2.209b; 2.207a, b)

XXV	$\{\omega_a - \bar{\omega}, \lambda_a - \lambda\} \neq \{0, 0\}$ $f \sim \exp\left[(i\omega_a - \lambda_a)t\right]$	yes	attractor	yes-no	2.8.4	—	—	(2.214b, c)	(2.212a, b)	—	—
XXVI	$\omega_a = 0$ $f \sim f_a \exp\left[(i\omega_a - \lambda_a)t\right]$	yes	attractor	yes-no	2.8.4	—	—	(2.215b, c)	—	—	—
XXVII	$\omega_a - \bar{\omega} = 0 \neq \lambda - \lambda_a$ $f \sim f_a \exp\left[(i\omega_a - \lambda_a)t\right]$	yes	attractor	yes-no	2.8.5	—	—	(2.214b, c)	(2.216c,d)	—	—
XXVIII	$\lambda_a - \lambda = 0 \neq \omega_a - \bar{\omega}$ $f \sim f_a \exp\left[(i\omega_a - \lambda_a)t\right]$	yes	attractor	yes-no	2.8.5	—	—	(2.217c, d)	—	—	—
XXIX	$\lambda_a - \lambda = 0 = \omega_a - \omega_0$ $f \sim f_a \exp\left[(i\omega_a - \lambda_a)t\right]$	yes	attractor	yes-no	2.8.5	—	—	(2.218c, d)	—	—	—
XXX	$\omega_a - \bar{\omega} = 0 = \lambda_a - \lambda$ $f \sim f_a \exp\left[(i\omega_a - \lambda_a)t\right]$	yes	attractor	yes-yes	2.8.6	—	—	(2.221c, d)	—	—	—
XXXI	$\omega_0 \neq \lambda = 0 \neq f$ $f \sim t^n$	yes-no	attractor	(10.37b)	E.10.3.1	—	—	(10.40a, b)	—	—	—
XXXII	$\omega_a \neq \omega_0 \neq \lambda = 0 \neq f$ $f \sim t\cos(\omega_a t)$	yes-no	attractor	(10.37c)	E.10.3.1	—	—	(10.42a–c)	—	—	—
XXXIII	$\omega_a = \omega_0 \neq \lambda = 0 \neq f$ $f \sim t\cos(\omega_a t)$	yes-yes	attractor	(10.37c)	E.10.3.1	—	—	(10.43a–c)	—	—	—
XXXIV	$0 \neq \omega_0, \lambda, f$ $f \sim t$	yes-no	attractor	(10.38a)	E.10.3.2	—	—	(10.46)	—	—	—
XXXV	$\omega_a \neq \omega_0, \lambda, f \neq 0$ $f \sim t\cos(\omega_a t)$	yes-no	attractor	(10.38b)	E.10.3.2	—	—	(10.48)	—	—	—
XXXVI	$\omega_a = \omega_0, \lambda, f \neq 0$ $f \sim t\cos(\omega_a t)$	yes-yes	attractor	(10.38b)	E.10.3.2	—	—	(10.49a, b)	—	—	—
XXXVII	$\lambda - \omega_0 = 0 \neq f$ $f \sim t$	critical	attractor	yes	2.9.2–2.9.3	—	—	(2.237a–c)	—	—	—
XXXVIII	$\lambda = 0 \neq \omega_0, f$ $f \sim t\cos(\omega_a t)$	no	attractor	yes	2.9.1, 2.9.3	—	—	(2.239b)	—	—	—

(Continued)

TABLE 2.1 *(Continued)*

Case	Conditions	Damping Amplification	Attractor or Repeller	Forcing Resonance	Section	Figure	Phase Plane	Displacement Velocity	Amplitude Phase	Energies Activity Dissipation	Time Average
XXXIX	$\lambda - \omega_0 > 0 \neq f$ $f \sim t\cos(\omega_a t)$	supercritical	attractor	yes	2.9.1, 2.9.3	—	—	(2.241b)	—	—	—
XL	$\lambda - \omega_0 < 0 \neq f$	subcritical	attractor	yes	2.9.1, 2.9.3	—	—	(2.243b)	—	—	—
XLI	$f = const \equiv f_0$	all	attractor	(2.246a)	2.9.4	—	—	(2.246b, 2.247b)	—	—	—
XLII	$\lvert f(t) \rvert \leq f_{mass}$	all	attractor	(2.254a)	2.9.5	—	—	(2.254b)	—	—	—
XLIII	$\lambda = 0 \neq \omega_0 - m\omega_a$	no	attractor	yes-no	N.2.4	—	—	(2.257b)	—	—	—
XLIV	$\lambda = 0 = \omega_0 - m\omega_a$	no	attractor	yes-yes	N.2.4	—	—	(2.258b)	—	—	—
XLV	$\lambda = 0 \neq \omega_0 - m\omega_a$	yes	attractor	yes-no	N.2.4	—	—	(2.261b)	—	—	—
XLVI	$\lambda = 0 = \omega_0 - m\omega_a$	yes	attractor	yes-no	N.2.4	—	—	(2.262b)	—	—	—
XLVII	$\lambda = 0 \neq f$	yes	attractor	spectrum	N.2.5	—	—	(2.270)	—	—	—
XLVIII	$\lambda - \omega_0 = 0 \neq f$	no	attractor	spectrum	N.2.6	—	—	(2.275)	—	—	—
XLIX	$\lambda - \omega_0 > 0 \neq f$	yes	attractor	spectrum	N.2.7	—	—	(2.281)	—	—	—
L	$\lambda - \omega_0 < 0 \neq f$	yes	attractor	spectrum	N.2.8	—	—	(2.285)	—	—	—
LI	$\lambda = 0$, $f = f_a \exp(-t^2/T^2)$	no	attractor	Gaussian	N.2.12	—	—	(2.313b)	—	—	—
LII	$\lambda = 0$, $f = \frac{f_a}{\sigma\sqrt{2\pi}} \exp \left[-\frac{(t-\mu)}{2\sigma^2} \right]$	no	attractor	Gaussian	N.2.12	—	—	(2.317b)	—	—	—

Note: Fifty-two cases of the linear second-order system with constant coefficients including: (i) undamped unforced attractor (repeller) in cases I (II); (ii) damped (amplified) unforced oscillator in cases III–VI (VII–XIV); (iii) degenerate cases XV–XIX like small mass; (iv) forcings either sinusoidal (cases XX–XXIV) with decay (cases XXV–XXX) and other time dependences (cases XXXI–XXXVI); (v) forcing by arbitrary ordinary or generalized functions of time (cases XXXVII–LII) in Table 2.2.

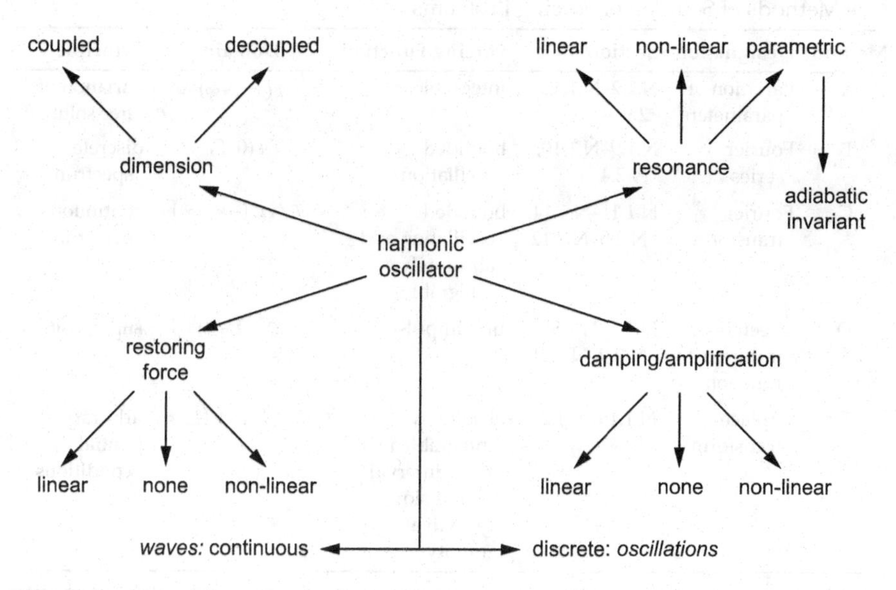

DIAGRAM 2.2
The linear second-order system with constant coefficients (Diagram 2.1) may be generalized to non-linear systems with variable coefficients that may be discrete (vibrations) or continuous (waves), and have several degrees of freedom and couplings.

be lifted subsequently. The equation of motion (2.15) is linear (i), excluding large displacements and velocities; the case of non-linear restoring and/or friction forces is first considered in chapter 4. The coefficients in the linear equation of motion (2.15) are assumed to be constant (ii), that is, independent of time except for slow variations in the case of the adiabatic invariant (subsection 2.2.3); in the case of coefficients a fast functions of time, such as coefficients periodic functions of time, for example, a spring with oscillating support leads to parametric resonance (section 4.3). The differential equation of motion, even linear with constant coefficients, lead (iii) to singular points on the phase plane (for example, center, saddle point, spiral sink or source, etc.), through which pass no curves or several curves; other possibilities of singular points occur for linear (chapter 4, sections 5.1–5.2) and non-linear cases. The oscillator is discrete, that is a point mass (iv) whose position depends on time; in the case of continuous systems, the independent variable is position, for example, for the deflection of a string (chapter III.2) or a bar or beam (chapter III.4).

The equation of motion is of the second-order (v), because the highest order derivative is the acceleration, that is, the second-order derivative of the displacement with regards to time; higher-order systems can be considered,

TABLE 2.2

Five Methods of Solution of Forcing Problems

Method	Designation	Section	Forcing Function	Domain	Principle
A	variation of parameters	N.1.2–N.1.4; 2.9	integrable	$\mathcal{E}(-\infty,+\infty)$	variation of free solution
B	Fourier series	N.1.9–N.1.10; N.2.4	bounded oscillation	$\mathcal{F}(0,T)$	discrete spectrum
C	Fourier transform	N.1.11–N.1.14; N.2.5–N.2.12	bounded oscillation and absolutely integrable	$\mathcal{F} \cap \mathcal{L}^1(-\infty,+\infty)$	continuous spectrum
D	Green or influence function	N.1.5–N.1.8; N.2.9–N.2.11	unit impulse	$\mathcal{C}(-a,+b)$	superposition
E	Laplace transform	N.1.15–N.1.27	absolutely integrable in a finite interval and of slow growth at infinity	$\mathcal{L}^1(0,L) \cap \underline{\mathcal{V}}(L,\infty)$	arbitrary initial conditions

Note: Five approaches to the calculation of the response of a linear second-order system with constant coefficients to forcing by arbitrary ordinary or generalized functions of time.

such as the elastic instability of a beam (sections 6.1–6.3) that is, a case of a continuous fourth-order system. The oscillator has a single degree-of-freedom (vi), namely, it is specified by a displacement satisfying an ordinary differential equation; the case of several degrees-of-freedom, for example, vibrations of a rigid body (sections 8.3–8.8), there are several dependent variables (discrete coordinates) and one independent variable (time) that leads to coupled systems of ordinary differential equations (chapter 7). A single independent variable was considered (vii), namely, time; the case of several independent variables, for example, multidimensional deformations, or dependence on position and time, for example, waves and diffusion, leads to partial differential equations (p.d.e.s).

Combinations of several of the features (i) to (vii) are also considered, such as non-linear waves. These extensions of the harmonic oscillator are indicated in Diagram 2.2. The methods used to study the basic harmonic oscillator (Diagram 2.1) are the basis for the extension to higher-order discrete or continuous systems with more independent and dependent variables (Diagram 2.2). The cases of unforced and forced motions (Table 2.1) are completed by considering (note 3.3) the five methods applicable to arbitrary forcing (Table 2.2).

NOTE 2.3: Five Methods for Forced Systems

The linear second-order system with constant coefficients is used next (notes 2.4–2.9) to illustrate five methods (Table 2.2) of obtaining the displacement due to forcing by an arbitrary function of time; these methods apply to linear ordinary differential equations with constant coefficients of any order (notes 1.1–1.28 and notes III.3.1–III.3.18). The method B applies if the forcing function has bounded oscillation over a finite interval; it can be repeated periodically outside the interval, leading to a representation by a Fourier series (notes 1.9–1.10 and section II.5.7), corresponding to a discrete spectrum consisting of an applied frequency and its multiplies or harmonics (note 2.4); by the superposition principle that applies to a linear oscillator each frequency corresponds to a forcing, without (with) damping with: (i) no resonance [case XLII (XLV)] if the applied frequency and all its harmonics do not coincide with the natural frequency; (ii) if the applied frequency or one of its harmonics coincides with the natural frequency there is resonance only for that term [case XLIV (XLVI)].

The method C concerns a forcing function absolutely integrable and with bounded oscillation over an infinite interval; it can be represented by a Fourier integral (notes 1.11–1.14) corresponding to a continuous spectrum. In this case, the calculation of the response involves the inversion of the Fourier integral by residues (notes III.3.1–III.3.18) and distinguishes four cases of (XLVII) no damping, (XLVII) critical damping, and [XLIX (XL)] of super(sub)critical damping, respectively, in the notes 2.5 to 2.8. The method E uses the Laplace transform (notes 1.15–1.28) for a function absolutely integrable in a finite interval of the positive real line and of slow growth at infinity. The method D uses the influence or Green function (notes 1.5–1.8) that is, the response to a unit impulse (chapters III.1, 3, 5, 7) and can be calculated: (i) using as initial conditions zero displacement with unit velocity; (ii)(iii) either the Fourier (note 2.9) or the Laplace transform. The influence function together with the superposition principle specifies the forcing by an arbitrary function. The method D of the influence function leads to the same result as the method A of variation of parameters (note 1.3) applied to the harmonic oscillator (section 2.9 and note 2.9).

The method C of the Fourier transform applied to a function that vanishes on the negative real line leads to the same result as the method E of the Laplace transform with the same initial conditions of zero displacement and unit velocity. The method E of the Laplace transform has two advantages: (i) it allows arbitrary initial displacement and velocity as initial conditions; (ii) since the forcing functions is restricted to positive real arguments it can be more general, that is absolutely integrable in a finite integral of slow growth at infinity (instead of absolutely integrable and of bounded fluctuation for the Fourier transform). The second disadvantage disappears extending the Fourier transform and the Laplace transform from ordinary (volumes I and II) to generalized functions (volume III). The Fourier transform may be easier to invert by contour integration, which applies also to the Laplace transform. In the sequel are used the Fourier series (transform) to consider the forcing of a harmonic oscillator by a discrete (continuous) spectrum [note(s) 2.4 (2.5–2.8)]; this leads to the influence function (note 2.9) and confirms (note 2.10) the results (note 2.11) of the method of variation of parameters (section 2.9). The Gaussian forcing (section 2.12) is considered via its continuous spectrum, which can be extended to Gaussian noise (note 2.13).

NOTE 2.4: **Non-Resonant/Resonant Forcing by a Discrete Spectrum**

Consider the forcing of an undamped harmonic (2.255b) oscillator with natural frequency ω_0 by a function with bounded oscillation, (2.255a) ≡ (1.539a–d), in a finite interval:

$$f \in \mathcal{F}(-T,+T): \quad \ddot{x} + \omega_0^2 x = f(t) = \mathrm{Re}\left\{\sum_{n=-\infty}^{+\infty} f_n e^{in\pi t/T}\right\} = \sum_{n=-\infty}^{+\infty} f_n \cos\left(\frac{\pi n t}{T}\right), \tag{2.255a–c}$$

that can be represented by a Fourier series, (2.255c) ≡ (1.540a–c), corresponding to: (i) an applied frequency (2.256a) and its multiples (2.256b) or **harmonics**: (ii) the associated amplitudes (2.256c):

$$\omega_a = \frac{\pi}{T}, \quad \omega_{an} = n\omega_a = \frac{n\pi}{T}: \qquad f_n = \frac{1}{2T}\int_{-T}^{+T} f(t)\cos\left(\frac{n\pi t}{T}\right)dt. \tag{2.256a–c}$$

The forcing function $f(t)$ may be defined in the interval $(0,T)$ and: (i) extended symmetrically $f(-t) = f(t)$ to the interval $(-T,+T)$; (ii) repeated periodically outside the interval $f(t+2nT) = f(t)$. This leads to an even periodic function of bounded oscillation that has a cosine series (subsection III.5.7.6). Since the differential equation (2.255c) is linear the principle of superposition applies, and the response: (i) is (2.168b) ≡ (2.257b) in (problem 51) the non-resonant case (2.168a) when (case XLII) the natural frequency is not a multiple of the applied frequency (2.257a):

$$\omega_0 \neq \frac{m\pi}{T}: \quad x_*(t) = \sum_{n=-\infty}^{+\infty} \frac{f_n}{\omega_0^2 - \omega_{an}^2}\cos(\omega_{an} t) = \sum_{n=-\infty}^{+\infty} \frac{f_n T^2}{\omega_0^2 T^2 - n^2\pi^2}\cos\left(\frac{n\pi t}{T}\right); \tag{2.257a, b}$$

$$\begin{aligned} \omega_0 = \frac{m\pi}{T}: \quad x_*(t) &= \frac{f_m t}{2\omega_{am}}\sin(\omega_{am} t) + \sum_{\substack{n=-\infty \\ n\neq m}}^{+\infty} \frac{f_n}{\omega_0^2 - \omega_{an}^2}\cos(\omega_{an} t) \\ &= \frac{f_n T t}{2m\pi}\sin\left(\frac{m\pi t}{T}\right) + \sum_{\substack{n=-\infty \\ n\neq m}}^{+\infty} \frac{f_n T^2}{\omega_0^2 T^2 - n^2\pi^2}\cos\left(\frac{n\pi t}{T}\right), \end{aligned} \tag{2.258a, b}$$

(ii) resonance occurs (2.175a, b) if (problem 52) the natural frequency equals a multiple of the applied frequency (2.258a), in which case (XLIV) all terms in (2.257b) with $n \neq m$ are unchanged except for the resonant term $n = m$ in (2.257b) that is replaced by (2.176b) in (2.258b).

The extension (2.22) from the undamped (2.255b) to the damped (2.259b) oscillator forced by a function of bounded variation (2.259a) in a finite interval $(-T,+T)$ is:

$$f \in \mathcal{F}(-T,+T): \quad \ddot{x} + 2\lambda\dot{x} + \omega_0^2 x = f(t) = \operatorname{Re}\left\{\sum_{n=-\infty}^{+\infty} f_n e^{in\pi/T}\right\} = \sum_{n=-\infty}^{+\infty} f_n \cos\left(\frac{n\pi t}{T}\right). \tag{2.259a, b}$$

The presence of damping changes the response to (2.198a) ≡ (2.260):

$$x_*(t) = f_a \frac{\left(\omega_0^2 - \omega_{an}^2\right)\cos(\omega_{an} t) + 2\omega_{an}\lambda \sin(\omega_{an} t)}{\left(\omega_0^2 - \omega_{an}^2\right)^2 + 4\lambda^2\omega_{an}^2}, \tag{2.260}$$

from (2.257a, b) with (2.256a–c) to (2.261):

$$\bar{\omega} \neq \frac{n\pi}{T}: \quad x_*(t) = \sum_{n=-\infty}^{+\infty} \frac{F_n T^2}{\left(\omega_0^2 T^2 - n^2\pi^2\right)^2 + 4\pi^2 n^2 \lambda^2 T^2}$$
$$\left[\left(\omega_0^2 T^2 - n^2\pi^2\right)\cos\left(\frac{n\pi t}{T}\right) + 2n\pi\lambda T \sin\left(\frac{n\pi t}{T}\right)\right], \tag{2.261a, b}$$

that is valid both in: (i) the (case XLV) non-resonant (2.257a) damped (problem 53) case (2.261a, b); (ii) the resonant (2.262a) damped case (XLVI) that (problem 54) simplifies the n-th term in (2.261b) to (2.262b):

$$\bar{\omega} = \frac{m\pi}{T}: \quad x_*(t) = \frac{f_m T}{2\pi m\lambda} \sin\left(\frac{m\pi}{T}\right) + \sum_{\substack{n=-\infty \\ n\neq m}}^{+\infty} \frac{f_n T^2}{\left(\omega_0^2 T^2 - n^2\pi^2\right)^2 + 4\pi^2 n^2 \lambda^2 T^2}$$
$$\left[\left(\omega_0^2 T^2 - n^2\pi^2\right)\cos\left(\frac{n\pi t}{T}\right) + 2n\pi\lambda T \sin\left(\frac{n\pi t}{T}\right)\right]. \tag{2.262a, b}$$

It has been shown that *the forcing by a function of time of bounded oscillation, (2.255a) ≡ (2.259a), in a finite interval represented by a Fourier series (2.255a–c; 2.256a–c) leads to the displacement specified in the non-resonant, (2.257a) ≡ (2.261a) [resonant (2.258a) ≡ (2.262a)], case given: (i) by (2.261b) [(2.262b)] for a damped oscillator (2.259b): (ii) by (2.157b) [(2.158b)] for the undamped oscillator (2.255b). Resonance occurs when the natural frequency is a multiple of the applied frequency (2.256a, b) and can apply only to one term of the Fourier series, namely, (2.258a) [(2.262a)] without (with) damping.*

NOTE 2.5: Forcing of an Undamped Oscillator by a Continuous Spectrum

A forcing function of bounded oscillation (and absolutely integrable) on a finite interval (2.255a) [the real line (2.263a)] can be represented by a Fourier series (2.255c) [integral (2.263b)] corresponding to a discrete (continuous) spectrum with amplitudes (2.256c) [Fourier transform (2.263c):

$$f(t)\in \mathcal{L}^1 \cap \mathcal{F}(|R): \quad \ddot{x}+\omega_0^2 x = f(t) = \int_{-\infty}^{+\infty} \tilde{f}(\omega) e^{i\omega t}\, d\omega, \quad \tilde{f}(\omega) \equiv \frac{1}{2\pi}\int_{-\infty}^{+\infty} f(t) e^{-i\omega t}\, dt. \tag{2.263a–c}$$

In (2.263b) is considered (problem 55) an undamped oscillator; critical and super (sub) critical cases will be considered in the sequel (respectively in the notes 2.6 to 2.8). In all cases the displacement may be represented by a Fourier integral (1.549a) ≡ (2.264a):

$$x(t) = \int_{-\infty}^{+\infty} \tilde{x}(\omega) e^{i\omega t}\, d\omega: \qquad \ddot{x}+\omega_0^2 x = \int_{-\infty}^{+\infty} \left(\omega_0^2-\omega^2\right) \tilde{x}(\omega) e^{i\omega t}\, d\omega, \tag{2.264a, b}$$

implying (2.264b) under the assumptic that (2.264a) is uniformly convergent with regards to time and hence (I.13.40) the time derivatives can be taken inside the integrand. Equating (2.264b) ≡ (2.263b) leads to the algebraic relation between the forcing $\tilde{f}$ and displacement $\tilde{x}$ spectra (2.265a):

$$\left(\omega_0^2-\omega^2\right)\tilde{x}_*(\omega) = \tilde{f}(\omega); \qquad x_*(t) = \int_{-\infty}^{+\infty} \frac{\tilde{f}(\omega)}{\omega_0^2-\omega^2} e^{i\omega t}\, d\omega, \tag{2.265a, b}$$

solving (2.265a) for $\tilde{x}$ and substituting in (2.264a) specifies the displacement as a function of time (2.265b).

The integral (2.265b) can be evaluated (section I.17.5) closing the path of integration along the real axis (Figure 2.24a) by a half-circle in the upper (lower) complex-ω half-plane for $t>0 (t<0)$, and the integral over the half-circle vanishes (I.17.29) if the condition (2.266a, b) is met:

$$\operatorname{Im}(\omega) >< 0: \qquad \lim_{|\omega|\to\infty} \tilde{f}(\omega) = 0; \quad x_*(t) = -\int_{-\infty}^{+\infty} \frac{\tilde{f}(\omega)}{(\omega-\omega_0)(\omega+\omega_0)} e^{i\omega t}\, d\omega, \tag{2.266a–c}$$

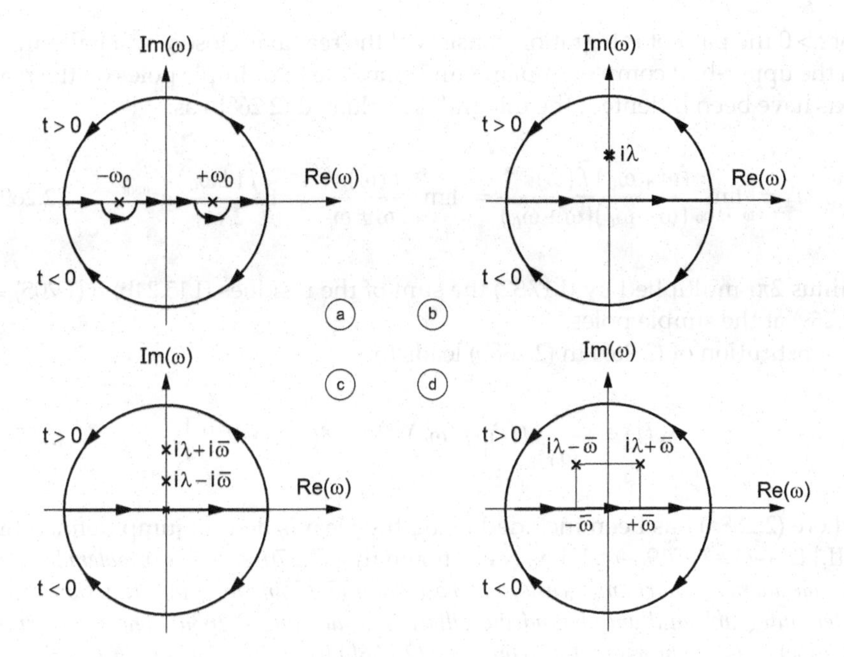

FIGURE 2.24
The Fourier transform is one of the five methods (Table 2.2) to determine the response of a linear second-order system with constant coefficients to an arbitrary function of time that is: (i) either an ordinary function absolutely integrable and of bounded fluctuation for all time; (ii) or a generalized function over test functions of the class (i). The response is specified by a Fourier integral that may be evaluated by contour integration in the complex frequency plane, assuming that the Fourier spectrum of the forcing decays to zero at infinity. The contour integration is specified by the residues at the poles of the integrand, leading to four cases: (i) two simple poles on the real axis indented by deformation of the path of integration in the undamped case (Figure 2.24a); (ii) a double pole on the imaginary axis for critical damping (Figure 2.24b); (iii) two simple poles on the imaginary axis for supercritical damping (Figure 2.24c); (iv) two simple poles outside the real and imaginary axis for subcritical damping (Figure 2.24d).

the exponential factor in the Fourier integral (2.266c) vanishes at infinity (2.267a):

$$\lim_{|\omega|\to\infty}\left|e^{i\omega t}\right| = \lim_{|\omega|\to\infty}\left|e^{it\,\mathrm{Re}(\omega)}e^{-t\,\mathrm{Im}(\omega)}\right| = \lim_{|\omega|\to\infty} e^{-t\,\mathrm{Im}(\omega)} = 0 \Rightarrow t\,\mathrm{Im}(\omega) > 0, \qquad (2.267\text{a, b})$$

if the upper (lower) half-circle is chosen for $t > 0 (t < 0)$. For $t < 0$, the path of integration consisting of the real axis closed by the half-circle in the lower-half complex-ω plane, contains no poles, and the integral (2.266c) is zero (2.268a):

$$x_*(t) = \begin{cases} 0 & \text{if} \quad t > 0; & (2.268\text{a}) \\ -2\pi i\left(T_+ + T_-\right) & \text{if} \quad t < 0, & (2.268\text{b}) \end{cases}$$

for $t > 0$ the path of integration consists of the real axis closed by a half-circle in the upper-half complex ω-plane, and since the two simple poles on the real axis have been indented, the integral is evaluated (2.268b) as:

$$T_{\pm} = \lim_{\omega\to\pm\omega_0} \frac{(\omega \mp \omega_0)\tilde{f}(\omega)e^{i\omega t}}{(\omega-\omega_0)(\omega+\omega_0)} = \lim_{\omega\to\pm\omega_0} \frac{\tilde{f}(\omega)e^{i\omega t}}{\omega \pm \omega_0} = \pm\frac{\tilde{f}(\pm\omega_0)}{2\,\omega_0}e^{\pm i\omega_0 t}. \tag{2.269}$$

minus $2\pi i$ multiplied by (I.17.32) the sum of the residues (I.15.24b) ≡ (1.205) ≡ (2.269) at the simple poles.

Substitution of (2.269) in (2.268b) leads to:

$$x_*(t) = -\frac{i\pi}{\omega_0}H(t)\left[\tilde{f}(\omega_0)e^{i\omega_0 t} - \tilde{f}(-\omega_0)e^{-i\omega_0 t}\right], \tag{2.270}$$

where (2.268a) has been included using the Heaviside unit jump defined by (III.1.28a–c) ≡ (1.519a–c). It has been shown that *(2.270) specifies (problem 55) the displacement of a harmonic (case XLVI) oscillator (2.263b) forced by a function absolutely integrable and with bounded oscillation for all time (2.263a), whose spectrum (2.263c) satisfies the asymptotic condition (2.266b) in all directions in the complex-ω plane (2.266a).*

NOTE 2.6: Spectral Forcing of a Critically Damped Oscillator

In the case of a forced harmonic oscillator (2.22) with (problem 56) critical damping, (2.84a–c) ≡ (2.271a), for a continuous spectrum (2.263a, c) then (2.263b) is replaced by (2.271b):

$$\lambda = \omega_0: \qquad \ddot{x} + 2\lambda\dot{x} + \lambda^2 x = f(t) = \int_{-\infty}^{+\infty} \tilde{f}(\omega)e^{i\omega t}\,d\omega. \tag{2.271a, b}$$

The Fourier transform of (2.271a) is (2.272):

$$\tilde{f}(\omega) = \left(\lambda^2 + 2i\omega\lambda - \omega^2\right)\tilde{x}(\omega) = (\lambda + i\omega)^2\,\tilde{x}(\omega) = -(\omega - i\lambda)^2\,\tilde{x}(\omega). \tag{2.272}$$

Substitution of (2.272) in (2.264a) leads to (2.273a):

$$x_*(t) = -\int_{-\infty}^{+\infty} \frac{\tilde{f}(\omega)e^{i\omega t}}{(\omega - i\lambda)^2}\,d\omega = -2\pi i H(t)\lim_{\omega\to i\lambda}\frac{\partial}{\partial\omega}\left[\tilde{f}(\omega)e^{i\omega t}\right], \tag{2.273a, b}$$

where: (i) the integrand has a double pole at $\omega = i\lambda$ in the upper-half complex-ω plane (Figure 2.24b); (ii) if the asymptotic condition (2.266a, b) is met in the lower-half complex-ω plane, the integral is zero because there is no pole in the interior; (iii) this corresponds to the introduction of the Heaviside unit function of time, (III.1.28a–c) ≡ (1.519a–c), as a factor in (2.273b); (iv) the integral along the real axis closed by a half-circle in the upper-half complex-ω plane (2.273a), which is evaluated (2.273b) as $2\pi i$ times (I.15.45) the residue at the double pole (I.15.33b) ≡ (1.210) that involves:

$$\frac{\partial}{\partial\omega}\left[\tilde{f}(\omega)e^{i\omega t}\right]=e^{i\omega t}\left[it\,\tilde{f}(\omega)+\tilde{f}'(\omega)\right]; \tag{2.274}$$

(v) substitution of (2.274) in (2.273b) leads to:

$$x_*(t)=2\pi H(t)e^{-\lambda t}\left[t\tilde{f}(i\lambda)-i\tilde{f}'(i\lambda)\right]. \tag{2.275}$$

It has been shown that *(2.275) specifies the displacement of (problem 56) a critically damped (case XLVIII) oscillator (2.271a, b) forced by a function absolutely integrable and with bounded oscillation for all time (2.263a), whose spectrum (2.263c) satisfies the asymptotic condition (2.266b) in all directions in the complex-ω plane (2.266a).*

NOTE 2.7: Spectral Forcing of a Supercritically Damped Oscillator

In the case of a damped oscillator (2.22) in the (problem 57) general non-critically damped (2.276a), instead of (2.271b) is used (2.276b):

$$\lambda\neq\omega_0:\qquad \ddot{x}+2\lambda\dot{x}+\omega_0^2x=f(t)=\int_{-\infty}^{+\infty}\tilde{f}(\omega)e^{i\omega t}d\omega. \tag{2.276a, b}$$

The Fourier transform of (2.276b) is (2.277):

$$\tilde{f}(\omega)=\left[\omega_0^2-\omega^2+2i\lambda\omega\right]\tilde{x}(\omega)=-(\omega-\omega_+)(\omega-\omega_-)\tilde{x}(\omega), \tag{2.277}$$

where $\omega_\pm$ are given by (2.92a–c) ≡ (2.278b, d) in the case of supercritical damping (2.278a, c):

$$\lambda>\omega_0:\qquad \bar{\omega}\equiv\left|\lambda^2-\omega_0^2\right|^{1/2}<\lambda,\qquad \omega_\pm=i\lambda\pm i\bar{\omega}. \tag{2.278a–d}$$

Substitution of (2.277) in (2.264a) gives:

$$x_*(t)=-\int_{-\infty}^{+\infty}\frac{\tilde{f}(\omega)e^{i\omega t}}{(\omega-i\lambda-i\bar{\omega})(\omega-i\lambda+i\bar{\omega})}d\omega, \tag{2.279}$$

where the integrand has simple poles (2.278d) in (Figure 2.24c) the upper-half complex-ω plane (2.278a).

Thus, closing the real line on the lower-half ω-plane with the asymptotic condition (2.266a, b), the integral (2.279) vanishes because there are no poles; this corresponds to inserting the Heaviside unit jump, (III.1.28a–c) ≡ (1.519a–c), as a factor and evaluating the integral (2.279) on the real line closed on the upper-half complex-ω plane as $2\pi i$ times (I.15.45) the sum (2.280a) of the residues (2.280b) at the two simple poles:

$$x_*(t) = -H(t)\,2\pi i\,(R_+ + R_-):$$

$$R_\pm = \lim_{\omega \to i\lambda \pm i\bar{\omega}} \frac{(\omega - i\lambda \mp i\bar{\omega})\tilde{f}(\omega)\,e^{i\omega t}}{(\omega - i\lambda - i\bar{\omega})(\omega - i\lambda + i\bar{\omega})} = \pm\frac{\tilde{f}(i\lambda \pm i\bar{\omega})\,e^{-\lambda t \mp \bar{\omega} t}}{2i\bar{\omega}};$$

(2.280a, b)

substitution of (2.280b) in (2.280a) leads to:

$$x_*(t) = \frac{\pi}{\bar{\omega}} H(t) e^{-\lambda t}\left[\tilde{f}(i\lambda - i\bar{\omega})e^{\bar{\omega} t} - \tilde{f}(i\lambda + i\bar{\omega})e^{-\bar{\omega} t}\right]. \qquad (2.281)$$

It has been shown that *the forcing of (problem 57) an (case XLIX) supercritically (2.278a–d) damped oscillator (2.276a, b) by: (i) a function of time absolutely integrable and of bounded oscillation on the real line (2.263a); (ii) whose spectrum (2.263c) satisfies the asymptotic condition (2.266b) on the whole complex ω-plane (2.266a); (iii) leads to the displacement (2.281) corresponding to a decay in time with amplitudes specified by the spectrum (2.263a) at (2.278d).*

NOTE 2.8: Spectral Forcing of a Subcritically Damped Oscillator

The remaining case (problem 58) of a subcritically damped oscillator is similar to the preceding (2.276a, b) except that the condition (2.278a) is reversed to (2.282a):

$$\lambda < \omega_0: \qquad \bar{\omega} \equiv \left|\omega_0^2 - \lambda^2\right|^{1/2} < \omega_0, \qquad \omega_\pm = i\lambda \pm \bar{\omega}, \qquad (2.282\text{a–d})$$

so that (2.105a–c) the simple poles are now at (2.282d), that is, in the upper-half complex ω-plane but outside the imaginary axis (Figure 2.24d). The displacement is given by (2.283a):

$$x_*(t) = -\int_{-\infty}^{+\infty} \frac{\tilde{f}(\omega)\,e^{i\omega t}}{(\omega - \omega_+)(\omega - \omega_-)}\,d\omega$$

$$= -H(t)\int_{-\infty}^{+\infty} \frac{\tilde{f}(\omega)\,e^{i\omega t}}{(\omega - i\lambda - \bar{\omega})(\omega - i\lambda + \bar{\omega})}\,d\omega = -H(t)\,2\pi i\,(S_+ + S_-),$$

(2.283a–c)

where: (i) assuming the asymptotic condition (2.266a, b) and closing the path of integration along the real axis in the lower-half ω-plane gives zero because there are no poles there, hence the Heaviside unit function, (III.1.28a–c) ≡ (1.519a–c), as factor in (2.283b); (ii) closing the path of integration by a half-circle in the upper-half complex-ω plane evaluates (I.15.45) the integral as $2\pi i$ times the sum of the residues at the simple poles (2.238c) given, (I.15.24b) ≡ (1.105), by:

$$S_\pm = \lim_{\omega\to i\lambda\pm\bar{\omega}} \frac{(\omega - i\lambda \mp \bar{\omega})\tilde{f}(\omega)e^{i\omega t}}{(\omega - i\lambda - \bar{\omega})(\omega - i\lambda + \bar{\omega})} = \pm\frac{e^{-\lambda t}}{2\bar{\omega}}\tilde{f}(i\lambda \pm \bar{\omega})e^{\pm i\bar{\omega}t}. \tag{2.284}$$

Substitution of (2.284) in (2.283c) specifies:

$$x_*(t) = H(t)\frac{\pi}{i\bar{\omega}}e^{-\lambda t}\left[\tilde{f}(i\lambda + \bar{\omega})e^{i\bar{\omega}t} - \tilde{f}(i\lambda - \bar{\omega})e^{-i\bar{\omega}t}\right], \tag{2.285}$$

the displacement of a subcritically (case L) damped (2.282a–d) harmonic oscillator (2.276a, b) forced (problem 58) by a function absolutely integrable and with bounded oscillation over all time (2.263a) whose spectrum (2.263c) satisfies the asymptotic condition (2.266a, b) in all directions in the complex ω-plane.

NOTE 2.9: Influence Function Due to Impulsive Forcing

The **influence or Green function** *for the damped harmonic oscillator is the displacement due to forcing by a unit impulse:*

$$\ddot{G} + 2\lambda\dot{G} + \omega_0^2 G = \delta(t). \tag{2.286}$$

The preceding results concerning forcing by an arbitrary function also apply to forcing by the unit impulse, using its Fourier transform. The **unit impulse** *is defined by the property, (III.3.15a) ≡ (1.513a,b) ≡ (2.287b), over the set of continuous test functions (2.287a):*

$$f \in C(|R): \qquad \int_{-\infty}^{+\infty} \delta(t) f(t)\,dt = f(0); \tag{2.287a, b}$$

thus, *the spectrum of the unit impulse is a constant:*

$$\tilde{\delta}(\omega) \equiv \frac{1}{2\pi}\int_{-\infty}^{+\infty} \delta(t) e^{-i\omega t}\,dt = \frac{1}{2\pi}, \tag{2.288}$$

corresponding to **white noise,** *that is, it excites all frequencies with the same amplitude.* This may be applied to the four subcases of the linear second-order system.

Substituting (2.288) in (2.275) for (problem 59), the case of the critically damped oscillator (2.289a), leads to (2.294b):

$$\lambda = \omega_0: \qquad G(t) = H(t)e^{-\lambda t}t. \qquad (2.289a, b)$$

In the (problem 60) case (2.290a) of the subcritically damped oscillator (2.285), substitution of (2.288) leads to (2.290b):

$$\lambda < \omega_0: \qquad G(t) = H(t)\frac{e^{-\lambda t}}{2i\bar{\omega}}\left(e^{i\bar{\omega}t} - e^{-i\bar{\omega}t}\right) = H(t)e^{-\lambda t}\frac{\sin(\bar{\omega}t)}{\bar{\omega}}. \qquad (2.290a, b)$$

In the (problem 61) case (2.291a) of the supercritically damped oscillator (2.281), substitution of (2.288) leads to (2.291b):

$$\lambda > \omega_0: \qquad G(t) = H(t)\frac{e^{-\lambda t}}{2\bar{\omega}}\left(e^{\bar{\omega}t} - e^{-\bar{\omega}t}\right) = H(t)e^{-\lambda t}\frac{\sinh(\bar{\omega}t)}{\bar{\omega}}. \qquad (2.291a, b)$$

In the (problem 62) case of the undamped oscillator (2.292a), substitution of (2.288) in (2.270) leads to (2.292b):

$$\lambda = 0: \qquad G(t) = \frac{H(t)}{2i\omega_0}\left(e^{i\omega_0 t} - e^{-i\omega_0 t}\right) = H(t)\frac{\sin(\omega_0 t)}{\omega_0}, \qquad (2.292a, b)$$

in agreement with (2.290a, b) for $\lambda = 0$, hence $\bar{\omega} = \omega_0$.

NOTE 2.10: Unit Initial Velocity with Zero Initial Displacement

Collecting the preceding four results (2.289a, b; 2.290a, b; 2.291a, b; 2.292a, b) it follows that *the influence or Green function for the linear second-order system (2.286) is given by:*

$$G(t) = H(t) \times \begin{cases} \dfrac{\sin(\omega_0 t)}{\omega_0} & \text{if} \quad \lambda = 0, & (2.293a) \\ \dfrac{e^{-\lambda t}}{\bar{\omega}}\sin(\bar{\omega}t) & \text{if} \quad \lambda < \omega_0, & (2.293b) \\ te^{-\lambda t} & \text{if} \quad \lambda = \omega_0, & (2.293c) \\ \dfrac{e^{-\lambda t}}{\bar{\omega}}\sinh(\bar{\omega}t) & \text{if} \quad \lambda > \omega_0, & (2.293d) \end{cases}$$

in the case of: (i) the undamped harmonic oscillator, (2.292a,b) ≡ (2.293a); (ii) the subcritically damped oscillator, (2.290a,b) ≡ (2.273b); (ii) the critically damped oscillator, (2.289a,b) = (2.293c); (iv) the supercritically damped oscillator, (2.291a,b) ≡ (2.293d).

The influence or Green function is identically specified by: (a) forcing by a unit impulse (2.286); (b) a free oscillation (2.294a) with zero initial displacement (2.294b), and unit initial velocity (2.294c):

$$G(0)=0, \quad G'(0)=1: \qquad \ddot{G}+2\lambda\dot{G}+\omega_0^2 G=0. \tag{2.294a–c}$$

The statement (a) has already been proved (note 2.9); the equivalence with the statement (b) is proved next by showing that (2.294a–c) leads to the same four cases (2.293a–d). In the case of the undamped harmonic oscillator, (2.56a, b) ≡ (2.295a,b), the initial conditions (2.294a, b) lead to (2.295c, d):

$$\lambda=0: \quad G(t)=C_1\cos(\omega_0 t)+C_2\sin(\omega_0 t), \quad 0=G(0)=C_1, \quad 1=\dot{G}(0)=C_2\omega_0; \tag{2.295a–d}$$

substitution of (2.295c, d) in (2.295b) yields (2.293a). In the case of the subcritically damped oscillator, (2.106a, b) ≡ (2.296a, b):

$$\lambda<\omega_0: \qquad G(t)=e^{-\lambda t}\left[C_1\cos(\bar{\omega}t)+C_2\sin(\bar{\omega}t)\right], \tag{2.296a,b}$$

the initial conditions (2.294a, b) lead to (2.296c, d):

$$0=G(0)=C_1, \qquad 1=\dot{G}(0)=-\lambda C_1+C_2\bar{\omega}=C_2\bar{\omega}; \tag{2.296c, d}$$

substitution of (2.296c, d) in (2.296b) gives (2.293b). In the case of the critically damped oscillator, (2.85a, b) ≡ (2.297a, b), the initial conditions (2.294a, b) lead to (2.297c, d):

$$\lambda=\omega_0: \quad G(t)=(C_1+C_2 t)e^{-\lambda t}, \quad 0=G(0)=C_1, 1=\dot{G}(0)=C_2-\lambda C_1=C_2; \tag{2.297a–d}$$

substituting (2.297c, d) in (2.297b) yields (2.293c). In the case of the supercritically damped oscillator, (2.93a,b) ≡ (2.298a,b):

$$\lambda>\omega_0: \qquad G(t)=e^{-\lambda t}\left[C_1\cosh(\bar{\omega}t)+C_2\sinh(\bar{\omega}t)\right], \tag{2.298a, b}$$

the initial conditions (2.294a, b) lead to (2.298c, d):

$$0=G(0)=C_1, \qquad 0=\dot{G}(0)=\bar{\omega}C_2-\lambda C_1=\bar{\omega}C_2; \tag{2.298c, d}$$

substitution of (2.298c, d) in (2.298b) leads to (2.293d), completing the four cases of influence function for the linear second-order system. The proofs made in (2.295a–d; 2.296a–d; 2.297a–d; 2.298a–d) with two amplitudes (C_1, C_2) could also be made, respectively, from (2.56a, b; 2.106a, b; 2.85a, b; 2.93a, b) with amplitude and phase (a, α).

NOTE 2.11: Arbitrary Forcing for a Damped Harmonic Oscillator

The fundamental property, (III.3.15a) ≡ (2.287b) ≡ (2.299b), of the unit impulse relative to a continuous test function, (2.287a) ≡ (2.299a), is:

$$f \in C(|R): \qquad f(t) = \int_{-\infty}^{+\infty} f(t-s) \quad \delta(s) ds. \qquad (2.299\text{a, b})$$

Comparing the displacement (2.271b) [influence function (2.286)] of a damped harmonic oscillator forced by a continuous function (2.299a) [a unit impulse (2.299b)] of time leads to:

$$\left\{ \frac{d^2}{dt^2} + 2\lambda \frac{d}{dt} + \omega_0^2 \right\} x_*(t) = f(t) = \int_{-\infty}^{+\infty} f(t-s) \quad \delta(s) ds$$
$$= \left\{ \frac{d^2}{dt^2} + 2\lambda \frac{d}{dt} + \omega_0^2 \right\} \int_{-\infty}^{+\infty} f(t-s) G(s) ds, \qquad (2.300)$$

where it is assumed that the integrals are uniform with regards to the parameter t, thus allowing (section I.13.8) differentiation to be taken out of the integral sign. From (2.300) follows that *the displacement of a damped harmonic oscillator (2.271b) due to forcing by a continuous function, (2.299a) ≡ (2.301a), is (problem 63) specified, (2.300) ≡ (2.301b), by a* **convolution integral** *(section III.7.5) with the influence function:*

$$F \in C(|R): \qquad x_*(t) = \int_{-\infty}^{+\infty} f(t-s) G(s) ds \equiv f * G(t). \qquad (2.301\text{a, b})$$

and hence is given: (i) by (2.302b) for (problem 64) an undamped oscillator, (2.293a) ≡ (2.302a):

$$\lambda = 0: \qquad x(t) = \int_0^{+\infty} f(t-s) \frac{\sin(\omega_0 s)}{\omega_0} ds; \qquad (2.302\text{a, b})$$

(ii) by (2.303b) for (problem 65) a subcritically damped oscillator, (2.293b) ≡ (2.303a):

$$\lambda > \omega_0: \qquad x(t) = \int_0^{+\infty} f(t-s) e^{-\lambda t} \frac{\sinh(\bar{\omega} s)}{\bar{\omega}} ds; \qquad (2.303a, b)$$

(iii) by (2.304b) for (problem 66) a critically damped oscillator, (2.293c) ≡ (2.304a):

$$\lambda = \omega_0: \qquad x(t) = \int_0^{+\infty} f(t-s) s e^{-\lambda t} ds; \qquad (2.304a, b)$$

(iv) by (2.305b) for (problem 67) a supercritically damped oscillator, (2.293d) ≡ (2.305a):

$$\lambda > \omega_0: \qquad x(t) = \int_0^{+\infty} f(t-s) e^{-\lambda s} \frac{\sin(\bar{\omega} s)}{\bar{\omega}} ds. \qquad (2.305a, b)$$

These results (note 2.10) coincide with those obtained by the method of variation of parameters (section 2.9), as shown next, using (2.306a) the symmetry property of the convolution integral, (III.7.56a) ≡ (2.306b):

$$u \equiv t-s: \qquad f * g(t) \equiv \int_0^{+\infty} f(t-s) g(s) ds = \int_{-\infty}^{t} f(u) g(t-u) du = g * f(t).$$

(2.306a, b)

Thus, the displacement due to forcing by an integrable function can be obtained by the method of variation of parameters (subsections 2.9.1–2.9.3) [the superposition principle applied to the influence function (note 2.11)] in all four cases of: (i) undamped oscillator, (2.239a, b) ≡ (2.302a, b); (ii) critical damped oscillator, (2.237a–c) ≡ (2.304a, b); (iii) supercritically damped oscillator, (2.241a, b) ≡ (2.303a, b); (iv) subcritically damped oscillator, (2.243a, c) ≡ (2.305a, b). The pairs of integrals mentioned above (i–vi) have the same integrand and differ in the limits of integration, namely indefinite integral at t [lower limit $-\infty$ in (2.299b)]; thus, they may differ by a set of terms satisfying the unforced equation, that is, a free oscillation may always be added to the forced oscillation. In all cases the forcing function must ensure the convergence of the integrals (notes 2.5–2.11) and series (note 2.4); the convergence may be taken in the sense of ordinary (chapter I.21) or generalized (chapter III.1, 3.5 and notes 1.23–1.28) functions.

NOTE 2.12: Forcing by a Gaussian Function of Time

As an example, distinct from the preceding, consider a damped harmonic oscillator forced (problem 68) by a Gaussian function of time with time scale T:

$$\ddot{x} + 2\lambda\dot{x} + \omega_0^2 x = f(t) = f_a \exp\left(-\frac{t^2}{T^2}\right). \tag{2.307}$$

The Gaussian function (2.307): (i) has oscillation $2f_a$ on the real line (2.308a) and hence, is of bounded oscillation:

$$\mathcal{F}\left(f_a\, e^{-t^2/T^2}; -\infty, +\infty\right) = 2f_a; \qquad \int_{-\infty}^{+\infty} \exp\left(-\frac{t^2}{T^2}\right) dt = T\sqrt{\pi}, \tag{2.308a, b}$$

(ii) is positive and integrable on the real line, (III.1.10b) ≡ (2.308b), and hence, it is absolutely integrable. It follows (2.263a) that it has (2.263c) a Fourier transform (2.309):

$$\tilde{f}(\omega) = \frac{f_a}{2\pi}\int_{-\infty}^{+\infty} \exp\left(-i\omega t - \frac{t^2}{T^2}\right) dt = \frac{f_a T}{2\sqrt{\pi}} \exp\left(-\frac{\omega^2 T^2}{4}\right), \tag{2.309}$$

where in (2.309) was used:

$$\alpha = \frac{1}{T^2}, \quad \beta = -\omega: \qquad \int_{-\infty}^{+\infty} \exp\left(i\beta x - \alpha x^2\right) dx = \sqrt{\frac{\pi}{\alpha}} \exp\left(-\frac{\beta^2}{4\alpha}\right), \tag{2.310a–c}$$

the integral, (I.1.13) ≡ (2.310c), with (2.310a, b).

Thus, *the* (Figure 2.25a) *Gaussian function (2.311a) has* (Figure 2.25b) *a Gaussian spectrum (2.311b):*

$$f(t) = f_a \exp\left(-\frac{t^2}{T^2}\right), \qquad \tilde{f}(\omega) = \frac{f_a T}{2\sqrt{\pi}} \exp\left(-\frac{\omega^2 T^2}{4}\right). \tag{2.311a, b}$$

A narrower forcing in time (2.311a), which is smaller T in Figure 2.25a, *leads to a broader spectrum (2.311b), which is larger 2 / T in* Figure 2.25b; *the limit of the unit impulse as input (2.287a) is white noise as spectrum (2.288). The displacement of a damped harmonic oscillator (2.307) forced by a Gaussian function of time (2.311a)*

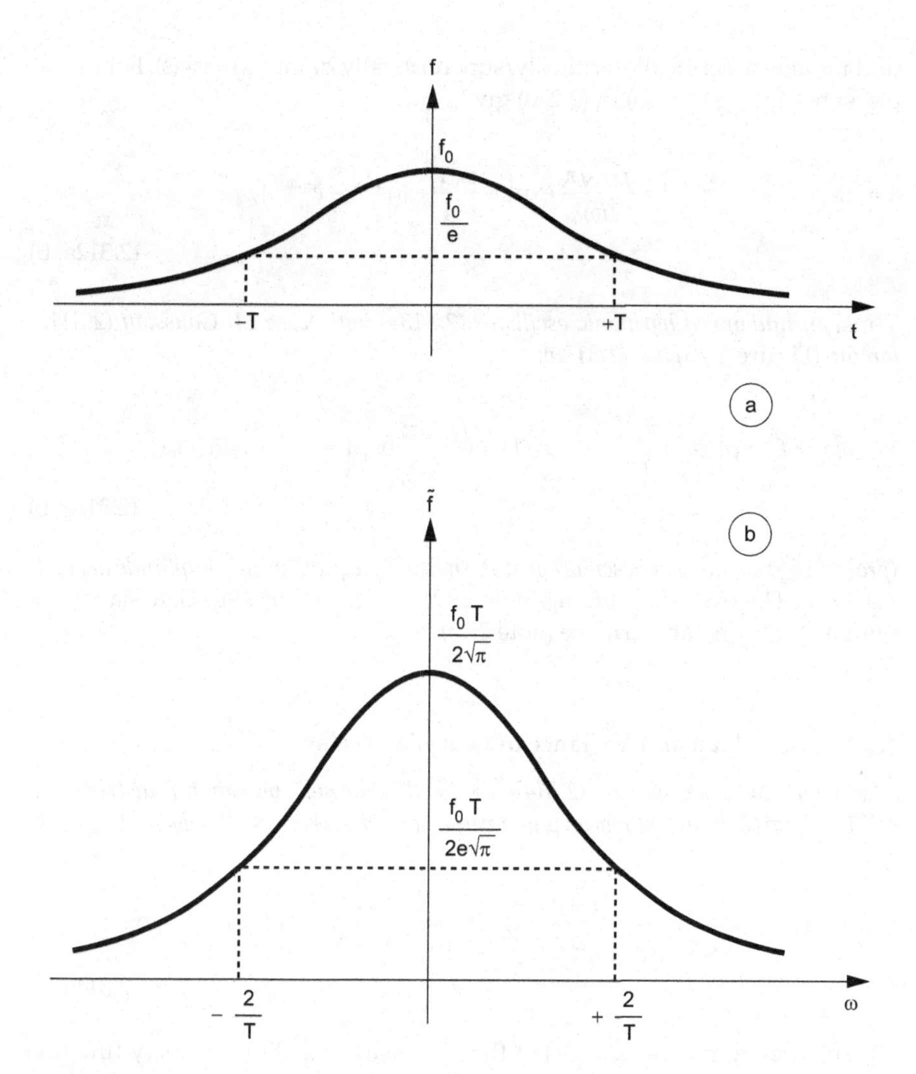

FIGURE 2.25
The Gaussian function (Figure 2.25a) represents the probability density of a Gaussian random process with given: (i) mean value; (ii) variance σ^2 or root mean square (r.m.s.) value σ. It represents random forcing by a normal probability distribution, and its Fourier transform is the characteristic function of the random process, and corresponds to the spectrum (Figure 2.25b), which is also a Gaussian function.

is specified substituting the spectrum (2.311b) in (2.270) [(2.285)/(2.275)/(2.281)], respectively in the undamped (subcritically/critically/supercritically) damped case(s). The same result would be obtained substituting the Gaussian (2.311a) forcing (2.307) function and performing the integrations in (2.302b) ≡ (2.239b) [(2.305b) ≡ (2.243b)/(2.304b) ≡ (2.237b)/(2.303b) ≡ (2.241b)], respectively, in the undamped (subcritically/critically/supercritically damped) case(s). For example, substituting (2.311b) in (2.270) gives:

$$\lambda = 0: \qquad x_*(t) = \frac{f_a T \sqrt{\pi}}{2i\omega_0} \exp\left(-\frac{\omega_0^2 T^2}{4}\right)\left(e^{i\omega_0 t} - e^{-i\omega_0 t}\right); \tag{2.312a, b}$$

Thus, *an undamped harmonic oscillator (2.313a) with (case LI) Gaussian (2.311a) forcing* (Figure 2.25) *has (2.313b):*

$$\ddot{x} + \omega_0^2 x = f_a \exp\left(-\frac{t^2}{T^2}\right): \qquad x_*(t) = \frac{f_a T \sqrt{\pi}}{\omega_0} \exp\left(-\frac{\omega_0^2 T^2}{4}\right)\sin(\omega_0 t), \tag{2.313a, b}$$

(problem 68) a sinusoidal oscillation at the natural frequency with amplitude depending on ω_0. The Gaussian forcing (note 2.12) can be extended to Gaussian noise with arbitrary mean variance (note 2.13).

NOTE 2.13: Mean and Variance of Gaussian Noise

The Gaussian corresponds (2.314b–d) to the normal probability distribution, (III.1.120a) ≡ (2.314a), with mean μ *and variance* σ^2 *and changes of variable (2.314a–d):*

$$f(t) = \frac{f_0}{\sigma\sqrt{2\pi}} \exp\left[-\frac{(t-\mu)^2}{2\sigma^2}\right]; \quad f_a \to \frac{f_1}{\sigma\sqrt{2\pi}}, t \to t - \mu, \quad T = \sigma\sqrt{2}. \tag{2.314a–d}$$

The Fourier transform (2.263c) of the Gaussian probability density function (2.314a) corresponds to the characteristic function of the random process (III.1.133) and is evaluated (2.315b) using the change of variable (2.315a) and the integral (2.310c):

$$\begin{aligned} s = t - \mu: \qquad \tilde{f}(\omega) &= \frac{f_0}{2\pi\sigma\sqrt{2\pi}} \int_{-\infty}^{+\infty} \exp\left[-\frac{(t-\mu)^2}{2\sigma^2} - i\omega t\right] dt \\ &= \frac{f_0\, e^{-i\omega\mu}}{2\pi\sigma\sqrt{2\pi}} \int_{-\infty}^{+\infty} \exp\left(-\frac{s^2}{2\sigma^2} - i\omega s\right) ds \\ &= \frac{f_0}{2\pi} \exp\left(-i\omega\mu - \frac{\sigma^2\omega^2}{2}\right). \end{aligned} \tag{2.315a, b}$$

Substitution of (2.315b) in (2.270) leads to:

$$x_*(t) = \frac{f_0}{2i\omega_0} \exp\left(-\frac{\sigma^2\omega_0^2}{2}\right)\left[e^{i\omega_0(t-\mu)} - e^{-i\omega_0(t-\mu)}\right], \tag{2.316}$$

which simplifies to (2.317b):

$$\ddot{x} + \omega_0^2 x = \frac{f_0}{\sigma\sqrt{2\pi}} \exp\left[-\frac{(t-\mu)^2}{2\sigma^2}\right]: \quad x_*(t) = \frac{f_0}{\omega_0} \exp\left(-\frac{\sigma^2\omega_0^2}{2}\right) \sin\left[\omega_0(t-\mu)\right], \tag{2.317a, b}$$

that coincides with (2.313b) with the substitutions (2.314b–d). Thus, *(2.317b) specifies (problem 69) the response of a harmonic oscillator with natural frequency* ω_0 *to (2.317a) normal random forcing (case LII) with mean* μ *and root mean square value* σ. The response of the undamped harmonic oscillator (2.307) to Gaussian forcing (2.311a, b) can also be obtained direct from the convolution integral (2.302b) with the influence function (2.293c):

$$\begin{aligned} x_*(t) &= \frac{f_a}{\omega_0} \int_{-\infty}^{+\infty} \exp\left(-\frac{s^2}{T^2}\right) \sin\left[\omega_0(t-s)\right] ds \\ &= \frac{f_a}{\omega_0} \operatorname{Im}\left\{\exp(i\omega_0 t) \int_{-\infty}^{+\infty} \exp\left(-\frac{s^2}{T^2} - i\omega_0 s\right) ds\right\} \\ &= \frac{f_a}{\omega_0} T\sqrt{\pi} \exp\left(-\frac{\omega_0^2 T^2}{4}\right) \operatorname{Im}\left[\exp(i\omega_0 t)\right] \\ &= \frac{f_a T\sqrt{\pi}}{\omega_0} \exp\left(-\frac{\omega_0^2 T^2}{4}\right) \sin(\omega_0 t), \end{aligned} \tag{2.318}$$

in agreement with (2.318) ≡ (2.313b).

Conclusion 2

The example of damped or amplified oscillators with forcing include the analogous mechanical system (electrical circuits) [Figure 2.1 (2.3)]. For the mechanical system, the potential energy (Figure 2.2) is: (i) (ii): quadratic positive (negative) for a linear spring about a position $x = 0$ of stable (unstable) equilibrium [Figure 2.2a (b)]; (iii) with an inflexion at the position $x = 0$ of unstable equilibrium (Figure 2.2c); (iii) fourth order allowing stable or metastable cases (Figure 2.2d). The undamped and unforced harmonic oscillator performs sinusoidal oscillations with constant frequency and amplitude (Figure 2.4), and corresponds to a suspended pendulum (Figure 2.7a) whose gravity potential has a minimum (Figure 2.5a) at the position of stable equilibrium, which is the center of elliptical paths in phase plane (Figure 2.5b) for a stable attractor. Perturbations of the natural frequency of the harmonic oscillator on a time scale large compared with the period deform the elliptical path in the phase plane while maintaining the area that is an adiabatic invariant (Figure 2.6). The inverted pendulum (Figure 2.7b) corresponds to an unstable repeller or saddle point in the phase plane (Figure 2.9b) at the position of unstable equilibrium (Figure 2.8), which is the maximum of the potential (Figure 2.9a). The oscillator with critical (overcritical) damping decays [Figure 2.10 (2.12)] monotonically or with a single extremum (always monotonically) towards the position of stable equilibrium, which is a tangential (parabolic) attractor in the phase plane [Figure 2.11 (2.13)]. The oscillator with subcritical damping has a decaying oscillation (Figure 2.14) towards the position of stable equilibrium, which is a spiral sink in the phase plane (Figure 2.15b) corresponding to the minimum of the potential (Figure 2.15a). The spiral source in the phase plane (Figure 2.15b) corresponds to an amplified oscillation; both the latter and monotonic amplification apply (Figure 2.18) to: (i) a mechanical circuit (Figure 2.16) on a conveyor belt with friction force (Figure 2.17); (ii) a Froude pendulum (Figure 2.19) with frictional torque (Figure 2.17) at the support; and (iii) an electric circuit with valve (Figure 2.20) with characteristic curve (Figure 2.21).

The undamped forced displacement is: (i) of constant amplitude and in-phase outside resonance (Figure 2.22a); (ii) of amplitude increasing linearly with time and out-of-phase by $\pi/2$ at resonance (Figure 2.22b); (iii) the approach to resonance corresponds to beats, with a slow sinusoidal modulation of the amplitude (Figure 2.22c). The damped forced displacement has: (i) an amplitude that increases as damping decreases, and is maximum at resonance (Figure 2.23a); (ii) a phase that increases with damping is $\pi / 2$ at resonance and tends to π for large frequencies (Figure 2.23b). In the case of forcing by an arbitrary ordinary or generalized function the response may be calculated using the Fourier transform with evaluation of the integral by residues at the poles in the complex frequency plane: (i) two simple poles indented on the real axis for the harmonic oscillator (Figure 2.24a); (ii)(iii) a double pole (two simple poles) on the imaginary axis for the critically (supercritically) damped oscillator [Figure 2.24b(c)]; (iv) two simple poles outside the axis for the subcritically damped oscillator (Figure 2.24d). An example is deterministic or random Gaussian forcing (Figure 2.25a), whose spectrum is another Gaussian (Figure 2.25b). The Fourier transform is one of the five methods applicable to the forcing of a damped harmonic oscillator (Table 2.2) that is included among the 52 cases (Table 2.1) of the second-order linear system with constant coefficients (Diagram 2.1); similar or generalized methods of analysis may be applied to the more general systems (Diagram 2.2).

Bibliography

The bibliography of the series *"Mathematics and Physics for Science and Technology"* is quite extensive since it covers a variety of subjects. In order to avoid overlaps, each volume contains only a part of the bibliography on the subjects most closely related to its content. The bibliography of earlier volumes is generally not repeated, and some of the bibliography may be relevant to earlier and future volumes. The bibliography covered in the four published volumes is:

- A. General
  - a. Overviews
    - 1. Mathematics: volume I
    - 2. Physics: volume II
    - 3. Engineering: volume III
  - b. Reference
    - 4. Collected works: volume IV
- B. Mathematics
  - c. Theory of functions
    - 7. Real functions: volumes I and II
    - 8. Complex analysis: volumes I and II
    - 9. Generalized functions: volume III
  - d. Differential and integral equations
    - 10. Ordinary differential equations: volume IV
    - 12. Non-linear differential and integral equations: volume IV
  - h. Higher analysis
    - 22. Special functions: volume IV
- C. Physics
  - j. Classical mechanics
    - 28. Material particles: volume IV
  - m. Solid mechanics
    - 37. Elasticity and plasticity: volume IV

This choice of subjects is explained next.

The general bibliography consists of overviews and reference works. The overviews have been completed with mathematics, physics, and engineering, respectively in the volumes I, II, and IV. The reference bibliography starts with the collected works of notable authors in section 1 of the present volume, IV. The bibliography on the theory of functions has appeared in the preceding volumes, I to III, and in the present volume, IV; sections 2 and 3 concern the ordinary differential functions in chapters 1, 3, 5, 7, and 9. The bibliography on special functions appears in section 4, as a complement to chapter 9. The main applications of ordinary differential equations have been to oscillators (chapters 2, 4, and 8) and elastic bars and plates (chapter 6) for which the bibliography is given in sections 5 and 6. The books in the bibliography that have influenced the present volume the most are marked with one, two, or three asterisks. In the first book of volume IV the bibliography concerns "ordinary differential equations."

Ordinary Differential Equations

Amann, H. *Ordinary Differential Equations.* Walter de Gruyer, Berlin, 1990.

Arnold, V. *Équations Différentielles Ordinaires.* Editions Mir, Moscow, 1974.

*Arnold V. *Chapitres Supplémentaires de la Théorie des Equations Différentielles Ordinaires.* Editions Mir, Moscow, 1980.

Arnold, V. *Mathematical Methods of Classical Mechanics.* Springer-Verlag, 1978, Editions Mir, Moscow, 1974.

Boole, G. *A Treatise on the Calculus of Finite Differences.* 1872, reprinted Cosimo, New York, 2007.

Brand, L. *Differential and Difference Equations.* Wiley, New York, 1966.

Braver, F. and Nohel, J. A. *The Qualitative Theory of Ordinary Differential Equations.* Benjamin, 1969, reprinted Dover, New York, 1989.

Brown, M. *Differential Equations and their Applications,* 3th ed., Springer Verlag, Heideberg, 1983.

Coddington, E. A. *Ordinary Differential Equations.* Prentice-Hall, 1961, Englewood Cliffs, New Jersey, reprinted Dover, New York, 1989.

Coddington, E. A. and Carlson, R. *Linear Ordinary Differential Equations.* Society for Industrial and Applied Mathematics, New York, 1997.

Costa, F. P. *Equações Differencias Ordinárias.* IST Press, Lisbon, 1998.

Fadell, A.G. *Vector Calculus and Differential Equations.* Van Nostrand, New York, 1968.

*Forsyth, A. R. *Theory of Differential Equations.* 6 vols., Cambridge University Press, Cambridge, 1899–1904.

**Forsyth, A. R. *Treatise of Differential Equations.* Macmillan, 1885, 6th ed., London, 1929.

Franklin, P. *Differential Equations for Engineers.* 1933, reprinted Dover, New York, 1960.

Goldstein, M. E. & Braun, W. H. *Advanced Methods for the Solution of Differential Equations.* National Aeronautics and Space Administration, SP-316, Lewis Research Center, Ohio.

Greenspan, D. *Theory and Solution of Ordinary Differential Equations.* Macmillan, New York, 1960.

Hille, E. *Ordinary Differential Equations in the Complex Domain.* Wiley, 1976, New York, reprinted Dover, New York, 1997.

Hochstadt, H. *Differerential Equations.* Constable, 1963, reprinted Dover, New York, 1975.

**Ince, E. L. *Ordinary Differential Equations.* Longmans, 1936, London, reprinted Dover, New York, 1956.

Jones, D. S., Plank, M. J., and Sleeman, B. D. *Differential Equations and Mathematical Biology.* CRC Press, London, 2009.

**Kamke, E. *Differentialgleichungen.* 2 vols., Teubner, 1944, reprinted Chelsea, Leipzig, 1974.

Kaplan, W. *Ordinary Differential Equations.* Addison-Wesley, Reading, Massachusetts, 1958.

Kartsatos, A. G. *Advanced Ordinary Differential Equations.* Mariner Publishing, Tampa, Florida, 1980.

Kells, L. M. *Elementary Differential Equations.* McGraw-Hill, New York, 1932.

Lanczos, C. *Linear Differential Operators.* Van Nostrand, New York, 1961.

Leighton, W. *Ordinary Differential Equations.* Wadsworth, Belmont, California, 1963.

Martin, W. T. *Elementary Differential Equations.* Addison-Wesley, 1961, reprinted Dover, New York, 1986.

Miller, K. S. *Linear Differential Equations in the Real Domain.* Norton, New York, 1963.

*Milne-Thomson, L. M. *The Calculus of Finite Differences.* Macmillan, London, 1933, reprinted Chelsea, New York, 1981.

Moulton, F. R. *Differential Equations.* Macmillan, London, 1930, reprinted Dover, New York, 1958.

Murphy, G. M. *Ordinary Differential Equations and their Solutions.* Van Nostrand, New York, 1960.

Piaggio, H. T. H. *Differential Equations.* Bell, London, 1920.

*Pontriaguine, L. *Équations Differentielles Ordinaires.* Editions Mir, Moscow, 1975.

*Poole, E. G. C. *Linear Differential Equations.* Oxford University Press, Oxford, 1936, reprinted Dover, New York, 1960.

Radihka, T. S. L., Ivengar, T. K. V., and Rani, T. R. *Approximate Analytical Methods for Solving Ordinary Differential Equations.* CRC Press, Boca Raton, Florida, 2015.

Rainville, E. D. and Bedient, P. E. *Differential Equations.* Macmillan, New York, 1969.

Reuter, G. E. H. *Elementary Differential Equations and Operators.* Free Press, Glencoe, Illinois, 1958.

Ross, S. L. *Differential Equations.* Blaisdell, New York, 1964.

Ross, S. L. *Ordinary Differential Equations,* 3rd ed. Wiley, New York, 1966, 1980.

Sagan, H. *Boundary and Eigenvalue Problems in Mathematical Physics.* Wiley, 1961, reprinted Dover, New York, 1989.

Spiegel, M. R. *Applied Differential Equations,* 3rd ed. Prentice-Hall, London, 1958, 1981.

Tenenbaum, M. and Pollard, H. *Ordinary Differential Equations.* Harper & Row, 1963, reprinted Dover, New York, 1985.

Tricomi, F. G. *Equazioni Differenziali.* Paolo Boringhieri, 1948, terza edizioni, Rome, 1961.

Rabenstein, A. L. *Ordinary Differential Equations.* Academic Press, New York, 1966.

Wright, W. S. and Wright, C. D. *Complete Solution Manual to Accompany Zill's,* PWS-Kent Publishing, Boston, 1989.

Zill, D. G. *A First Course in Differential Equations.* Wadsworth, 1986, 5th ed. Boston, 1992.

Zill, D. G. and Cullen, M. R. *Differential Equations with Boundary Value Problems.* Brooke/Cole Publishing, Pacific Grove, California, 1997.

Zwillinger, D. *Handbook of Differential Equations.* Academic Press, San Diego, California, 1989.

References

1691 Bernoulli, J. *Differentialrechnung*. Manuscript found in 1921.

1696 L'Hôspital, G. F. A. *Annalyse des Infinitement Petits pour l'Intelligence des Courbes*. Paris.

1762 D'Alembert, J. R. *Miscelanea Turinesia*, 381.

1765 Lagrange, J. L. *Miscelanea Turinesia* 3, 181 (Oeuvres 1,473).

1769 Euler, L. *Institutiones Calculis Integralis* **2**, 483.

1771 van der Monde, A. T. "Memoire sur la Resolutions des Équations." *Histoire de l'Académie des Sciences de Paris*, 365–416 (1774).

1772 van der Monde, A.T. "Mémoire sur l'Elimination." *Histoire de l`Académie des Sciences de Paris*, 516–532 (1776).

1812 Hoene-Wronski, J. *Refutation de la Théorie des Fonctions Analytiques de Lagrange*. Paris.

1815 Cauchy, A. A. "Mémoire sur les Fonctions qui ne Peuvent Obtenir que Deux Valeurs." *Journal de l'École Polytechnique* **17**, 29–107 (*Ouevres*, série 2, volume 1, 91–169, Gaultier-Villars, Paris, 1905).

1863 Maxwell, J. C. *Treatise of Electricity and Magnetism*. Clarendan Press, Oxford.

1866 Fuchs, J. L. "Zur Theorie der Linearen Differentialgleichungen mit Verändlichen Koefflizienten." *Journal pur Reine and Angewande Mathematik* **66**, 121–160.

1892 Poincaré, H. *Méthodes Nouvelles de la Mécanique Celeste*. Gauthier-Villars, Paris.

Index

Printed in the United States
by Baker & Taylor Publisher Services